Small Implants in Knee Reconstruction

Norberto Confalonieri • Sergio Romagnoli
Editors

Small Implants in Knee Reconstruction

Springer

Editors
Norberto Confalonieri
Orthopedic, Traumatology and Hand
Surgery Department
CTO Hospital
Milan, Italy

Sergio Romagnoli
Galeazzi Orthopedic Institute
Milan, Italy

ISBN 978-88-470-2654-4 ISBN 978-88-470-2655-1 (eBook)
DOI 10.1007/978-88-470-2655-1
Springer Milan Dordrecht Heidelberg London New York

Library of Congress Control Number: 2012951035

7 6 5 4 3 2 1 2012 2013 2014
Cover design: Ikona S.r.l., Milan, Italy
Typesetting: Grafiche Porpora S.r.l., Segrate (MI), Italy
Printing and binding: Grafiche Porpora S.r.l., Segrate (MI), Italy

Springer-Verlag Italia S.r.l. – Via Decembrio 28 – I-20137 Milan
Springer is a part of Springer Science+Business Media (www.springer.com)

Foreword

It is a huge pleasure to be participating in a book on knee reconstruction using small implants. Unlike previous publications, this book does not limit the possibility of modular replacement to a single compartment, whether tibiofemoral or patellofemoral, but offers the real possibility of articular replacement adapted to the specific type and location of the damage caused by degenerative disease. It provides surgeons with an opportunity to step back and reconsider the simplistic reasoning, all too commonly accepted, in which total knee replacement (TKR) is considered as the "gold standard" when damage to the joint is not limited to a single, isolated compartment. Since the time we spent with Leonard Marmor in 1974, we have never stopped defending, often in the face of a void of cosmic proportions, modular arthroplasty as the preferred reconstructive option, despite its frequent attack by the officially recognized theoreticians. It is perhaps worth pondering an old quotation from the eminent hand surgeon Professor Vilain: "Everything has already been written, but since we have not read everything, we may continue publishing". This appears more apropos than ever regarding the use of small implants in knee reconstruction. Indeed, it seems to have been forgotten that in 1972 Leonard Marmor was already promoting a new concept in total knee replacement, replacing the two tibiofemoral compartments at the same time in patients with osteoarthritis of the knee. Great visionary that he was, he considered that the overriding advantage of this new concept compared to the TKR technique in use at the time lay in the conservation of the ACL, sparing the soft tissues and preserving bone stock. It was only once this new concept was established that he began to consider that another, purely unicompartmental solution could be envisaged in cases where the opposite compartment was healthy.

Today, after performing over 3,000 combined or isolated modular knee replacements, we are able to assert that the functional results achieved are better than those of TKR, that revision procedures are often simpler and that, subject to correct fitting, this option should no longer be considered as a temporary solution pending an inevitable conversion to TKR.

Our commitment to the defense of these small implants over the last 40 years against the onslaught of the official naysayers would never have been possible without the precious support of European surgeons working towards the same aims. I take pleasure in thanking for their support: the Marseille school under J-M. Aubaniac and, later, J-N. Argenson; the Italian orthopedics school, whose worthy representatives are S. Romagnoli and N. Confalonieri, and the British school, specifically, J. Goodfellow and his students for their work on mobile bearings and J. Newman, one of the longest standing defenders of resurfacing fixed implants and mobile bearings.

Little streams come together to make big rivers, so let us hope that this reference work will enable the peaceful river of non-invasive surgeons to exist officially at last against the torrent of systematic proponents of TKR. With hindsight, there can be no question that modular knee surgery gives better results than TKR by maintaining knee proprioception and that it alone can re-establish physiological function without reverse roll-back during walking. On the other hand, it must be acknowledged that it is technically a more difficult operation and that in spite of the ancillary instruments available to facilitate fitting and computer-assisted surgery, knee reconstruction with small implants is more surgeon-dependent than TKR.

This obvious fact is no justification, however, for current attempts to simplify the fitting of these implants by moving the ancillaries towards those used for TKR, in order to replace resurfacing or minimal bone resection with a "half TKR" concept, with the fitting rules that this would entail. This is a commercial move aimed at reassuring surgeons who are just beginning to perform knee reconstructions using small implants and it is totally inconsistent with any possibility of respecting the philosophy of modular knee surgery.

Under no circumstances can it replace the need to complete an on-the-job apprenticeship alongside experts in teams trained to perform this type of surgery before beginning to fit these small implants. What would you prefer, a run-of-the-mill fast food or a dish that suits your palate? It is on this choice that your choice of prosthetic option and the experience of your patients will depend.

October 2012

Philippe Cartier
Hartmann Knee Institute
Clinique Hartmann
Neuilly-sur-Seine, France

Preface

In these last years, a new interest in less invasive reconstructive surgery has involved the entire orthopedic world. The shifting demographics of patients with localized knee arthritis, including younger, more active patients, is a major impetus for the growing interest in conservative surgical alternatives. Minimally invasive total knee replacement is increasing in popularity because of a theoretically reduced blood loss, faster recovery, and reduced economic costs. However, less invasive surgery has been often identified both by surgeons and prosthesis manufacturers, as a shorter surgical approach to the implantation of the same total prostheses used with traditional approaches. New, more conservative surgical approaches have been proposed, such as quad-sparing, mid-vastus, or sub-vastus. While these have the advantage that they spare skin and the quadriceps tendon, they may increase the risk of muscle and nerve damage, resulting in a biological contradiction. Giulio Bizzozero, an Italian biologist pioneer, already in the early years of the last century classified tissues and cells in three categories. He identified the "reproducible" tissues, such as epithelium (skin) and endothelium, the "stable" tissues, such as mesenchyma (tendons and ligaments) that recover very well following injury, and the "noble tissues", such as muscles and nerves, which should not be damaged as they are "perpetual" tissues.

On this purpose it has been hypothesized that real mini-invasive surgery should not be matched only with shorter incision but also with both a new respect for all the tissues and a preserved joint kinematics using new tools and smaller implants. This has led to a redefinition of mini-invasive surgery as tissue-sparing surgery.

Unicompartmental knee replacement (UKR) and patellofemoral replacement (PFR) are well-accepted surgical procedures for the treatment of knee arthritis. Furthermore, few surgeons in the world experienced the association of different small implants, matching a philosophy of real less invasive procedures.

Indeed, small implants and a preserved joint biomechanics could represent a new development in reconstructive surgery and the approaches described in this special issue highlight the attractive aspects of this strategy. In addition, the use of computer-assisted instruments may help the surgeon in reproducing this highly demanding surgery by standardizing the techniques.

We strongly believe that this "personalized on-time treatment" for each patient according to the severity of the disease and using different implant options could be one of the most interesting improvements in the coming years.

October 2012 The Editors

Contents

Contributors

Andrew A. Amis Department of Mechanical Engineering and Department of Surgery and Cancer, Imperial College London, London, UK

Jean-Noel Argenson Service de Chirurgie Orthopédique, Hôpital Sainte-Marguerite, Marseille, France

Jean-Manuel Aubaniac Service de Chirurgie Orthopédique, Hôpital Sainte-Marguerite, Marseille, France

David S. Barrett Trauma and Orthopaedics, Southampton General Hospital, Southampton, UK

Norberto Confalonieri Orthopedic, Traumatology and Hand Surgery Department, CTO Hospital, Milan, Italy

Michele Corbella Galeazzi Orthopedic Institute, Milan, Italy

Christopher A. F. Dodd Nuffield Department of Orthopaedics, Rheumatology and Musculoskeletal Sciences (NDORMS), University of Oxford, Nuffield Orthopaedic Centre, Headington, Oxford, UK

Jean Yves Jenny Hôpitaux Universitaires de Strasbourg, Centre de Chirurgie Orthopédique et de la Main, Illkirch, France

Alfonso Manzotti 1st Orthopedic Department, CTO Hospital, Milan, Italy

Anthony Miniaci Orthopedic Surgery, Cleveland Clinic Sports Health Center, Ohio, USA

David W. Murray Nuffield Department of Orthopaedics, Rheumatology and Musculoskeletal Sciences (NDORMS), University of Oxford, Nuffield Orthopaedic Centre, Headington, Oxford, UK

John Newman Litfield House Medical Centre, Bristol, UK

Matthieu Ollivier Service de Chirurgie Orthopédique, Hôpital Sainte-Marguerite, Marseille, France

Hermant G. Pandit Nuffield Department of Orthopaedics, Rheumatology and Musculoskeletal Sciences (NDORMS), University of Oxford, Nuffield Orthopaedic Centre, Headington, Oxford, UK

Sebastien Parratte Service de Chirurgie Orthopédique, Hôpital Sainte-Marguerite, Marseille, France

Lindsay Rolston Henry County Center for Orthopedic Surgery & Sports Medicine, New Castle, IN, USA

Sergio Romagnoli Galeazzi Orthopedic Institute, Milan, Italy

Dominique Saragaglia Clinique Universitaire de Chirurgie Orthopédique et de Traumatologie du Sport de l'Hôpital Sud de Grenoble, Échirolles, Cedex, France

Emmanuel Thienpont Department of Orthopedic Surgery, University Hospital Saint Luc, Brussels, Belgium

Francesco Verde Galeazzi Orthopedic Institute, Milan, Italy

Sam K. Yasen Trauma and Orthopaedics, Southampton General Hospital, Southampton, UK

Sara Zacchetti Galeazzi Orthopedic Institute, Milan, Italy

The Reason for a Choice

1

Norberto Confalonieri

Before starting to read this book the reader should know what it is going to explore. Nowadays, in the orthopedic world osteoarthritis, prosthesis, mini-invasive surgery, tissue-saving surgery, small implants, etc. are "hot" topics approached from a multitude of perspectives, which ultimately run the risk of becoming repetitive [1-4].

Thus, let's first of all try to create order in these many topics, considering that the philosophy underlying the writing of this book is to repair the degenerative arthritic knee disease of our patients. But which patients? And, what type of arthritis?

In our practice, we have come to realize that our patients have progressively changed: they are younger, smarter, more sensitive to pain, more informed, more demanding, and often have an intact or surgically reconstructed anterior cruciate ligament (ACL) [2, 3, 5]. Likewise, even the arthritic knees of our own generation have changed: we see fewer and fewer knees destroyed by an advanced primary arthritis but we increasingly have to manage compartmental diseases. In many cases, these conditions are the results of sporting injuries, previous meniscectomies, plateau or condylar fractures, osteotomies, or prolonged overuse (Fig. 1.1).

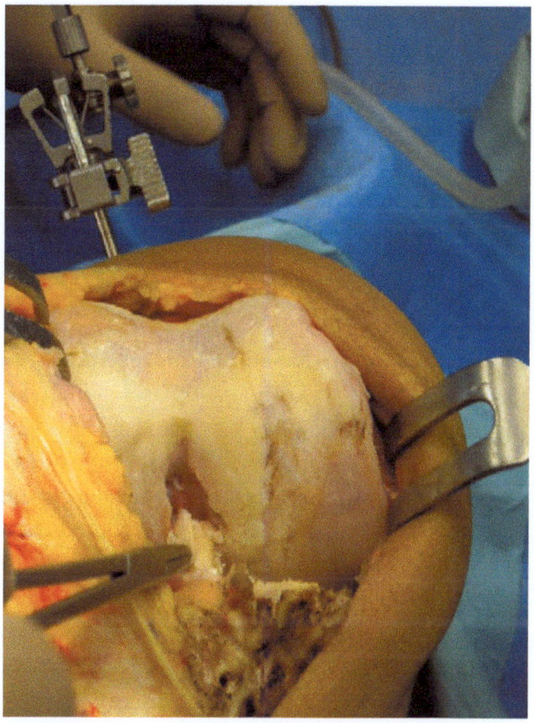

Fig. 1.1 Bicompartmental post-traumatic arthritis in a young man with an intact anterior cruciate ligament

Nevertheless, almost 90% of surgeons worldwide still implant a total prosthesis in these knees, firstly resecting ACL and often, even the posterior cruciate ligament [6-8]. In many cases, in order to maintain the promise of a MIS (mini invasive surgery) to the patients, a small incision is performed, often with higher risks of damages of the noble tissue under skin, a sort of "key-hole" surgery [9-14].

We propose a totally different strategy: tissue sparing surgery (TSS), which does not consider the length of the incision to be more important

N. Confalonieri (✉)
Orthopedic, Traumatology and Hand Surgery Department
CTO Hospital
Milan, Italy
E-mail: norberto.confalonieri@icp.mi.it

N. Confalonieri, S. Romagnoli (eds.), *Small Implants in Knee Reconstruction*,
DOI 10.1007/978-88-470-2655-1_1, © Springer-Verlag Italia 2013

than the size of the prosthesis [15, 16]. This prosthetic reconstruction, whether uni- or bi-compartmental, saves the two ligaments, which are the true fulcrum of joint biomechanics [17-19]. It involves the minimal removal of bone tissue from the tibia, femoral cartilage removal, sparing of the central pivot, and a small skin incision without damaging the extensor apparatus. It is clear that this surgical solution offers a genuinely minimally invasive surgery of the knee. Nonetheless, there are several considerations that are still matters of debate, including the indications, surgical technique and medium-term results [20-24]. Yet, there is no doubt that with the most recent technological developments, the increasingly precise surgical tools, computer assistance, and more convincing experience with unilateral knee replacement (UKR) [17, 20-22, 25, 26], positive, sometimes exciting, the short term results are possible [18, 27] and have led to very intense interest in this surgical approach to knee arthritis (Fig. 1.2).

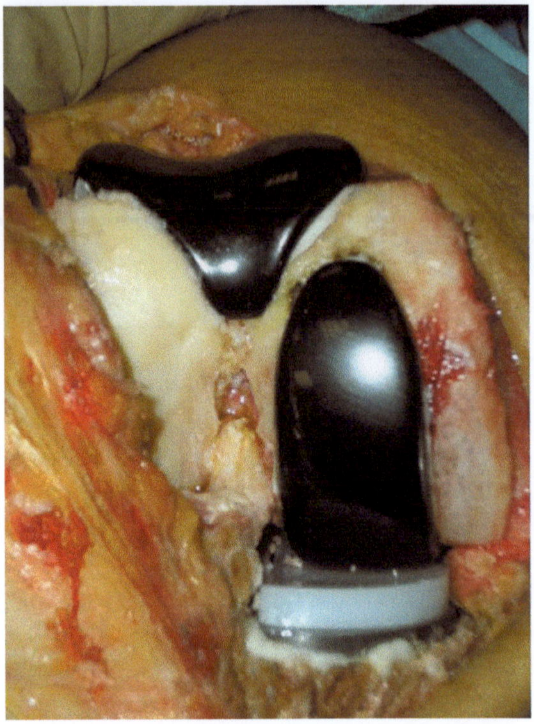

Fig. 1.2 Bicompartmental reconstruction: unicompartmental and patellofemoral computer-assisted arthroplasty

In fact, it represents a "historical return," because the history of knee arthroplasty starts with uni- and bi-uni condylar procedures. However, inaccurate instrumentation, incorrect indications and, consequently, less success guided the choice to a total prosthesis, which was considered easier to implant because it sacrificed everything to achieve a balanced design [5-7].

It is important to know that the three compartments of the knee joint are anatomically different and that each has its own specific biomechanics [31-34]. Thus, reconstructive knee surgery requires a vision of the joint that considers not only the anatomical structures but also the biomechanics as a whole, including muscle forces and ligament constraints. Thus, total knee replacement (TKR) is not a "biological" replacement but instead creates a new "artificial" joint with new, albeit abnormal kinematics [31, 35, 36]. Despite new and sophisticated prosthetic designs (gender-specific, one or two radius curvatures, mobile-bearing, etc.), TKR sacrifices the cruciate ligaments, changes the anatomy of the compartments, and in the majority of cases includes medial and lateral condyles of the same size. In addition, it has been widely emphasized that the results of TKR depend on the use of guides, which can lead to significant errors in reconstruction of the mechanical axis of the lower limbs based on the absence of data on proper soft-tissue balancing of the ligaments, thereby affecting both the functionality and the durability of the system [5, 37, 38].

From a surgical point of view, surgical compartmental reconstruction (UKR, UKR + PFA, bi-UKR) is considerably less invasive than total replacement: the ligamentous apparatus remains undamaged, does not require the use of intramedullary tools, and permits a three-dimensional correction of an arthritis deformity [15, 39]. Moreover, it preserves bone stock and, in case of failure, can be more easily revised with traditional total arthroplasty [40, 41].

In addition to these "surgical" advantages, there are also several practical ones, even for the patient [35, 36, 42, 43]:

- Reduced blood loss, with less need for a blood transfusion, even in the case of simultaneous bilateral implants.

- Lower risk of deep-vein thrombosis and sepsis.
- Improved indications for loco-regional anesthesia.
- Reduced incidence of lift-off of the lateral compartment compared to TKR because it is ACL-sparing.
- Option of using all-polyethylene tibial implant with lower stresses between bone and prosthesis.
- Option of using different prosthetic sizes and models for each compartment, thus respecting the knee's natural anatomy and biomechanics.
- Absence of posterior polyethylene wear (edge-loading), since the ACL is retained, which prevents posterior subluxation of the femur.
- Integrity of joint proprioception.
- Shorter hospital stay and quicker recovery of the joint, based on the better function compared to TKR.

These advantages also play a role in treatment for special indication such as in patients with neurological problems (e.g. Parkinson's disease), in whom a total replacement leads to a worsening of the underlying disease whereas compartmental reconstruction avoids the effect of somato-agnosy (loss of sensation of a body part) [44, 45]. Last but not least, there is an obvious savings in health costs, an advantage in terms of the management of economic resources.

In conclusion we must point out that these results are possible only with a rigorous selection of patients and the use of a rigorous surgical technique. These two factors will provide such patients with an almost complete recovery of the range of motion in "normal" joint biomechanics.

In this volume, the reader will become familiar with all of these aspects as well as others in this extensive discussion of TSS by leading international experts. Our hope is to encourage a consideration of compartmental knee reconstruction as a valid alternative to total knee replacement.

References

1. Choong PF, Dowsey MM (2011)Update in surgery for osteoarthritis of the knee. Int J Rheum Dis 14(2):167-74
2. Dieppe P, Lim K, Lohmander S (2011) Who should have knee joint replacement surgery for osteoarthritis? Int J Rheum Dis 14(2):175-80
3. Chapple CM, Nicholson H, Baxter GD, Abbott JH (2011) Patient characteristics that predict progression of knee osteoarthritis: a systematic review of prognostic studies. Arthritis Care Res (Hoboken) 63(8):1115-25
4. Pandit H, Aslam N, Pirpiris M, Jinnah R (2006)Total knee arthroplasty: the future. J Surg Orthop Adv 15(2):79-85
5. Archibeck MJ, White RE Jr (2006) What's new in adult reconstructive knee surgery. J Bone Joint Surg Am 88(7):1677-86
6. Pavone V, Boettner F, Fickert S, Sculco TP (2001). Total condylar knee arthoplasty: a long term follow-up. Clin Orthop 388:18-25
7. Dennis MG, Di Cesare PE (2003)Surgical management of the middle age arthritic knee. Bull Hosp Jt Dis 61(3-4):172-8
8. Pagnano MW, Clarke HD, Jacofsky DJ, Amendola A, Repicci JA (2005) Surgical treatment of the middle-aged patient with arthritic knees. Instr Course Lect 54:251-9
9. Berger RA, Sanders S, Gerlinger T, Della Valle C, Jacobs JJ, Rosenberg AG (2005) Outpatient total knee arthroplasty with a minimally invasive technique. J Arthroplasty 20 7(Suppl 3):33-8
10. Haas SB, Cook S, Beksac B (2004) Minimally invasive total knee replacement through a mini midvastus approach: a comparative study. Clin Orthop Relat Res 428:68-73
11. Laskin RS (2005) Minimally invasive total knee arthroplasty: the results justify its use. Clin Orthop Relat Res. Nov 440:54-9
12. Lonner JH (2006) Minimally invasive approaches to total knee arthroplasty: results. Am J Orthop 35 (7 Suppl):27-33
13. Berend KR, Lombardi AV Jr (2005) Avoiding the potential pitfalls of minimally invasive total knee surgery. Orthopedics 28(11):1326-30
14. Dalury DF, Dennis DA (2005) Mini-incision total knee arthroplasty can increase risk of component malalignment. Clin Orthop Rel Res 440:77-81
15. Confalonieri N, Manzotti A, Montironi F, Pullen C (2008) Tissue sparing surgery in knee reconstruction: unicompartmental (UKA), patellofemoral (PFA), UKA + PFA, bi-unicompartmental (Bi-UKA) arthroplasties. J Orthop Traumatol 9(3):171-7

16. Confalonieri N, Manzotti A, Pullen C (2007) Navigated shorter incision or smaller implant in knee arthritis? Clin Orthop Relat Res 463:63-7
17. Confalonieri N, Manzotti A (2005) Mini-invasive computer-assisted bi-unicompartimental knee replacement. Int J Med Robot 1(4):45-50
18. Confalonieri N, Manzotti A, Cerveri P, De Momi E (2009) Bi-unicompartmental versus total knee arthroplasty: a matched paired study with early clinical results. Arch Orthop Trauma Surg. Sep 129(9):1157-63
19. Heyse TJ, Khefacha A, Cartier P.Tria AJ Jr (2010) Bicompartmental arthroplasty of the knee. Instr Course Lect. 59:61-73 UKA in combination with PFR at average 12-year follow-up. Arch Orthop Trauma Surg 130(10):1227-30
20. O'Rourke MR, Gardner JJ, Callaghan JJ, Liu SS, Goetz DD, Vittetoe DA, Sullivan PM, Johnston RC (2005) The John Insall Award: unicompartmental knee replacement: a minimum twenty-one-year followup, end-result study. Clin Orthop Relat Res 440:27-37
21. Swienckowski JJ, Pennington DW (2004) Unicompartmental knee arthroplasty in patients sixty years of age or younger. J Bone Joint Surg 86-A Suppl 1(Pt 2):131-42
22. Newman J, Pydisetty RV, Ackroyd C (2009) Unicompartmental or total knee replacement: the 15-year results of a prospective randomised controlled trial. J Bone Joint Surg Br 91(1):52-7
23. Heyse TJ, Khefacha A, Cartier P (2010) UKA in combination with PFR at average 12-year follow-up. Arch Orthop Trauma Surg 130(10):1227-30
24. Parratte S, Pauly V, Aubaniac JM, Argenson JN (2010) Survival of bicompartmental knee arthroplasty at 5 to 23 years. Clin Orthop Relat Res 468(1):64-72
25. Konyves A, Willis-Owen CA, Spriggins AJ (2010) The long-term benefit of computer-assisted surgical navigation in unicompartmental knee arthroplasty. J Orthop Surg Res 31 5:94
26. Jenny JY (2008) Navigated unicompartmental knee replacement. Sports Med Arthrosc 16(2):103-7
27. Rolston L, Siewert K (2009) Assessment of knee alignment after bicompartmental knee arthroplasty. J Arthroplasty 24(7):1111-4
28. Buechel FF, Pappas MJ (1984). New Jersey low contact stress knee replacement system. Ten-year evaluation of meniscal bearings. Orthop Clin North Am 20(2):147-77
29. Lewallen DG, Bryan RS, Peterson LF (1984). Polycentric total knee arthroplasty. A ten-year follow-up study. J Bone Joint Surg Am 66(8):1211-8
30. Cloutier JM, Sabouret P, Deghrar A (1999)Total knee arthroplasty with retention of both cruciate ligaments. A nine to eleven-year follow-up study. J Bone Joint Surg Am 81(5):697-702
31. Andriacchi TP, Andersson GB, Fermier RW, Stern D, Galante JO (1980) A study of lower-limb mechanics during stair-climbing. J Bone Joint Surg Am 62(5):749-57
32. Freeman MA, Pinskerova V (2005) The movement of the normal tibio-femoral joint. J Biomech 38(2):197-208
33. Martelli S, Pinskerova V (2002) The shapes of the tibial and femoral articular surfaces in relation to tibiofemoral movement. J Bone Joint Surg Br 84(4):607-13
34. Pinskerova V, Samuelson KM, Stammers J, Maruthainar K, Sosna A, Freeman MA (2009) The knee in full flexion: an anatomical study. J Bone Joint Surg Br 91(6):830-4
35. Banks SA, Frely BJ, Boniforti F, Reischmidt C, Romagnoli S (2005) Comparing in vivo kinematics of unicondylar and bi-unicondylar knee replacement. . Knee Surg Sports Traumatol Arthrosc 13:551-6
36. Fuchs S, Tibesku CO, Frisse D, Genkinger m, Laaß H, Rosenbaum D (2005) Clinical and functional of uni-and bicondylar sledge prostheses. Knee Surg Sports Traumatol Arthrosc 13:197-202
37. Fehring TK, Odum S, Griffin WL, Mason JB, Nadaud M (2001) Early failures in total knee arthroplasty. Clin Orthop Relat Res (392):315-8
38. Rand JA, Coventry MB (1988) The accuracy of femoral intramedullary guides in total knee arthroplasty. Clin Orthop 232:168-173
39. Zanasi S (2011)Innovations in total knee replacement: new trends in operative treatment and changes in peri-operative management. Eur Orthop Traumato 2(1-2):21-31
40. Springer BD, Scott RD, Thornhill TS (2006) Conversion of failed unicompartmental knee arthroplasty to TKA. Clin Orthop Relat Res 446:214-20
41. Châtain F, Richard A, Deschamps G, Chambat P, Neyret P (2004) Revision total knee arthroplasty after unicompartmental femorotibial prosthesis: 54 cases. Rev Chir Orthop Reparatrice Appar Mot 90(1):49-57
42. Weale AE, Halabi OA, Jones PW, White SH (2001) Perceptions of out-comes after unicompartmental and total knee replacements. Clin Orthop 382:143-153
43. Patil S, Colwell CW, Ezet KA, D'Lima DD (2005) Can normal knee kinematics be restored with unicompartmental knee replacement? J Bone Joint Surg 87A:332-338
44. Fast A, Mendelsohn E, Sosner J (1994) Total knee arthroplasty in Parkinson's disease. Arch Phys Med Rehabil 75(11):1269-70
45. Macaulay W, Geller JA, Brown AR, Cote LJ, Kiernan HA (2010) Total knee arthroplasty and Parkinson disease: enhancing outcomes and avoiding complications. J Am Acad Orthop Surg 18(11):687-94

Bicompartmental Arthroplasty: Past, Present, and Future

2

Emmanuel Thienpont

2.1 Introduction

Bicompartmental osteoarthritis (OA) affects both the medial tibiofemoral and the patellofemoral compartment, in which case it is called medio-patellofemoral (MPF) osteoarthritis [1]. Selective resurfacing of either the medial or the patellofemoral compartment has been reported to be safe and efficient [2, 3]. It tends to be more controversial if the arthritis is limited to two compartments of the knee and there is no significant deformity, excellent motion, and intact cruciate ligaments. These patients are thus candidates for bicompartmental resurfacing [4].

Bicompartmental knee arthroplasty (BKA) is a type of resurfacing surgery in which the medial tibiofemoral and patellofemoral joints are both replaced but the lateral compartment of the native knee is conserved [5]. It is used to bridge the gap between unicompartmental knee arthroplasty (UKA) and total knee arthroplasty (TKA) [6]. High tibial osteotomy and/or tibial tubercle transposition, unicompartmental arthroplasty with neglect of the patellofemoral joint, if painless, and total knee arthroplasty are well known alternatives to treat bicompartmental arthritis [7-9]. In TKA, both the unaffected lateral compartment and at least one or both cruciate ligaments are sacrificed, leading to altered biomechanics of the knee joint [1,10].

In BKA, the anterior and posterior cruciate ligaments are preserved, yielding important advantages in terms of enhanced stability, decreased shear force at the implant-bone interface, more physiological tibiofemoral kinematics, and maintenance of proprioception [5]. Thus, not only the restoration of normal kinematics, but also the preservation of bone stock must be considered in resurfacing surgery [6].

Today, BKA can be accomplished by two theoretically different femoral component designs: (1) separate modular unlinked components individually positioned; (2) a single monolithic design with a fixed relationship between patello- and tibiofemoral components [5, 11, 12].

2.2 The Past

Orthopedic surgery has a tendency to evolve in cycles, reconsidering ideas from the past in a new light. This cyclical pattern is frequently driven by technological or material developments that become available to solve long-standing problems. This is also the case in bicompartmental arthroplasty, performed ever since the origin of knee arthroplasty. Likewise, multi-compartmental arthroplasty with discrete components has a long history that begins with bi-unicompartmental implants [13, 14]. Indeed, the term bicompartmental arthroplasty was initially used to describe implants that replaced the tibiofemoral joint medially and laterally, without addressing the patellofemoral joint. Many of these designs were of

E. Thienpont (✉)
Department of Orthopedic Surgery
University Hospital Saint Luc
Brussels, Belgium
E-mail: emmanuel.thienpont@uclouvain.be

N. Confalonieri, S. Romagnoli (eds.), *Small Implants in Knee Reconstruction*,
DOI 10.1007/978-88-470-2655-1_2, © Springer-Verlag Italia 2013

the hinged or spacer type but in many cases were associated with early failure in rheumatoid patients [15-17].

Within this same concept of native tissue appreciation, the importance of conserving both the anterior and posterior cruciate ligaments in TKA, to prevent posteromedial wear, has been incorporated in total condylar designs [18, 19]. Patients who were recently asked which implant they preferred still chose an ACL-PCL conserving design as their preferred knee [20]. Excellent results have been published regarding modern type designs of unicompartmental arthroplasty in a bi-uni setting, often navigation-assisted [21-24].

2.3 The Present

Knee OA typically affects joints in a non-uniform manner, with the medial compartment of the knee most frequently affected in both men and women [11, 25]. The three most common areas of knee OA distribution are medial compartment, patellofemoral compartment, and medial/patellofemoral compartment overlap [26].

Cadaveric and radiographic studies of normal age-associated wear of the knee cartilage indicated that structural changes typically progress from the medial condyle to the patellofemoral compartment [27, 28]. Four main patterns (a–d) of cartilage lesions in knee osteoarthritis were identified by Bae et al., with the lesion size varying from small to large in distinct regions. Pattern a consists of relatively small lesions (area of 2–3% in each region) and is the most abundant pattern (prevalence of 58%). Three sub-patterns were also described: (a1) 'mixed small' with small lesions (area of 1%) in all locations, (a2) medial femoral condyle (MFC) small (area of 6–7%), and (a3) patellofemoral groove (PFG) small. Pattern b has a predominant lesion (23% area) in the MFC and smaller (< 3% area) lesions elsewhere (prevalence 23%). Pattern c involves predominant lesions in the lateral femoral condyle (area of 19%), MFC (area of 10%), and PFG (area of 5%). In pattern d the predominant lesion is in the PFG (area of 15%), with smaller lesions in the MFC (area of 6%) and LFC (area of 2%). Three distinct patterns emerged from cluster analysis: MFC degeneration, posterior LFC degeneration also involving smaller lesions in the central PFG and the lateral aspect of the MFC; and PFG degeneration accompanied by small lesions in the lateral aspect of the MFC [29]. A radiological study found 60% medial, 15% lateral, and 25% patellofemoral OA, similar to the pattern distribution of 60% pattern b, 20% pattern c, and 20% pattern d [29, 30].

Arno et al. used the Weidow grading scale to visually assess cartilage integrity in the resected bones of 97 patients with varus TKA. They also reviewed the operative reports for possible contraindications to early intervention procedures. Healthy lateral compartment cartilage was found in 61% of the patients [31].

The Oxford group examined the patellofemoral joints (PFJ) of 824 knees of 793 patients undergoing medial UKA for OA. Full-thickness cartilage loss on the trochlear surface was observed in 13%, on the medial facet of the patella in 9%, and on the lateral facet in 4% of the knees. Full-thickness cartilage loss at any location was found in 16% of the knees. The authors concluded that OA of the medial facet of the PFJ is not a contraindication to UKA, but they recommended greater caution in case of lateral patellofemoral degeneration [32, 33]. This finding was recently confirmed by Munk et al., who reported inferior results in a group of patients undergoing unicompartmental arthroplasty, with lateral subluxation of the patella [34]. In particular, flexion contracture and varus deformity of the knee with lateralization of the patella are aggravating factors for patellofemoral symptoms in medial OA of the knee [35].

The radiological prevalence of patellofemoral OA was studied by Davies et al. Patellofemoral arthritis was present in about one-third of subjects after 60 years. An isolated lateral radiograph was poor for the detection of patellofemoral OA, with a sensitivity of only 66%. Instead, proper assessment requires a skyline view [30]. Chang et al. found that patellar translation and obliteration of the joint space were associated with anterior knee pain and that translation was significantly associated with difficulty in rising from a chair

[36]. This is in contrast with osteophyte formation, which should not necessarily influence function or be associated with symptoms [37].

In 2009, a nationwide anonymous survey was performed in Germany regarding the indications of unicompartmental arthroplasty: 43.4% of responders felt that bicompartmental arthroplasty is an option in case of additional affection of the PFJ [38].

Despite the many new and sometimes different knee designs on the market and the never ending efforts of surgeons to implant these devices as functionally as possible, TKA results are certainly not as perfect as we would wish. Patients with TKA still experience substantial functional impairment compared with their age- and gender-matched peers, especially with respect to biomechanically demanding activities. In fact, 52% of the patients who had TKAs reported some degree of limitation in performing functional activities [39]. Bourne et al. published a study of 1703 primary total knee patients, in which 1 in 5 TKA patients were dissatisfied with the outcome [40]. Thus, especially younger, more active, high-demand patients may be eligible for this type of resurfacing surgery. It should be considered also as an option in a patient with a well-functioning unicompartmental arthroplasty who develops arthritis in another compartment [4].

Smaller implants can be considered as true minimally invasive surgery because these procedures are tissue-sparing knee surgery, an important aspect in this younger patient population. The ultimate goals of true minimally invasive surgery are: (1) the avoidance of fat embolism; (2) the use of smaller incisions; (3) a faster and less painful rehabilitation; (4) a reduced hospital stay with a fast return to the normal activities of daily living; (5) an improved range of motion; (6) a reduced need for analgesics; and (7) to obtain a durable, well-aligned, highly functional implant [23].

2.4 Kinematics and Proprioceptive Function

Patient preference for ACL-PCL conserving TKAs as the preferred implant probably reflects the better feeling of stability conferred by these prostheses. In addition, the ACL-PCL prostheses may provide superior proprioception and greater leverage for the extensor mechanism by preventing anterior slide and shortening of the quadriceps lever/arm [10, 20]. Other arguments for kinematic preservation can be found in the literature [4]. In vivo studies have shown that relatively normal kinematics of the knee are not achieved by retention of the PCL alone because posterior femoral rollback in flexion did not occur in the knees studied or, if it did, it was erratic [41]. Another in vivo study showed that preservation of both cruciates was the only way to eliminate paradoxical anterior translation following TKA during deep knee bends [42]. According to Komistek et al., preservation of the ACL and PCL restored normal axial rotation during normal walking [43]. In vivo kinematics have demonstrated that preserving both cruciate ligaments in bi-unicondylar knee arthroplasty maintains several of the basic features of normal knee kinematics and stability, comparable to the native knee [44, 45].

In gait studies, the knees in which both cruciate ligaments were retained were the only ones that had normal flexion when the patients ascended and descended stairs [46]. Wang et al. analyzed gait kinematics in BKA patients 1 year postoperatively. Less isokinetic knee extensor strength was observed than in the normal limb from the control group. There was no difference in knee extensor moment at push-off among the BKA versus the control limbs; however, the maximum knee extensor strength of the BKA limb was still less than the control. No differences in peak knee adduction angle and moment were observed between BKA and controls, suggesting that BKA had resulted in good frontal plane knee mechanics during walking. Finally, level walking was well performed by the BKA group, with similar walking speed and similar joint and gait kinematics between BKA and non-involved limbs [25].

Wunschel et al. analyzed kinematics after different types of arthroplasty. Only slight internal rotation was observed during flexion in TKA. The importance of ACL integrity in BKA was evidenced by the fact that there was no difference in tibial rotation, leading to the assumption that the ACL does influence tibial rotation during simulated weight-bearing flexion. However, significant anterior movement of the tibia occurred when the ACL was sectioned, due to the flat tibial plateau in BKA, which is not able to compensate for the missing ACL [5]. Better functional results have been ascribed to the preservation of the ACL and its mechanoreceptors [47]. Patients with TKA have worse proprioceptive results than normal age-matched controls [48-50] but better proprioceptive abilities than age-matched OA controls [51].

Laidlaw et al. found better roll back on lateral radiographs in patients with bicompartmental arthroplasty compared to those with a PCL-retaining implant [52].

Use of a monolithic femoral component for trochlear-MFC resurfacing has several challenges. The varus-valgus alignment of the component is determined by the apposition of the lateral transitional edge of the trochlear component with the lateral femoral condyle. The location of the transition zone is based on the rotational orientation of the cutting block, the depth of the femoral cut, and the valgus orientation of the distal femoral cut [4, 53]. Rotational alignment is based on Whiteside's line. The depth of the distal femoral resection is set to 9 mm [53]. Given the variability in coronal alignment and the morphology of the distal femur, there will be concomitant variability in the alignment of the implant needed to ensure that the lateral edge of the trochlear prosthesis is flush with the lateral femoral condyle [54]. The positioning of this component remains challenging, since even with the use of patient-specific instruments (PSI) rotational malalignment occurred in 20% of the cases [55].

In modular bicompartmental resurfacing, the size of the gap between the transitional edge of the trochlear component and the proximal edge of the femoral component of the UKA may vary. The distance may be as short as 1 mm or as long as 15 mm, depending on the shape and size of the distal femur. Problems with the transitional gap have not occurred with independent resurfacing, provided that the implants are appropriately positioned, i.e., flush with or recessed approximately 1 mm relative to the articular cartilage. Implant edge prominence can result from technical errors or implant design flaws [56].

Banks et al. examined the morphology of the reconstructed CT scans of 117 knees and found that the anteroposterior (AP) and proximodistal (PD) relationships between the condylar and trochlear arc centers were highly variable. There was no significant correlation between the AP femur size and the AP distance from the condylar to the patellofemoral (PF) arc centers or between the mediolateral (ML) femur size and the AP distance from the condylar to the PF arc centers. The standard errors for these regressions were at least 4.5 mm. There were statistically significant relationships between the AP and ML femur size and the PD distance from the condylar to the PF arc centers, but the standard errors were also at least 4 mm. These data show that the geometric relationship between the femoral condyles and patellar trochlea is highly variable and that modular components are probably the better choice [57].

2.5 Functional Results

Clinical arguments for tissue-sparing surgery come from the superior functional performance of patients with UKA compared to those treated with TKA [58, 59]. UKA patients were also reported to have better functional outcomes and an increased likelihood of returning to normal functional activity [3]. Patients undergoing UKA are also more likely to return to low-impact sports [60]. Patients with bilateral TKAs preferred retention of both their cruciate ligaments over both postero-stabilized and PCL-retaining designs [10, 20].

For modular BKA designs, Argenson et al. reported on a series of 183 patellofemoral arthroplasties (PFA), 104 of which were performed in conjunction with UKA between 1972 and 1990. Outcomes were satisfactory in 84% of the overall results but the subset of patients who underwent PFA-UKA was not distinguished in the overall clinical results [61].

Cartier et al. reported on a series of 72 PFAs, 36 of which were performed in conjunction with UKA (30 medial, 6 lateral). Although 85% of the overall results were good or excellent, the data did not specifically address the group that underwent bicompartmental arthroplasty [62].

Paratte et al. published improved Knee Society (KS) knee and function scores ranging from 42 ± 8 (range, 17–59) to 88 ± 2 (range, 58–100) and from 35 ± 9 (range, 10–57) to 79 ± 15 (range, 58–100) at a minimum follow-up of 5 years (mean, 12 years; range, 5–23 years). Mean active flexion improved from 118° ± 9° (range, 100–150°) preoperatively to 134° ± 6° (range, 120–153°) at final follow-up [6].

In patients who underwent modular BKA performed by the method of Cartier, Heyse et al. determined an improvement of the KS score from a preoperative 68.8 ± 26.2 to 175.5 ± 22.9 at an average follow-up of 11.8 ± 5.4 years (range, 4–17 years). The function score increased from 30.0 ± 8.9 to 82.8 ± 17.5. Other results were: WOMAC 18.3 ± 8.6, average pain score 3.2 ± 4.1, stiffness score 2.4 ± 2.6. Range of motion (ROM) improved from 107 ± 12.1° to 121.1° ± 14.3°. Within the clinical review and evaluation, none of the patients reported instability with walking. Three patients suffered from light pain when rising from a seated position. No patient described swelling of the operated joint. Only one patient reported occasional pain of the patella. Six patients had difficulties with squatting and kneeling [1].

Finally, Lonner et al. examined a series of 12 consecutive modular bicompartmental arthroplasties implanted with robotic arm assistance. The mean knee ROM significantly improved from 100° of flexion preoperatively to a mean of 126° of flexion. Improvements in WOMAC scores and KS scores were also statistically significant [4].

For the monolithic femoral components, less convincing clinical results were obtained. Palumbo et al. reported a mean functional KS of 65.4 (range, 30–100). Excellent results (80–100 points) were achieved in 11 out of 36 (31%) knees; 6 (17%) had a good result (70–79), 5 (14%) had a fair result (60–69), and 14 (39%) had a poor result. The mean WOMAC score was 75.8 (range, 50–97) which is a poor result compared to historical TKA WOMAC scores. The mean ROM improved from 113° (range, 87–130°) to 120° (range, 110–135°) at latest follow-up. The mean pain score improved from 8.7 (range, 5–10) to 4.0 (range, 0–8) postoperatively. Only 19% of the patient's knees were painless after Deuce BKA. Sixteen patients (44%) stated that they were completely satisfied with the surgery, whereas 9 (25%) rated their satisfaction as partial and 11 (31%) stated that they were unsatisfied with the procedure. Nineteen patients (53%) stated they would not repeat the surgery [54].

Morrison et al. compared functional scores between 21 BKA Journey-Deuce knees and 33 TKA knees. At 3 months postoperatively, both cohorts achieved significant improvements over baseline SF-12 physical and WOMAC pain and physical function scores. The BKA cohort was able to achieve a significant improvement in WOMAC stiffness at 3 months whereas in the TKA cohort this was not the case until 1 year postoperatively. The TKA cohort had a significant improvement in SF-12 mental status at 3 months, whereas for the BKA cohort this was not achieved even by the 2-year follow-up end point. When both cohorts were compared at follow-up, the BKA cohort had significantly better WOMAC pain and physical function scores at 3 months. There was no significant difference in SF-12 or WOMAC subscores between cohorts at 1 or 2 years postoperatively. The postoperative ROM was the same in both cohorts despite a lower preoperative flexion in the TKA cohort. Thus, according to these findings, although both BKA and TKA result in less pain and improved physical function in the early postoperative period, BKA does so to a greater extent. These advantages over TKA do not persist past 1 year postoperatively; and when adjusting for age, sex, BMI, and baseline status, the early postoperative advantages offered by BKA are minimal. In the early postoperative period, patients experienced a more rapid and drastic reduction in stiffness after BKA [63].

2.6 Radiological Results

Restoration of the mechanical axis to the center of the tibial plateau is reportedly achieved in 95% of BKA procedures [64].

Palumbo et al. observed no lucencies of the patellar or femoral component in any of their Deuce cases. Progressive radiolucencies at the tibial bone-cement interface were seen in 22 (61%) knees. Seventeen (47%) tibial trays showed grade I radiolucencies, and 5 (14%) demonstrated grade II. The incidence and location of lucencies were consistent with those in previous reports of unicompartmental devices. It was thus not clear whether they represented component loosening. The authors postulated that the increased tibial baseplate bone–cement interface strain led to micromotion, resulting in instability of the fibrocartilaginous zone and subsequently to a high incidence of knee pain, poor clinical outcome, and even a fractured tibial baseplate [54].

In the group of Heyse et al., two patients developed radiolucent lines at the tibial component (< 1 mm) that were not progressive with time. There was one osteolysis around the tibial fixation screw in an uncemented component of a male active and sportive patient. Radiolucent lines at the femoral component were found in one patient. Two patella onlays showed radiolucent lines, and one patient had polyethylene wear on the lateral side. Five tibial polyethylene inlays showed signs of wear [1].

Paratte et al. found 25 knees (15.5%) with radiolucencies (< 1 mm) at the tibial bone–cement interface without any sign of progression after 5 years of follow-up. No femoral lucencies were observed. The mean AP axis of the tibial component was ± 89° ± 3° (range, 85–90°) on the medial side. Mean tibial slope was 3° ± 4° (range, 0–8°). The mean femoral AP axis was 92° ± 7° (range, 86–94°) [6].

Lonner et al. found no evidence of loosening, polyethylene wear, or progressive lateral compartment degenerative arthritis in a group of 12 robotics-assisted bicompartmental arthroplasties at short-term follow-up [4].

2.7 Complications

Patients with monolithic femoral components are more likely to suffer early complications, specifically, persistent pain requiring revision arthroplasty [54]. Morrison et al. reported one manipulation under anesthesia and two patellar problems (one subluxation and one inferior patellar fracture). They concluded that patients undergoing BKA are more likely to suffer early complications, especially persistent pain requiring revision arthroplasty. The overall complication rate was 28.6% compared to 6.1% in the TKA cohort ($p = 0.045$; odds ratio, 6.2). These revisions may have been related to poor patient selection, according to the authors [63].

Heyse et al. reported two knees manipulated within 3 weeks postoperatively, due to stiffness. It was unclear to the authors whether this was related to the type of implant used [1].

2.8 Revision

Bicompartmental arthroplasty can be considered a bone-stock-sparing procedure. The total amount of bone removed on the femur and the tibia using a standard TKA implant is 3.5 times greater than the amount removed using a bicompartmental onlay implant and 4 times greater than the amount removed when using an inlay implant (data on file at MAKO). In all the published papers on BKA revision, primary TKA was used to revise the failed BKAs [6, 54, 63].

For combined femoral components, Heyse et al. reported no surgical revisions after an average follow-up of 11.8 ± 5.4 (4–17) years in a group of patients with an average age of 64 ± 5 years [1].

Paratte et al. published the results of their BKA revisions: 27 out of 28 knees were revised for aseptic loosening. In 20 knees there was isolated loosening of the patellofemoral implant (15 uncemented and 5 cemented) while seven knees had loosening of the tibial plateau related to polyethylene wear. The relatively high revision rate in the medial UKA/PFA group could be explained by the use of early-generation implants. The authors concluded that improved results may be obtained with enhanced instrumentation and techniques, better polyethylene, and contemporary designs. In this group, 20 of the 27 failures were related to aseptic loosening of an uncemented patellofemoral implant. Bone stock was preserved and revision was considered easier than a revision performed after TKA. All revisions were done with conventional postero-stabilized TKA [6].

Palumbo et al. converted 5 (14%) of their 36 Journey-Deuce knees to TKA due to persistent pain at the anterior medial aspect of the proximal tibia. The mean time to conversion was 19 months (range, 15–26 months). All revisions were performed using primary, cemented TKA components. Intra-operatively, all tibial baseplates were grossly loose and easily explanted. In one patient, the baseplate was found to be fractured transversely through its center, between the two pegs [54].

Morrison et al. revised three of their 21 Journey-Deuce BKA to TKA due to persistent pain after 1 year postoperatively and found a nearly significant trend of an increased revision rate ($p = 0.054$) at 2 years of follow-up [63].

2.9 Disease Progression of the Third Compartment

One mechanism of long-term failure after unicompartmental resurfacing is the development or progression of arthritis in the non resurfaced compartment.

Khan et al. found that 7% (2/30) of the patients with UKA developed patellofemoral arthritis within 10 years. In the series of Berger et al., patellofemoral arthritis developed in 1.6% of the treated knees within 10 years and 10% within 15 years [65].

Cartier et al. found that 10% (8/79) of PFA patients developed tibiofemoral arthritis at a mean follow-up of 10 years [66]. Nicol et al. reported a 12% revision rate to TKA of 103 PFAs for symptomatic tibiofemoral arthritis after a mean of 55 months (range, 14–95 months) [67]. Kooijman et al. noted that 21% (12/56) of PFAs required additional surgery to address progressive tibiofemoral arthritis at a mean of 15.6 years (range, 10–21 years) [68]. Argenson et al. reported that 25% of PFAs were revised to TKA at a mean of 7.3 years (range, 1–12 years) because of progressive and painful tibiofemoral arthritis [69].

According to Paratte, isolated asymptomatic disease progression in the lateral compartment occurred in 6 out of 77 knees, with 17 years follow-up. This low rate of OA progression is related to proper preoperative screening. Quantitative evaluation of the cartilage status using modern dedicated tools such as T2 mapping may be helpful in optimizing patient selection [6]. Heyse et al. published the results of nine knees, five of which showed degenerative changes in the lateral tibiofemoral compartment. As categorized with the Kellgren score (0-4), two knees were Kellgren 1, two were Kellgren 2, and one was Kellgren 4. However this did not lead to complaints and none of the patients required therapy at the time the report was published [1]. Lonner et al. found no lateral compartment degeneration at short term follow-up [4].

2.10 Survivorship

Maintaining the anterior cruciate ligament in bi- and tricompartmental knee arthroplasty may be advantageous in terms of survivorship [18, 70]. Bicompartmental arthroplasty demonstrated a durability of 54% (95% confidence interval, 0.47-0.61), with a 17-year survival to revision, radiographic loosening, or disease progression [6]. The authors concluded that the results were inferior to TKA but determined several risk factors for these results, such as implant design, patient selection, absent instrumentation and component malalignment [6].

Heyse et al. published an average follow-up after BKA of 11.8 ± 5.4 (4–17) years on nine knees in eight females and 1 male with 100% survivorship of the implants. The average age at index operation was 64 ± 5 years [1].

Confalonieri et al. reported briefly on 12 cases of BKA in which a computer-assisted technique was used; there was no case of failure at 2 years follow-up [23].

Morrison et al. observed a near significant trend of an increased rate of revision arthroplasty ($p = 0.054$) at 2 years follow-up for a monolithic femoral component [63].

2.11 The Future

The underlying principles of soft-tissue-sparing surgery and the retention of native structures are appealing to many surgeons. The dilemma is often how to evaluate the remaining compartment to avoid early cartilage degeneration leading to implant failure and the risk of a more complex surgery to link individual components in the correct position.

In the future, available technology will help surgeons to assess the patient indications and to properly execute the procedure. Some of these new technologies are already available but are sure to undergo modifications once they are used by mainstream orthopedic surgeon and not only in excellence centers.

Computer navigation is now a daily practice tool for many knee surgeons. Its pros and cons have been extensively discussed in recent years, as has its value for the implantation of combined bi-unicompartmental arthroplasties [21, 24], Moreover, navigation systems can be used preoperatively to analyze the alignment and soft-tissue aspects of the knee as well as the stability of the joint, guiding the surgeon in making frontal and sagittal incisions [71-73]. Nonetheless, the absolute value of navigation for rotational alignment has not been proven yet [74].

For several years now, PSI for TKA have been in use [75-77]. Recently, several devices have been developed for unicompartmental resurfacing. The excellent control of frontal and sagittal alignment and the greater safety ensured while making the bone cuts substantially add to the value of this system. As an extra feature, T2 cartilage mapping of the entire joint is available, allowing the surgeon during surgical planning to evaluate the cartilage thickness in each compartment. Typically, an anteromedial wear pattern is observed in which cartilage is absent on both the tibial and femoral surfaces but especially in the anterior zones. A shift of the wear pattern more posteriorly is suggestive of an ACL deficiency. Both the patellofemoral joint and the lateral side can be evaluated; if greater lateral wear of the patella is observed then bicompartmental arthroplasty is appropriate. In case of tricompartmental disease, TKA planning for PSI-assisted surgery can be performed without the need for new imaging.

Patient-matched implants have been used by ConforMIS based on the same technology. Magnetic resonance imaging is used to analyze the anatomy of the individual patient and to design PSI and implants. The advantage of this system is clearly the patient-tailored anatomical reconstruction of the individual joint surfaces [78].

Finally, robotics have been introduced with great success in optimizing selective resurfacing of the knee. Current robotic systems can be classified as autonomous (RoboDoc, Sacramento, CA) , teleoperated (da Vinci, Intuitive Surgical, Sunnyvale, CA) or haptic-surgeon-guided (Acrobot Sculptor by Acrobot, London, UK, and MAKO TGS System, MAKO Surgical, Fort Lauderdale, FL).

In surgeon-guided systems, the surgeon provides the power needed for instrument motion while the robot constrains the position and/or orientation of the instrument within a given anatomically registered volume. The surgeon-guided robotic system provides virtual cutting guides for bone removal with either a saw or burr. This capability enables accurately sculpted, patient-specific, free-form bone resection in which less bone is removed than in traditional piecewise resections with a saw and cutting jigs [79-81]. Haptic robotics consist of a systems approach to the design of a minimally invasive modular knee arthroplasty. The classic designs of implants can be abandoned, making them more anatomical and bone sparing [82].

2.12 Conclusions

Bicompartmental arthroplasty with modular components is a valid treatment option for medio-patellofemoral OA in appropriately selected patients with limited deformity, intact cruciate ligaments, and a good ROM. Good functional results and better biomechanics are obtained, with low rates of revision or disease progression. Thus far, the long-term results suggest the need for caution but in these early adaptations this was probably related to instrumentation and tribology issues. Newer implant designs and improved instrumentation should ameliorate these results. The upcoming generation of surgical tools will improve the positioning of the individual components, making an anatomical reconstruction of the joint possible for most knee surgeons practicing today.

References

1. Heyse T, Khefacha A, Cartier P (2010) UKA in combination with PFR at average 12-year follow-up. Arch Orthop Trauma Surg 130:1227-1230
2. Lustig S, Magnussen RA, Dahm DL, Parker D (2012) Patellofemoral arthroplasty, where are we today? Knee Surg Sports Traumatol Arthrosc Epub Mar 10
3. Saccomanni B (2010) Unicompartmental knee arthroplasty: a review of literature. Clin Rheumatol 29:339-346
4. Lonner J (2009) Modular bicompartmental knee arthroplasty with robotic arm assistance. Am J Orthop (Belle Mead NJ) 38:28-31
5. Wünschel M, Lo J, Dilger T, Wülker N, Müller O (2011) Influence of bi-and tri-compartmental knee arthroplasty on the kinematics of the knee joint. BMC Musculoskeletal Disorders 12:29-35
6. Paratte S, Pauly V, Aubaniac JM, Argenson JN (2010) Survival of bicompartmental knee arthroplasty at 5 to 23 years. Clin Orthop Relat Res 468:64-72
7. Carr AJ, Robertsson O, Graves S, Price AJ, Arden NK, Judge A, Beard DJ (2012) Knee replacement. Lancet 379:1331-1340
8. Deschamps G, Chol C (2011) Fixed-bearing unicompartmental knee arthroplasty. Patients' selection and operative technique. Orthop Traumatol Surg Res 97:648-661
9. Gomoll AH (2011) High tibial osteotomy for the treatment of unicompartmental knee osteoarthritis: a review of the literature, indications, and technique. Phys Sportsmed 39:45-54
10. Pritchett JW (2004) Patient preferences in knee prostheses. J Bone Joint Surg Br 86:979-982
11. Rolston L, Bresch J, Engh G, Franz A, Kreuzer S, Nadaud M, Puri L, Wood D (2007) Bicompartmental knee arthroplasty: a bone-sparing, ligament-sparing, and minimally invasive alternative for active patients. Orthopedics 30:70-73
12. Zanasi S (2011) Innovations in total knee replacement: new trends in operative treatment and changes in peri-operative management. Eur Orthop Traumatol 2:21-31
13. Laskin RS. (1976) Modular total knee-replacement arthroplasty. A review of eighty-nine patients. J Bone Joint Surg Am 58:766-773
14. Stockley I, Douglas DL, Elson RA (1990) Bicondylar St. Georg sledge knee arthroplasty. Clin Orthop Relat Res. 255:228-234
15. Callahan CM, Drake BG, Heck DA, Dittus RS (1995) Patient outcomes following unicompartmental or bicompartmental knee arthroplasty. A meta-analysis. J Arthroplasty 10:141-150
16. Swanson AB, De Groot Swanson G, Powers T, Khalili MA, Maupin BK, Mayhew DE, Moss SH (1985) Unicompartmental and bicompartmental arthroplasty of the knee with a finned metal tibial-plateau implant. J Bone Joint Surg Am 67:1175-1182
17. Woodburn KR, Braidwood AS (1990) GUEPAR total knee prosthesis. J R Coll Surg Edinb 35: 56-60
18. Cloutier JM, Sabouret P, Deghrar A (1999) Total knee arthroplasty with retention of both cruciate ligaments. A nine to eleven-year follow-up study. J Bone Joint Surg Am 81:697-702
19. Lewis P, Rorabeck CH, Bourne RB, Devane P (1994) Posteromedial tibial polyethylene failure in total knee replacements. Clin Orthop 299:11-17
20. Pritchett JW (2011) Patients prefer a bicruciate-retaining or the medial pivot total knee prosthesis. J Arthroplasty 26:224-228
21. Confalonieri N, Manzotti A (2005) Mini-invasive computer-assisted bi-unicompartmental knee replacement. Int J Med Robot 1:45-50
22. Confalonieri N, Manzotti A, Pullen C (2007) Navigated shorter incision or smaller implant in knee arthritis? Clin Orthop Relat Res 463:63-67
23. ConfalonieriN,ManzottiA,MontironiF,PullenC(2008) Tissue sparing surgery in knee reconstruction: unicompartmental (UKA), patellofemoral (PFA), UKA+ PFA, bi-unicompartmental (Bi-UKA) arthroplasties. J Of Orthopaedics and Traumatology 9:171-177
24. Confalonieri N, Manzotti A, Cerveri P, De Momi E (2009) Bi-unicompartmental versus total knee arthroplasty: a matched paired study with early clinical results. Arch Orthop Trauma Surg 129:1157-1163
25. Wang H, Dungan E, Frame J, Rolston L. (2009) Gait analysis after bicompartmental knee replacement. Clin Biomech 24:751-754
26. McAlindon TE, Cooper C, Kirwan JR, Dieppe PA (1992) Knee pain and disability in the community. Br J Rheumatol 31:189-192
27. Miller R, Kettelkamp DB, Laubenthal KN, Karagiorgos A, Smidt GL (1973) Quantitative correlations in degenerative arthritis of the knee. J Bone Joint Surg Am 55:956-962
28. Temple MM, Bae WC, Chen MQ (2007) Age-and site-associated biomechanical weakening of human articular cartilage of the femoral condyle. Osteoarthritis Cartilage 15:1042-1052
29. Bae WC, Payanal MM, Chen AC, Hsieh-Bonassera ND, Ballard BL, Lotz MK, Coutts RD, Bugbee WD, Sah RL (2010) Topographic patterns of cartilage lesions in knee osteoarthritis. Cartilage 1:10-19
30. Davies AP, Vince AS, Shepstone L, Donell ST, Glasgow MM (2002) The radiologic prevalence of patellofemoral osteoarthritis. Clin Orthop Relat Res 402:206-212

31. Arno S, Maffei D, Walker PS, Schwarzkopf R, Desai P, Steiner GC (2011) Retrospective analysis of total knee arthroplasty cases for visual, histological, and clinical eligibility of unicompartmental arthroplasties. J Arthroplasty 26:1396-1403
32. Beard DJ, Pandit H, Gill HS, Hollinghurst D, Dodd CA, Murray DW (2007) The influence of the presence and severity of pre-existing patellofemoral degenerative changes on the outcome of the Oxford medial unicompartimental knee replacement. J Bone Joint Surg 89:1597-1601
33. Beard DJ, Pandit H, Ostlere S, Jenkins C, Dodd CA, Murray DW (2007) Pre-operative clinical and radiological assessment of the patellofemoral joint in unicompartmental knee replacement and its influence on outcome. J Bone Joint Surg 89:1602-1607
34. Munk S, Odgaard A, Madsen F, Dalsgaard J, Jorn LP, Langhoff O, Jepsen CF, Hansen TB (2011) Preoperative lateral subluxation of the patella is a predictor of poor early outcome of Oxford III medial unicompartmental knee arthroplasty. Acta Orthop 82:582-588
35. Inaba Y, Numazaki S, Koshino T, Saito T (2003) Provoked anterior knee pain in medial osteoarthritis of the knee. Knee 10:351-355
36. Chang CB, Han I, Kim SJ, Seong SC, Kim TK (2007) Association between radiological findings and symptoms at the patellofemoral joint in advanced knee osteoarthritis. J Bone Joint Surg Br 89:1324-1328
37. Han I, Chang CB, Choi JA, Kang YG, Seong SC, Kim TK (2007) Is the degree of osteophyte formation associated with the symptoms and functions in the patellofemoral joint in patients undergoing total knee arthroplasty? Knee Surg Sports Traumatol Arthrosc 15:372-377
38. Köck FX, Weingärtner D, Beckmann J, Anders S, Schaumburger J, Grifka J, Lüring C (2011) Operative treatment of the unicompartmental knee arthritis-results of a nationwide survey in 2008. Z Orthop Unfall 149:153-159
39. Noble PC, Conditt MA, Cook KF, Mathis KB (2010) The John Insall Award: Patient expectations affect satisfaction with total knee arthroplasty: who is satisfied and who is not? Clin Orthop Relat Res 468:57-63
40. Bourne RB, Chesworth BM, Davis AM, Mahomed NN, Charron KD (2010) Patient satisfaction afer total knee arthroplasty: who is satisfied and who is not? Clin Orthop Relat Res 468:57-63
41. Dennis DA, Komistek RD, Colwell CE Jr, Ranawat CS, Scott RD, Thornhill TS, Lapp MA (1998) In vivo anteroposterior femorotibial translation of total knee arthroplasty: a multicenter analysis. Clin Orthop 356:47-57
42. Stiehl JB, Komistek RD, Cloutier JM, Dennis DA (2000) The cruciate ligaments in total knee arthroplasty: a kinematic analysis of 2 total knee arthroplasties. J Arthroplasty 15:545-550
43. Komistek RD, Allain J, Anderson DT, Dennis DA, Goutallier D (2002) In vivo kinematics for subjects with and without an anterior cruciate ligament. Clin Orthop Relat Res 404:315-325
44. Banks SA, Fregly BJ, Boniforti F, Reinschmidt C, Romagnoli S (2005) Comparing in vivo kinematics of unicondylar and bi-unicondylar knee replacements. Knee Surg Sports Traumatol Arthrosc 13:551-556
45. Lo J, Müller O, Dilger T, Wülker N, Wünschel M (2011) Translational and rotational knee joint stability in anterior and posterior cruciate-retaining knee arthroplasty Knee 18:491-495
46. Andriacchi TP, Galante JO, Fermier RW (1982) The influence of total knee-replacement design on walking and stair-climbing. J Bone Joint Surg Am 64:1328-1335
47. Hogervorst T, Brand RA (1998) Mechanoreceptors in joint function. J Bone Joint Surg Am 80:1365-1378
48. Barrack RL, Skinner HB, Cook SD, Haddad RJ Jr (1983) Effect of articular disease and total knee arthroplasty on knee joint-position sense. J Neurophysiol 50:684-687
49. Fuchs S, Thorwesten L, Niewerth S (1999) Proprioceptive function in knees with and without total knee arthroplasty. Am J Phys Med Rehabil 78:39-45
50. Skinner HB, Barrack RL, Cook SD, Haddad RJ Jr (1984) Joint position sense in total knee arthroplasty. J Orthop Res 1:276-283
51. Barrett DS, Cobb AG, Bentley G (1991) Joint proprioception in normal, osteoarthritic and replaced knees. J Bone Joint Surg Br 73:53-56
52. Laidlaw MS, Rolston LR, Bozic KJ, Ries MD (2010) Assessment of tibiofemoral position in total knee arthroplasty using the active flexion lateral radiograph. Knee 17:38-42
53. Engh G (2007) A bi-compartmental solution: what the Deuce? Orthopedics 30:770
54. Palumbo BT, Henderson ER, Edwards PK, Burris RB, Gutierrez S, Raterman SJ (2011) Initial experience of the Journey-Deuce bicompartmental knee prosthesis. J Arthroplasty 26:40-45
55. Tibesku CO, Innocenti B, Wong P, Salehi A, Labey L (2011) Can CT-based patient-matched instrumentation achieve consistent rotational alignment in knee arthroplasty? Archives of Orthopaedic and Trauma Surgery 132:171-177
56. Lonner JH (2008) Patellofemoral arthroplasty: the impact of design on outcomes. Orthop Clin North Am 39:347-354
57. Banks SA, Abbasi A, Van Vorhis RL, Chen R, Otto J, Conditt MA (2010) Morphology of the distal femur for bicompartmental arthroplasty. AAOS Annual Meeting Podium Presentation, New Orleans, USA
58. McAllister CM (2008) The role of unicompartmental knee arthroplasy versus total knee arthroplasty in providing maximal performance and satisfaction J Knee Surg 21:286-292
59. Willis-Owen C, Brust K, Alsop H, Miraldo M, Cobb JP (2009) Unicondylar knee arthroplasty in the UK National Health Service: An analysis of candidacy, outcome and cost efficiency. The Knee 16:473-478
60. Hopper G, Leach W (2008) Participation in sporting activities following knee replacement: total versus

unicompartmental. Knee Surg Sports Traumatol Arthrosc 16:973-979

61. Argenson JN, Guillaume JM, Aubaniac JM (1995) Is there a place for patellofemoral arthroplasty? Clin Orthop 321:162-167
62. Cartier P, Sanouiller JL, Greisamer R (1990) Patellofemoral arthroplasty: 2-12 year follow-up study. J Arthroplasty 5:49-55
63. Morrison TA, Nyce JD, Macaulay WB, Geller JA (2011) Early adverse results with bicompartmental knee arthroplasty: a prospective cohort comparison to total knee arthroplasty. J Arthroplasty 26:35-39
64. Rolston L, Siewert K (2009) Assessment of knee alignment after bicompartmental knee arthroplasty. J Arthroplasty 24:1111-1114
65. Khan OH, Davies H, Newman JH, Weale AE (2004) Radiological changes ten years after St. Georg Sled unicompartmental knee replacement. Knee 11:403-407
66. Cartier P, Sanouiller JL, Khefacha A (2005) Long-term results with a first patellofemoral prosthesis. Clin Orthop 436:47-54
67. Nicol SG, Loveridge JM, Weale AE, Ackroyd CE, Newman JH (2006) Arthritis progression after patellofemoral joint replacement. Knee 13:290-295
68. Kooijman HJ, Driessen AP, van Horn JR (2003) Long-term results of patellofemoral arthroplasty. A report of 56 arthroplasties with 17 years of follow-up. J Bone Joint Surg Br 85:836-840
69. Argenson JN, Flecher X, Paratte S, Aubaniac JM (2005) Patellofemoral arthroplasty: an update. Clin Orthop 440:50-53
70. Goodfellow JW, O'Connor J (1986) Clinical results of the Oxford Knee: surface arthroplasty of the tibiofemoral joint with a meniscal bearing prosthesis. Clin Orthop Relat Res 205:21-42
71. Casino D, Martelli S, Zaffagnini S, Lopomo N, Iacono F, Bignozzi S, Visani A, Marcacci M (2009) Knee stability before and after total and unicondylar knee replacement: in vivo kinematic evaluation utilizing navigation. J Orthop Res 27:202-207
72. Casino D, Zaffagnini S, Martelli S, Lopomo N, Bignozzi S, Iacono F, Russo A, Marcacci M (2009) Intraoperative evaluation of total knee replacement: kinematic assessment with a navigation system. Knee Surg Sports Traumatol Arthrosc 17:369-373
73. Massin P, Boyer P, Hajage D, Kilian P, Tubach F (2010) Intra-operative navigation of knee kinematics and the influence of osteoarthritis. Knee 18:259-264
74. van der Linden-van der Zwaag HM, Bos J, van der Heide HJ, Nelissen RG (2011) A computed tomography based study on rotational alignment accuracy of the femoral component in total knee arthroplasty using computer-assisted orthopaedic surgery. Int Orthop 35:845-850
75. Mayer SW, Hug KT, Hansen BJ, Bolognesi MP (2012) Total Knee Arthroplasty in Osteopetrosis Using Patient-Specific Instrumentation. J Arthroplasty Epub Jan 26
76. Ng VY, DeClaire JH, Berend KR, Gulick BC, Lombardi AV Jr (2012) Improved accuracy of alignment with patient-specific positioning guides compared with manual instrumentation in TKA. Clin Orthop Relat Res 470:99-107
77. Nunley RM, Ellison BS, Zhu J, Ruh EL, Howell SM, Barrack RL (2012) Do patient-specific guides improve coronal alignment in total knee arthroplasty? Clin Orthop Relat Res 470:895-902
78. Fitz W (2009) Unicompartmental knee arthroplasty with use of novel patient-specific resurfacing implants and personalized jigs. J Bone Joint Surg Am 91 Suppl 1:69-76
79. Banks SA (2009) Haptic robotics enable a systems approach to design of a minimally invasive modular knee arthroplasty. Am J Orthop (Belle Mead NJ) 38:23-27
80. Dunbar NJ, Roche MW, Park BH, Branch SH, Conditt MA, Banks SA (2012) Accuracy of dynamic tactile-guided unicompartmental knee arthroplasty. J Arthroplasty 27:803-808
81. Lang JE, Mannava S, Floyd AJ, Goddard MS, Smith BP, Mofidi A, Seyler TM, Jinnah RH (2011) Robotic systems in orthopaedic surgery. J Bone Joint Surg Br 93:1296-1299
82. Cobb J, Henckel J, Gomes P, Harris S, Jakopec M, Rodriguez F, Barrett A, Davies B (2006) Hands-on robotic unicompartmental knee replacement: a prospective, randomised controlled study of the acrobot system. J Bone Joint Surg Br 88:188-197

Unicondylar Knee Replacement and the Cruciate Ligaments

3

Andrew A. Amis

3.1 Introduction

This chapter mainly addresses the way in which the actions of the cruciate ligaments affect the kinematics of the tibiofemoral joint after unicompartmental knee replacement (UKR). Although it is normal practise to excise one or both of the cruciate ligaments during total knee arthroplasty (TKA), this reflects the fact that, historically, TKA patients were severely disabled by their arthritis and so they did not demand high levels of function: pain relief was paramount. The degree of degenerative change in these osteoarthritic knees was such that the anterior cruciate ligament was usually absent, following a combination of soft-tissue degenerative changes associated with chronic inflammation and mechanical destruction mechanisms, such as sawing by the edges of the osteophytes that had formed around the antero-distal outlet of the femoral intercondylar notch. This has never been the case with UKR, as in these patients, who are often younger, only one compartment of the knee has arthritic damage severe enough to require arthroplasty. Therefore, the implants are required to work in harmony with the other structures of the knee and ideally with a high level of function.

A. A. Amis (✉)
Department of Mechanical Engineering
and Department of Surgery and Cancer,
Imperial College London,
London, UK
E-mail: a.amis@imperial.ac.uk

Although several reports of UKR have shown long-term survival statistics that rival those reported for TKA, it remains the case that some surgeons view the UKR as a means to 'buy time', perhaps for 10 years, before further degenerative changes in the knee make revision to a TKA inevitable. The approach in which the ligaments are preserved and the prosthesis is intended to allow the patient to return to relatively high levels of activity has recently started to influence the approach to TKA, with demands for higher knee flexion and joint function, given the greater confidence in the reliability of this procedure.

The scenario described above entails a difference of surgical strategy. The TKA, performed in a more damaged knee, allows the surgeon to concentrate on the restoration of limb alignment via the bone cuts. If there is a problem with the soft tissues, they are modified so that they will work as desired around the new metal-on-polyethylene articulation. Procedures such as 'soft-tissue releases' are intended to obtain the desired function of the TKA and usually result in one or the other of the collateral ligaments, most commonly the medial collateral ligament (MCL), being released from one bone attachment until the knee can be brought to its desired alignment. Although this method may de-function the ligament to some extent at the time of surgery, it usually heals back onto the surface of the tibia in a lengthened state, allowing both motion and stability for the TKA. In contrast, the UKR procedure demands greater respect for the ligaments and the prosthesis must work in harmony with them. Thus, it may be argued that a UKR is more demanding than a TKA as both higher levels of function and more subtle

N. Confalonieri, S. Romagnoli (eds.), *Small Implants in Knee Reconstruction*,
DOI 10.1007/978-88-470-2655-1_3, © Springer-Verlag Italia 2013

interactions between the prostheses and the ligaments are required. The aim of this chapter is to explore some of the underlying mechanisms of knee function relating to stability and kinematics, concentrating particularly on the roles of the cruciate ligaments but also considering the slope of the tibial plateau, which interacts with both the cruciate ligaments and the UKR.

3.2 Knee Kinematics and the Cruciate Ligaments

The anterior and posterior cruciate ligaments (ACL and PCL) are the primary restraints that control the anterior-posterior (AP) translation of the tibia in relation to the femur. Thus, by definition, they resist most of the load imposed on the knee in those directions, when the load tends to displace one bone anteriorly or posteriorly in relation to the other. In a classic experiment, Butler et al. [1] mounted intact knees in a materials testing machine, so that the femur was fixed and the tibia could be moved in an AP direction in relation to the fixed femur, and then measured the resulting forces. After the force needed to produce a 4-mm tibial anterior translation was measured, the ACL was cut and the movement was repeated. The drop in the force required showed that the ACL had resisted more than 90% of the applied load. A similar result was obtained for the PCL, with the notable difference that when the knee was tested near extension the contribution of the PCL fell and other structures, particularly the posterolateral and posteromedial soft tissues, took over more of the restraining action [2, 3]. This response occurs because the capsular soft tissues attach around the posterolateral and posteromedial aspects of the distal femur posterior to the flexion-extension axis, such that they are tensed by knee extension and contribute to preventing hyperextension, slackening when the knee flexes. In particular, this means that the medial compartment of the knee is stabilised by structures such as the posterior oblique ligament, which forms part of the posteromedial capsular structures, when the knee is extended [3]. This mechanism acts reciprocally with the PCL, the bulk of which slackens when the knee approaches full extension. If the capsular structures then fail to tighten it would allow posterior subluxation of the tibial component of a medial UKR. A lack of one or other of the cruciate ligaments frees the tibia to move away from its normal relationship to the femur when the knee is functioning, potentially resulting in a functional instability.

The restraint provided by the cruciate ligaments, at all angles of knee flexion, means that they must be attached to the bones in a way that allows them to remain relatively tight throughout the range of motion, implying that they must fit-in with the matching articular geometry. This cooperative mechanism imposes restraints on the geometry and position of the UKR components, as discussed below. The overall mechanism, consisting of the femur, the two cruciate ligaments and the tibia, forms what may be approximated to an engineering mechanism known as a 'four-bar linkage'. It is only an approximation because a classic four-bar linkage operates in a planar manner whereas the kinematics of the knee also include rotations out of the sagittal plane of flexion-extension motion. However, it remains a useful means to visualise the behaviour of the knee, as long as its limitations are recognised. The four-bar linkage mechanism of the cruciate ligaments was identified nearly 200 years ago [4] but was modelled by O'Connor et al. in a study published in 1989 [5]. It can be seen from this model (Fig. 3.1) that, as the knee flexes-extends, the cruciates swing around their attachments to the tibia while remaining (theoretically) at a constant length. Thus, the ACL starts out with a large angle of inclination above the tibial plateau when the knee is in extension and swings down towards the tibia as the knee flexes; the opposite is true for the PCL, which actually passes through vertical in deep knee flexion [6]. This mechanism imposes a fixed path of motion of the tibia in relation to the femur, which is usually shown as the femur 'rolling-back' across the tibial plateau when the knee flexes. This observation led to the use of mobile bearings in the Oxford type of UKR [7]. Although this simple model is superficially attractive, it misses some of the subtleties of the working of the knee, particularly the difference

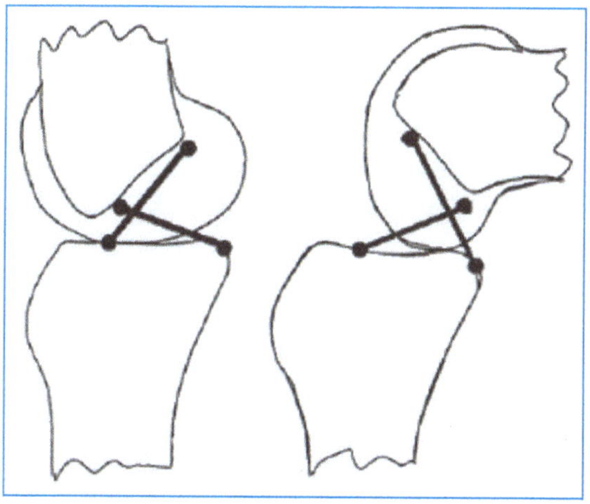

Fig. 3.1 The cruciate ligaments control the AP position of the femur in relation to the tibia: when the knee flexes, they cause the contact point to move posteriorly on the tibial plateau

in behaviour between the medial and lateral compartments, which is related to tibial internal-external rotation.

A more realistic way to visualise the loaded knee in vivo arose from the introduction of 'interventional' open-access magnetic resonance imaging (MRI), which allowed a living subject to have his or her knee scanned in a range of weight-bearing postures. It should be noted that the results were derived from a series of images of static positions, with the patient having to hold still during image acquisition. Nevertheless, these images revealed that the centre of the circular outline of the posterior part of the medial femoral condyle tended to remain almost stationary above the tibial plateau, while the lateral femoral condyle moved posteriorly [8]. The posterior movement of the lateral femoral condyle, while the medial one remained fixed, represents a tibial internal rotation during flexion of the loaded knee. Several lessons for the implementation of UKR may be drawn from these observations. In particular, it seems that the medial compartment should be less demanding biomechanically. In the natural knee, the medial tibial plateau has a slightly concave surface, and so it is inherently stable. During the most heavily loaded part of the walking gait cycle, when the leg is taking the load after the foot is planted on the ground, there is a force of several times the body weight acting to compress the medial compartment of the knee, such that the femoral condyle remains centred above it. Conversely, the extreme mobility of the femoral lateral condyle over the slightly convex tibial plateau is inherently less stable, and the adduction moment that occurs during the stance phase of gait unloads the lateral compartment, allowing relatively easy AP mobility of the femoral lateral condyle over the tibial plateau [9, 10]. The adduction moment is so high that there is a point during the gait cycle, just as the foot takes all the body weight, that 100% of the knee joint force is taken by the medial compartment and varus angulation is resisted by transient tension in the ilio-tibial tract [9, 10]. This loading mode is magnified in the typical patient with medial compartment osteoarthrosis, because the loss of medial cartilage thickness induces an increase in the varus misalignment of the tibia. That, of course, tends to increase the adduction moment acting on the knee during walking, hence increasing the loading on the medial compartment, thereby establishing a vicious circle. One of the roles of UKR in this situation is to use the thickness of the prosthetic components to realign the leg, to reduce the adduction moment acting on the knee and, hence, to reduce the forces acting on the medial UKR and its fixation.

Even in the absence of these displacing loads during dynamic activities, the cruciate mechanism induces 'femoral roll-back', which moves the contact point in the lateral compartment so far posteriorly in deep knee flexion that the posterior horn of the lateral meniscus is subluxated over the posterior lip of the plateau [11]. Thus, any prosthetic geometry will need to allow mobility and therefore be relatively unstable. In addition, the joint force will move towards the posterior edge, thus tending to edge-load the tibial component, rocking it on the bone and loosening the fixation. At the same time, the posterior motion of the lateral compartment, while the medial femoral condyle does not translate posteriorly during knee flexion, means that the medial UKR must have an articulation able to accommodate an internal-external rotational component during knee flexion-extension.

Observations of the mobility of the lateral compartment also help to explain why lateral UKR is more difficult than a medial procedure, because of the higher level of interaction with the guiding ligaments and therefore a fine tolerance between ligament tightness, which might limit motion and be painful, and ligament slackness, which might allow undesirable instability. In the natural knee, the lateral (fibular) collateral ligament (LCL) slackens significantly during knee flexion [12]. This is due to the fact that (1) the femoral attachment of the LCL is posterior to the axis of flexion and (2) the lateral tibial plateau slopes downwards posteriorly. Accordingly, there is greater coronal plane laxity in the lateral compartment than in the medial compartment of the normal knee [13]. This characteristic is a consequence of allowing an increasing mobility of the lateral compartment, and hence a greater range of tibial internal-external rotation as the knee flexes. It raises an interesting problem when setting-up a lateral UKR as this behaviour may tend to allow unwanted subluxation, yet over-control of soft tissue slackening (with an insufficient posterior slope, for example) may inhibit motion or cause pain.

3.3 Cruciate Ligament Deficiency and UKR

In an early review of the Oxford UKR, Goodfellow et al. [14] found that ACL deficiency led to a much higher rate of failure than in knees in which both of the cruciate ligaments were intact. That led to a recommendation that UKR was not indicated in knees with ACL deficiency—an interesting contrast to the situation with TKA, in which almost all of these patients have ACL excision as one of the early steps of the procedure. This situation has arisen because in the early days of TKA the patients had such severe arthritis that the ACL was degenerated or absent from most knees. A further factor is that preservation of the ACL entails setting-up the prosthesis so that it works in harmony with the cruciates, without causing abnormal ligament tension or blocking knee motion. There has been limited experience in which both cruciate ligaments were preserved in a TKA [15], but this approach has not become popular. However, if the instrumentation or navigational guidance can be improved, so that setting-up the ligaments becomes easier, then cruciate-preserving TKA opens the way to obtaining more physiological function from a TKA. Indeed, Komistek et al. [16] reported that a TKA in which the ACL was preserved resulted in kinematics closer to normal than a TKA in which the ACL was absent. When the situation with knee injuries in a younger population is contrasted with TKA, the opposite practise ensues: the ACL is the focus of surgical reconstruction while a PCL deficiency is often 'treated' conservatively. Several studies of knee kinematics after TKA have shown that aspects such as femoral roll-back and tibial internal-external rotation are not preserved [17, 18] whereas UKR seems to maintain relatively normal kinematics [19]. This is in contrast to the fact that the prosthetic articulation always has much greater frictional forces than in the natural knee, which could lead to abnormal patterns of rolling/sliding motion [20]. The situation is further complicated by noting the results of a study of TKA with mobile meniscal bearings [21]: the authors could not find a relationship between the AP laxity of the extended knee and its kinematics during weight-bearing flexion. It was therefore speculated that, during controlled activities, the kinematics are controlled by the muscle forces.

These differences of surgical practise raise questions of how best to deal with the cruciate ligaments in relation to UKR. There have been some studies of knee kinematics in the absence of the ACL, including two studies that used open-access MRI to examine weight-bearing knees in vivo [22, 23]. Both found that the pattern of movement of the medial compartment did not differ significantly from normal, i.e. the centre of the posterior medial femoral condyle remained almost stationary in the AP direction. However, the lateral compartment underwent significant anterior subluxation of the lateral tibial plateau compared with the ACL-intact knee. In the intact knee, Logan et al. [22] found that the centre of the posterior lateral femoral condyle moved posteriorly across the lateral tibial plateau with knee flexion, by 8 mm; when the ACL was absent, there is the same amount of movement but the lateral femoral condyle was consistently subluxed 6 mm posteriorly from the position with the ACL intact (Fig. 3.2). This caused the tibiofemoral articular contact point to be 6 mm further posterior than normal such that the tibia articulated in abnormal internal rotation, with the centre of the plateau approximately 3 mm anterior to the correct position. Nicholson et al. [23] also found that the lateral tibial plateau was subluxed anteriorly after ACL rupture, but reported that this was mainly near knee extension (8 mm at 0° flexion; 5 mm at 30°) and therefore not significantly different from intact kinematics at 60° and 90° flexion. The tibia tends further into abnormal internal rotation in deep knee flexion if the ACL is ruptured [24], which implies an extremely posterior edge-loading of the tibial component of a lateral UKR. There have also been gait analysis studies of the ACL-deficient knee; these have shown that the tibia moves with abnormalities of both anterior subluxation and internal rotation during normal activities [25, 26].

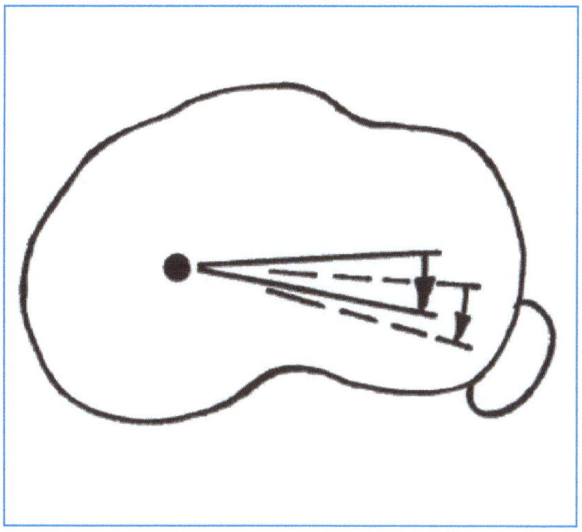

Fig. 3.2 The contact point does not move significantly in the medial compartment, which acts as though it is a pivot point. In the intact knee, the posterior movement of the contact point causes a secondary coupled tibial internal rotation (*solid lines*). After ACL rupture, the coupled rotation has the same magnitude, but is shifted further into internal rotation (*interrupted lines*), and so the contact point is further posterior on the lateral plateau

The PCL may also be injured, likewise altering the kinematics of the knee. Logan et al. [27] used the same open-access upright MRI method as in their study of ACL deficiency described above [22]. They found that loss of the PCL did not have a significant effect on the AP roll-back of the lateral compartment during weight-bearing knee flexion; however, it did affect the medial compartment as there was an approximately constant posterior shift of the medial tibial plateau of 5–6 mm at all angles of knee flexion examined, from 0° to 90°. Similar findings were reported by Chandasekaran et al. [28], from a conventional MRI study in which subjects pushed their feet against a weighted footrest while supine. The authors likewise found that the AP translation kinematics of the lateral compartment was not affected significantly by PCL deficiency; however, the medial tibial plateau showed a significant posterior subluxation across the range of flexion examined, reaching a maximum of approximately 3 mm at 75° knee flexion. The reduced size of the pathological shift compared with that reported by Logan et al. [27], may be related to the reduced load transmitted by the knee in the study by Chandasekaran et al. [28].

These observations from a range of studies in vivo and in vitro suggest that the largest pathological changes resulted from ACL deficiency, when the lateral tibial plateau subluxed anteriorly. They offer a clue as to why certain patterns of articular cartilage wear (as opposed to the damage induced during injury) are observed in chronic cases after one or the other cruciates has ruptured. The implications for UKR are more serious for the lateral compartment, suggesting that the abnormally large excursions of the contact point towards the posterior edge of the plateau may lead to loosening caused by an AP rocking effect, with the load then tending to crush the posterior supporting bone and to pull the fixation free in tension at the anterior edge. This has been suggested as a common mechanism of UKR failure. In addition to the loosening induced by abnormal articulation, cruciate ligament laxity may allow the joint to function with a chronic subluxation, which means that the articulation will not be working as intended, leading to increased wear due to the edge-loading [29].

3.4 Cruciate Ligament Reconstruction and UKR Bearing Design

The literature contains a number of papers in which it was concluded that UKR is not advisable if the ACL is deficient; this was sometimes an unrecognised problem in the early experience with UKR but it soon showed up as causing a greater rate of failure [14, 30]. At a mean follow-up of 7 years, a 25% failure rate among a series of 79 implants included 13 of the 15 knees in which there had been a pre-operative anterior laxity of 10 mm or more, implying that those knees had been ACL-deficient prior to surgery [30]. Similarly, the Oxford UKR resulted in a 21% rate of loosening failure at 2 years post-surgery if the ACL was deficient [14]. This lesson was learned rapidly, and it became accepted that UKR should not be performed in the ACL-deficient knee. The predominant cause of these failures was edge loading, which caused localised crushing of the supporting bone, accompanied by loosening.

More recently, as the joint-preserving ability of unicompartmental arthroplasty has become more established, surgeons have sought to expand the indications for its use, to include knees which are ACL-deficient. With arthroplasty spreading towards younger patients, a group of patients has been identified in which there is medial unicompartmental arthritis and ACL deficiency, yet also intact lateral and patellofemoral articulations. This group of patients is likely to expand, in view of both the increased risk of osteoarthritis of the medial compartment following ACL injury [31] and the further compounding of the likelihood of degenerative changes if the ACL deficiency then leads to meniscal damage [32]. In addition, this class of patients will often be relatively active, and wish to maintain their active lifestyle [33]. Although the above review of knee kinematics noted that the largest change following ACL rupture was in the lateral compartment, leading to localised wear of the articular cartilage from the posterior-lateral area of the tibial plateau, this injury has been shown to result in degeneration of the posterior part of the medial tibial plateau [34]. Reviews of clinical outcomes have shown that, compared with TKA patients, UKR patients have a larger range of knee flexion, knee kinematics that are closer to normal [35] and better functional outcome [36]. Thus, surgery that combines both ACL reconstruction and UKR (Fig. 3.3) may be an attractive option for patients who wish to maintain an active lifestyle.

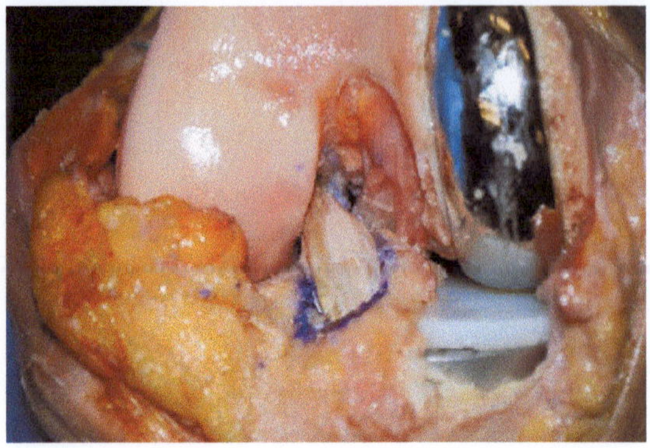

Fig. 3.3 A cadaveric knee with both a medial UKR and ACL reconstruction

There is a choice between fixed- or mobile-bearing UKR in conjunction with ACL reconstruction, and it may be argued that a fixed-bearing design will assist the reconstructed ACL in maintaining joint stability, as demonstrated in one series [33]. However, there have also been good clinical results published for patients who had ACL reconstruction combined with the Oxford mobile-bearing prosthesis [37], when the results of a group of patients with the combined procedure were the same as in a matched group with isolated UKR (Fig. 3.4). This is perhaps not surprising given that isolated ACL reconstruction is used mostly in a younger and more demanding population, and the grafts are unlikely to be stretched-out by the demands of the UKR population. Data from Oxford also suggest that the AP translation kinematics of the knee are similar to normal after the combined ACL plus UKR procedure, although the indirect measurement method used was relatively inaccurate and did not allow each of the two compartments to be

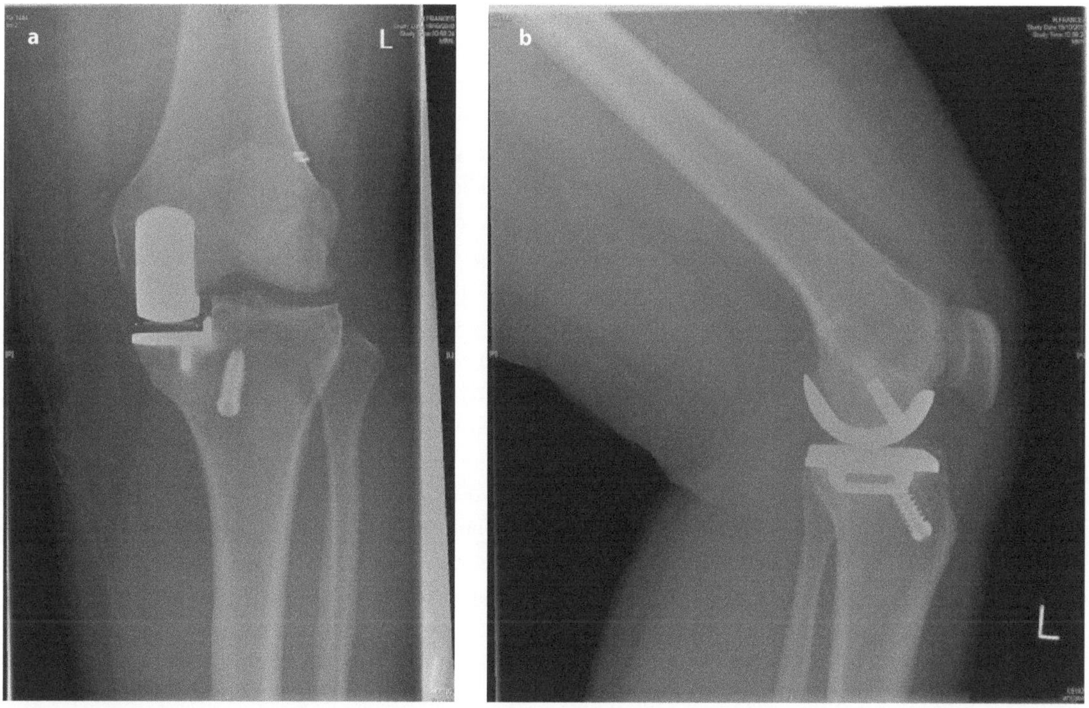

Fig. 3.4 Radiographs of an Oxford UKR combined with ACL reconstruction; antero-posterior (**a**) and lateral (**b**) views (with thanks to Dr. Dodd, of Oxford)

analysed, such that the tibial rotation could not be determined [38]. Both of the studies cited above used a standard four-strand hamstrings tendons graft, although the Oxford group noted in their discussion that they had started to use patellar tendon grafts because of their immediate strong bone-to-bone fixation [37]. Krishnan and Randle [39] used the medial third of the patellar tendon, which was accessible via their standard incision; they had been concerned that taking the central third, alongside the medial approach, may have led to devascularisation of the medial remnant. Their study also reported reliable restoration of knee stability after combined ACL plus UKR procedures. The maintenance of relatively normal kinematics in the mobile-bearing UKRs stabilised by an ACL reconstruction is supported by clinical results, which have not found the high rates of loosening that occurred when UKR was performed in ACL-deficient knees.

It is also likely that the kinematics of fixed-bearing UKR will not be much different from normal since in the absence of a mobile bearing, it is usual for the fixed bearing to have a flat or nearly flat articular surface on the tibial insert, in the AP direction. This is used to prevent the cruciate ligaments from 'fighting' the constraint imposed by a more conforming bearing geometry, if the position of the concavity is incompatible with both the kinematics of the reconstructed knee and the mechanics of the cruciate ligaments. In the past, that design philosophy sometimes led to the flat, or nearly-flat polyethylene bearing surface suffering severe localised plastic deformation and wear of the polyethylene [40], although more recent developments in the manufacture of polyethylene have ameliorated that concern. Argenson et al. [41], in a fluoroscopic study of the fixed-bearing M/G prosthesis (Zimmer, Warsaw, IN, USA), found that on average the contact point of the medial femoral condyle moved posteriorly by 0.8 mm, from 0° to 90° knee flexion, which was not significantly different than normal. They did note, however, that the mean behaviour included erratic kinematics, and that normal patterns of internal-external rotation appeared to have been lost.

3.5 Anterior-Posterior Slope of the Tibial Component

The AP slope of the tibial component in the sagittal plane has a profound effect on the mechanics of the normal knee and also on a UKR. As the mechanical effects are very strong, it is surprising that there has been little examination of the effects of changes in the posterior slope of the UKR on stability and kinematics. The literature contains many reports relating to both the natural knee and TKA, from which several lessons may be learned. The underlying mechanism arises because of the large axial compressive femorotibial joint forces allied with the extremely low coefficient of friction of the joint: this causes the femur to tend to 'slide downhill' across the slope of the tibial plateau. Since the normal knee has a tibial plateau that slopes distally/posteriorly, it follows that the femur tends to slide posteriorly across the plateau, which causes tibial anterior subluxation. The result is that this mechanism tenses the ACL.

There have been several studies of this mechanism in vitro, showing that the application of an axial load induced tibial anterior translation, which increased significantly if the ACL was deficient [42]. Liu-Barber et al. [43] found that application of a 1600N axial force (typical of walking loads) induced a tibial anterior translation of 8 mm when the ACL was intact. In the ACL-deficient knee, this anterior subluxation increased to 13 mm—an effect so powerful that it can induce rupture of the ACL. Meyer and Haut [44] found that an axial load acting alone could rupture the ACL, at a mean load of 5.4 kN, assuming an induction of a 12-mm anterior subluxation of the tibia. A load of 5.4 kN is a very large force, which may be reached when landing from a jump, or as an impact during skiing. Thus, a person with a large slope will be vulnerable to ACL strain; this helps to explain the prevalence of ACL ruptures in females, who often have a greater slope than males [45]. This factor is seen in an exaggerated form in quadrupedal animals, and the standard veterinary treatment for a rupture of the cranial cruciate ligament (the ACL) is a high tibial extension osteotomy aimed at reversing the large posterior slope found in many species [46].

The same mechanism may be related to the PCL and reduction or even reversal of the tibial slope. Two studies [47, 48] found that a change in slope of 4°–5°could reverse the pathological tibial subluxation resulting from cutting the PCL even under a joint force of only 200 N, which is only a small fraction of physiological loading.

Since most TKA procedures excise the ACL, it may be desirable to avoid an excessive posterior slope of the tibial tray in order to help to control anterior drawer laxity. However, along with a reversed slope leading to higher PCL tension, it has also been found that an increased posterior slope is related to a greater range of knee flexion [49] because it lowers the posterior rim of the tibial tray, thereby delaying posterior impingement [50]. This, however, may also lead to the femoral component articulating near to the posterior edge of the tibial polyethylene insert, causing abnormal wear [51]. For the UKR, this is clearly a sensitive situation, particularly if there is a low-conformity or a mobile bearing has been used, when the cruciate ligaments must control both tibiofemoral kinematics and stability. In this case, an inappropriate posterior slope may cause excessive ligament tension in use, potentially leading to creep elongation and ACL rupture. These powerful conflicting requirements mandate a precise control of the posterior slope.

The observations above were confirmed clearly in a clinical review of 99 UKRs at a mean follow-up of 16 years [52]. The AP relationship of the tibia to the femur was measured from true lateral radiographs of single-leg weight-bearing standing. In the 77 knees that had not been revised, there was a significant correlation between tibial anterior translation and the posterior slope. The slope was significantly less in these 77 knees without loosening than in those with loosening. Five knees had suffered a rupture of the ACL during follow-up, and their mean posterior slope was 13°. Furthermore, the original group of 99 UKRs included 18 cases in which the ACL was absent at the time of surgery: 11 of those had the UKR still in-situ at follow-up, with a mean slope of < 5°, while in the seven that had been revised the slope was > 8°. It was concluded that a posterior slope of > 7° should be avoided. Moller et al. [53] examined tibiofemoral contact points in both medial and lateral UKRs when loaded in vitro. Loss of the ACL led to the articulation moving approximately 6 mm posteriorly across the tibial plateau for both medial and lateral implantations. The authors also looked at the effect of increasing the posterior slope and found that the tibial anterior translation (inferred from the movement of the contact point) induced by cutting the ACL was similar whether the slope was 0° or 10°. A study in which cadaveric knees were loaded in a robotic test system that also included some muscle tension likewise found that the tibia translated anteriorly after ACL transection [54]. There was greater tension in the ACL near knee extension, when the changes in the kinematics are largest. Finally, and in line with the effects of changing the tibial posterior slope described above for the intact knee, it was shown that although tibial anterior laxity is increased following cutting of the ACL in a knee with a fixed-bearing medial UKR, the increase in laxity may be reversed by reducing the slope. An 8° reduction of tibial slope, from 12° to 4°, was able to reduce tibial anterior laxity by 5 mm during the Lachmann test [55].

3.6 Conclusions

Clinical reviews of UKR have shown that, in contrast to a TKA, it allows the knee to maintain normal kinematics during flexion-extension activities, resulting in a much closer match to the behaviour of the normal knee. This implies that in a UKR the cruciate ligaments are working in harmony with the prosthetic articulation. Evidence from older studies, in which the UKRs involved knees that were ACL-deficient, suggests that some of those knees were capable of surviving in-situ , as long as the posterior slope was < 7°. The slope of the tibial plateau has a profound effect on the articular behaviour of a UKR. Thus, although a larger slope may delay the onset of posterior impingement, a factor that limits the range of flexion of a TKA, it is associated with increased tibial anterior translation laxity in UKR and a larger load on the ACL. All of the evidence to date indicates that a combined UKR plus ACL reconstruction procedure is able to restore approximately normal knee kinematics and that it is reliable. These conclusions apply to both mobile- and fixed-bearing UKR designs. An increased posterior slope together with an ACL deficiency may allow the point where the femoral condyle rests on the tibial component to move posteriorly. This is of relevance because edge-loading is acknowledged in the literature as being the most-prevalent mechanism of loosening failure of a UKR.

References

1. Butler DL, Noyes FR, Grood ES (1980) Ligamentous restraints to anterior-posterior drawer in the human knee. A biomechanical study. J Bone Jt Surg (Am) 62-A:259-270
2. Race A, Amis AA (1996) Loading of the two bundles of the posterior cruciate ligament: an analysis of bundle function in A-P drawer. J Biomechs 29:873-879
3. Robinson JR, Bull AMJ, Thomas R deW, Amis AA (2006) The role of the medial collateral ligament and posteromedial capsule in controlling knee laxity. Am J Sports Med 34:1815-1823
4. Schindler OS (2012) Surgery for anterior cruciate ligament deficiency: a historical perspective. Knee Surg Sports Traumatol Arthrosc 20:5-47
5. O'Connor JJ, Shercliff TL, Biden E, Goodfellow JW (1989) The geometry of the knee in the sagittal plane. Proc Inst Mech Eng Pt H: Engng in Med 203:223-233
6. Komatsu T, Kadoya Y, Nakagawa S, Yoshida G, Takaoka K (2005) Movement of the posterior cruciate ligament during knee flexion – MRI analysis. J Orthop Res 23:334-339
7. O'Connor JJ, Goodfellow JW, Dodd CA, Murray DW (2007) Development and clinical application of meniscal unicompartmental arthroplasty. Proc Inst Mech Eng H 221:47-59
8. Johal P, Williams A, Wragg P, Hunt D, Gedroyc W (2005) Tibio-femoral movement in the living knee. A study of weight-bearing and non- weight-bearing knee linematics using 'interventional' MRI. J Biomech 38:269-276
9. Morrison JB (1968) Bioengineering analysis of force actions transmitted by the knee joint. Bio-Med Eng 3:164-170
10. Shelburne KB, Torry MR, Pandy MG (2005) Muscle,

ligament and joint-contact forces at the knee during walking. Med Sci Sports Ex 37:1948-1956
11. Vedi V, Williams A, Tennant SJ, Spouse E, Hunt DM, Gedroyc WM (1999) Meniscal movement. An in-vivo study using dynamic MRI. J Bone Jt Surg (Br) 81-B:37-41
12. Sugita T, Amis AA (2001). Anatomy and biomechanics of the lateral collateral and popliteofibular ligaments. Am J Sports Med 29:466-472
13. Okazaki K, Miura H, Matsuda S, Takeuchi N, Mawatari T, Hashizume M, Iwamoto Y (2006) Asymmetry of mediolateral laxity of the normal knee. J Orthop Sci 11:264-266
14. Goodfellow JW, Kershaw CJ, Benson MKd'A, O'Connor JJ (1988) The Oxford knee for unicompartmental osteoarthritis. The first 103 cases. J Bone Jt Surg (Br) 70:692-701
15. Cloutier J-M, Sabouret P, Deghrar A (1999) Total knee arthroplasty with retention of both cruciate ligaments. A nine to eleven-year follow-up study. J Bone Jt Surg (Am) 81-A:697-702
16. Komistek RD, Allain J, Anderson DT, Dennis DA, Goutallier D (2002) In vivo kinematics for subjects with and without an anterior cruciate ligament. Clin Orth Relat Res 404:315-325
17. Stiehl JB, Komistek RD, Dennis RD, Paxson RD, Hoff WA (1995) Fluoroscopic analysis of kinematics after posterior cruciate ligament retaining knee arthroplasty. J Bone Jt Surg (Am) 77:884-889
18. Stiehl JB, Dennis RD, Komistek RD, Crane HS (1999) In vivo determination of condylar lift-off and screw-home in a mobile-bearing total knee arthroplasty. J Arthrop 14:293-299
19. Patil S, Colwell CW, Ezzet KA, D'Lima DD (2005) Can normal knee kinematics be restored with unicompartmental knee replacement? J Bone Jt Surg (Am) 87:332-338
20. Wimmer MA, Andriacchi TP (1997) Tractive forces during rolling motion of the knee: implications for wear in total knee replacement. J Biomech 30:131-137
21. Ishii Y, Noguchi H, Matsuda Y, Takeda M, Walker SA, Komistek RD (2007) effect of knee laxity on in-vivo kinematics of meniscal-bearing knee prosthess. Knee 14:268-274
22. Logan M, Dunstan E, Robinson J, Williams A, Gedroyc W, Freeman M (2004) Tibiofemoral kinematics of the anterior cruciate ligament (ACL)-deficient weightbearing, living knee employing vertical access open "interventional" magnetic resonance imaging. Am J Sports Med 32:720-726
23. Nicholson JA, Sutherland AG, Smith FW, Kawasaki T (2012) Upright MRI in kinematic assessment of the ACL-deficient knee. Knee 19:41-48
24. Yamaguchi S, Gamada K, Sasho T, Kato H, Sonoda M, Banks SA (2009) In vivo kinematics of anterior cruciate ligament deficient knees during pivot and squat activities. Clin Biomech 24:71-76
25. Georgoulis AD, Papadonikolakis A, Papageorgiou CD, Mitsou A, Stergiou N (2003) Three-dimensional tibiofemoral kinematics of the anterior cruciate ligament-deficient and reconstructed knee during walking. Am J Sports Med 31:75-79
26. Knoll Z, Kocsis L, Kiss RM (2004) Gait patterns before and after anterior cruciate ligament reconstruction. Knee Surg Sports Traumatol Arthrosc 12:7-14
27. Logan M, Williams A, lavelle J, Gedroyc W, Freeman M (2004) The effect of posterior cruciate ligament deficiency on knee kinematics. Am J Sports Med 32:1916-1922
28. Chandrasekaran S, Scarvell JM, Buirski G, Woods KR, Smith PN (2012) Magnetic resonance imaging study of alteration of tibiofemoral joint articulation after posterior cruciate ligament injury. Knee 19:60-64
29. Bartley RE, Stulberg SD, Robb WJ, Sweeney HJ (1994) Polyethylene wear in unicompartmental knee arthroplasty. Clin Orthop Relat Res 299:18-24
30. Deschamps G, Lapeyre B (1987) Rupture of the anterior cruciate ligament: a frequently unrecognised cause of failure of unicompartmental knee prostheses: apropos of a series of 79 Lotus prostheses with a follow-up of more than 5 years. Rev Chir Orthop 73:544-551
31. Gillquist J, Messner K (1999) Anterior cruciate ligament reconstruction and the long-term incidence of gonarthrosis. Sports Med 27:143-156
32. McDermott I, Amis AA (2006) Review article: The consequences of meniscectomy. J Bone Jt Surg (Br) 88-B:1549-1556
33. Tinius M, Hepp, P, Becker R (2012) Combined unicompartmental arthroplasty and anterior cruciate ligament reconstruction. Knee Surg Sports Traumatol Arthrosc 20:81-87
34. Keyes GW, Carr AJ, Miller RK, Goodfellow JW (1992) The radiographic classification of medial gonarthrosis:correlation with operation methods in 200 knees. Acta Orthop Scand 63:497-501
35. Banks SA, Fregly BJ, Boniforti F, Rheinschmidt C, Romanoli S (2005) Comparing in vivo kinematics of unicondylar and bi-unicondylar knee replacements. Knee Surg Sports Traumatol, Arthrosc 13:551-556
36. Newman J, Pydisetty RV, Ackroyd C (2009) Unicompartmental or total knee replacement: the 15-year results of a prospective randomised controlled trial. J Bone Jt Surg (Br) 91-B:52-57
37. Pandit H, Beard DJ, Jenkins C, Kimstra Y, Thomas NP, Dodd CAF, Murray DW (2006) Combined anterior cruciate ligament and Oxford unicondylar knee arthroplasty. J Bone Jt Surg (Br) 88-B:887-892
38. Pandit H, Van Duren BH, Gallagher JA, Beard DJ, Dodd CA, Gill HS, Murray DW (2008) Combined anterior cruciate ligament reconstruction and Oxford unicondylar knee arthroplasty: in vivo kinematics. Knee 15:101-106
39. Krishnan SRSR, Randle R (2009) ACL reconstruction with unicondylar replacement in knee with functional instability and osteoarthritis. J Orthop Surg Res 4:43-47
40. Blunn GW, Joshi AB, Lilley PA, Engelbrecht E, Ryd L, Lidgren L, Hardinge K, Nieder E, Walker PS

(1992) Polyethylene wear in unicondylar knee prostheses. 106 retrieved Marmor, PCA, and St Georg tibial components compared. Acta Orthop Scand 63:247-255

41. Argenson JN, Komistek RD, Aubaniac JM, Dennis DA, Northcut EJ, Anderson DT, Agostini S (2002) In vivo determination of knee kinematics for subjects implanted with a unicompartmental arthroplasty. J Arthrop 17:1049-1054
42. Torzilli PA, Deng X, Warren RF (1994) The effect of joint-compressive load and quadriceps muscle force on knee motion in the intact and anterior cruciate ligament-sectioned knee. Am J Sports Med 22:105-112
43. Liu-Barba D, Hull ML, Howell SM (2007) Coupled motions under compressive load in intact and ACL-deficient knees: a cadaveric study. J Biomech Eng 129:818-824
44. Meyer EG, Haut RC (2008) Anterior cruciate ligament injury induced by internal tibial torsion or tibiofemoral compression. J Biomech 41:3377-3383
45. Hashemi J, Chandrashekar N, Gill B, Beynnon BD, Slaughterbeck JR, Schutt RC, Mansouri H, Dabezies E (2008) The geometry of the tibial plateau and its influence on the biomechanics of the tibiofemoral joint. J Bone Jt Surg Am 90-A:2724-2734
46. Kim SE, Pozzi A, Kowaleski MP, Lewis DD (2008) Review: Tibial osteotomies for cranial cruciate ligament insufficiency in dogs. Vet Surg 37:111-125
47. Agneskirchner JD,Hurschler C, Stukenborg-Colsman C, Imhoff AB, Lobenhoffer P (2004) Effect of high tibial flexion osteotomy on cartilage pressure and joint kinematics: a biomechanical study in human cadaveric knees. Arch Orthop Trauma Surg 124:575-584
48. Giffin JR, Stabile KJ, Zantop T, Vogrin TM, Woo SLY, Harner CD (2007) Importance of tibial slope for stability of the posterior cruciate ligament-deficient knee. Am J sports Med 35:1443-1449
49. Malviya A, Lingard EA, Weir DJ, Deehan DJ (2009) Predicting range of movement after knee replacement: the importance of posterior condylar offset and tibial slope. Knee Surg Sports Traumatol Arthrosc 17:491-498
50. Bellemans J, Robijns F, Duerinckx J, Banks S, Vandenneucker H (2004) The influence of tibial slope on maximal flexion after total knee arthroplasty. Knee Surg Sports Traumatol Arthrosc 13:193-196
51. Wasielewski RC, Galante JO, Leighty RM, Natarajan RN, Rosenberg AG (1994) Wear patterns on retrieved polyethylene tibial inserts and their relationship to technical considerations during total knee arthroplasty. Clin Orthop 299:31-43
52. Hernigou P, Deschamps G (2004) Posterior slope of the tibial implant and the outcome of unicompartmental knee arthroplasty. J Bone Jt Surg (Am) 86-A:506-511
53. Moller JT, Weeth RE, Keller JO, Nielsen S (1985) Unicompartmental arthroplasty of the knee. Cadaver study of the importance of the anterior cruciate ligament. Acta Orthop Scand 56:120-123
54. Suggs JF, Li G, Park SE, Sultan PG, Rubash HE, Freiberg AA (2006) Knee biomechanics after UKA and its relation to the ACL – a robotic investigation. J Orthop Res 24:588-594
55. Suero EM, Citak M, Cross MB, Bosscher RF, Ranawat AS, Pearle AD (2012) Effects of tibial slope changes in the stability of fixed bearing medial unicompartmental arthroplasty in anterior cruciate ligament deficient knees. Knee 19:365-9

4 Mobile and Fixed Bearings in Unicondylar Knee Resurfacing: Indications vs Osteotomies and Total Knee Replacements

David S. Barrett and Sam K. Yasen

4.1 Introduction

Whilst some indications for total knee replacement (TKR) are clear in patients with tricompartmental osteoarthritis (OA), limited flexion and significant deformity (Fig. 4.1a, b), the indications for osteotomy and unicompartmental knee resurfacing (UKR) continue to be variable [1, 2]. Moreover, the percentage of unicompartmental surgery performed varies from 10% [2] to 40% [3]. A similar variation is seen in the practice of corrective osteotomy for malalignment; for example, between the United Kingdom and Switzerland there are significant differences in training and experience along with patient expectations. These differences in indications relate to the surgical expertise and training available to perform osteotomy and UKR respectively.

Each technique, i.e. osteotomy [4], UKR [3] and TKR [5], produce reliable functional and long-term success but only in the correctly selected patient. Therefore a good understanding of the indications for each procedure is highly impor-

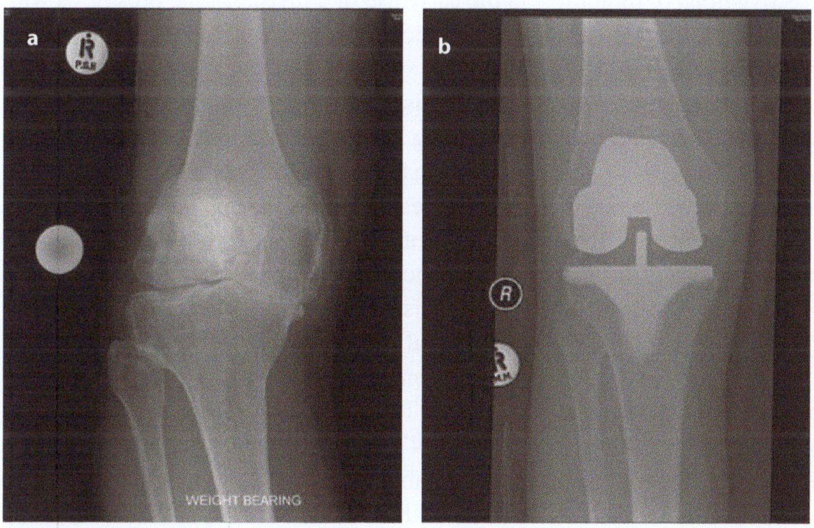

Fig. 4.1 **a, b** Pre and post-operative radiographs showing tricompartmental arthritis and good clinical result with a total knee replacement

D. S. Barrett (✉)
Trauma and Orthopaedics
Southampton General Hospital
Southampton, UK
E-mail: dbarrett1@aol.com

N. Confalonieri, S. Romagnoli (eds.), *Small Implants in Knee Reconstruction*,
DOI 10.1007/978-88-470-2655-1_4, © Springer-Verlag Italia 2013

tant in ensuring an excellent surgical outcome. There is considerable overlap in some cases regarding these indications. Where they are equally strong the surgeon should be guided by his or her personal experience and skills in each technique. It may be that surgeon A who is an experienced practitioner in osteotomy can attain a similar outcome as a surgeon B who is skilled in UKR.

4.2 Changing Indications

Previously, patients deemed "too young" or "too active" in manual occupations for TKR were offered osteotomy as a second option. Surgeons wary of the early poor performance of TKR in terms of early polyethylene failure, poor mobility and functional outcome often recommended osteotomy to "buy time" prior to eventual TKR, when the patient was older. The lack of effective revision prosthesis and techniques at that point also provoked caution in these patients, who might require up to three TKRs in their life time. This led to many younger patients with advanced OA, significant deformity and multi-compartment disease who underwent osteotomy. Nowadays, this group is regarded as being outside the current indications for corrective tibial or femoral osteotomy for malalignment and the early symptoms of premature osteoarthritic wear (Fig. 4.2) As a result, historically, in such cases osteotomy provided poor quality pain relief and functional results as well as a limited longevity of effect. Many revisions to TKR were performed before 7 years, during which pain relief was progressively incomplete [6]. Conversion to TKR has been shown to have an inferior outcome compared to a TKR performed as a primary procedure [7]. Therefore this group of younger patients had a poorly performing osteotomy with incomplete pain relief that often did not achieve the aim of a return to sports or manual activity [8], followed by a TKR that was functionally poorer than if the implant had been performed primarily.

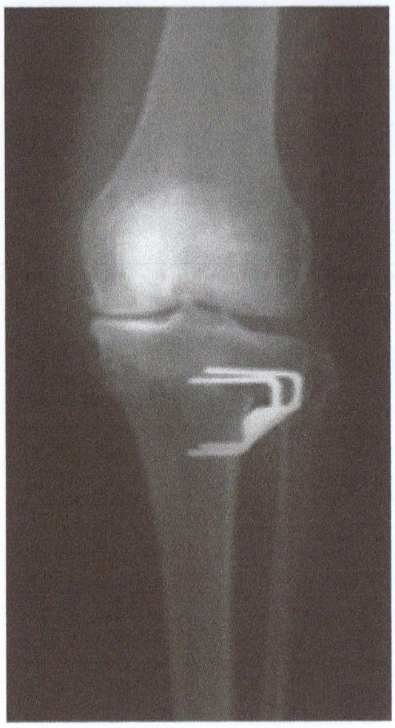

Fig. 4.2 Radiograph of failed high tibial osteotomy where indications were too advanced prior to original surgery

Similarly, in the early development of unicompartmental surgery, the indications were extremely narrow and the procedure was often described as a "pre knee" with conversion to a TKR being almost inevitable. Subsequent early failures required revisions. These were often complex, requiring a revision-type prosthesis and metal block augmentation, as deficiencies in UKR design and technique caused catastrophic failure with significant bone loss (Fig. 4.3a, b) Thus, in younger patients UKR surgery resulted in the early use of a revision-type prosthesis with poorer functional outcome, rather than a primary TKR.

The historically poor outcome and the disappointing functional result of revision in these younger patients treated with either osteotomy or UKR led many orthopedic surgeons to adopt a policy of delaying surgery as long as possible and then performing a primary TKR in this group. This method was particularly attractive to the general orthopedic surgeon who lacked specialist training in osteotomy or UKR but felt proficient in TKR. Willis-Owen et al. showed that although 47.6% of a group of 200 OA patients were suitable for UKR, surgeons still elected to perform TKR in the majority, offering UKR to only 8–15% [9]. However, functional results in young patients with TKR are disappointing and there is a significantly higher revision rate in this group than in older patients (Fig. 4.4) [5], leading yet again to early revision.

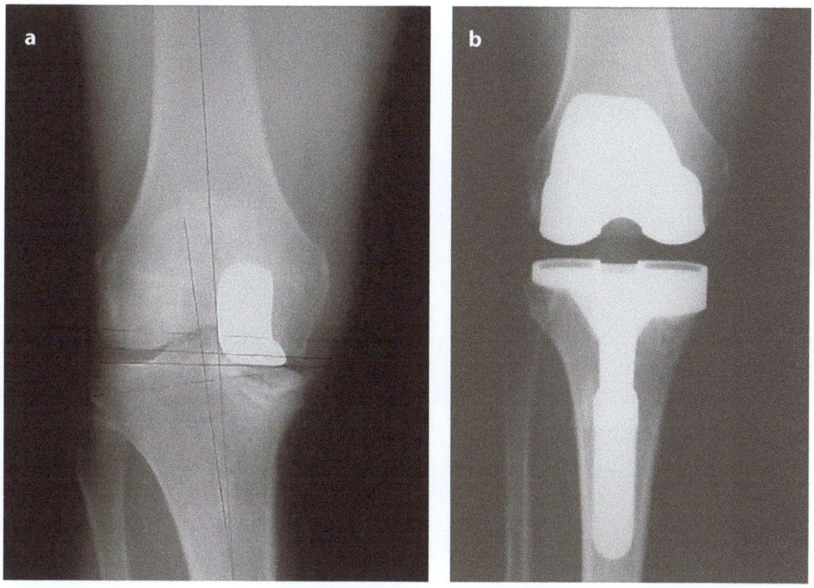

Fig. 4.3 a, b Pre and post-operative radiographs showing failure of UKR involving significant bone loss requiring use of revision prosthesis for primary revision

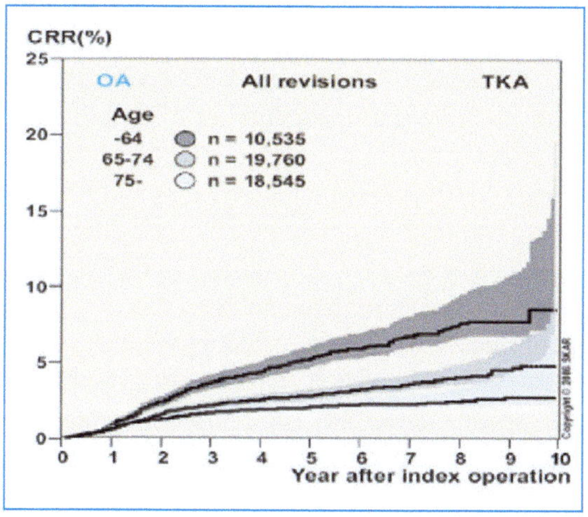

Fig. 4.4 Data taken from Swedish Knee Registry [5] showing increasing rates of revision of total knee replacement with decreasing patient age

Given the poor functional results and early revisions in this group with TKR, the indications, techniques and design of UKR and the planning, surgery and fixation of osteotomy have been re-evaluated. Consequently, UKR offers a better functional outcome than TKR on a more cost-effective basis [9] and the long-term results of properly indicated and performed tibial osteotomy have been shown to be much improved [4]. A revision of a well-performed tibial osteotomy to TKR can now be shown to provide similar results to those obtained in a primary TKR [7].

These findings have led to a reconsideration of the indications for the three procedures: osteotomy, UKR and TKR. Orthopedic perceptions have been significantly revised in response to both the changing osteoarthritic population and the recent advances in surgical technique and materials. Surgeons in this field need to ensure that they are fully aware of the changing indications in order to allow their patients the full benefits of these procedures.

Moreover, not only the orthopedic techniques but also the patients themselves are changing. They are younger and heavier [10], with an increasing number in the 40- to 59-year age group; indeed, in this group knee surgery is predicted to increase by 20% [11] (Fig. 4.5). This age group poses considerable challenges in terms of the much higher activity of these individuals, which in turn influences the wear potential of the implants. A higher range of movement coupled with up to seven times the number of cycles per year may lead to a wear rate in excess of six times normal for standard designs with standard polyethylene inserts [12]. These patients are not prepared to wait until they reach an acceptable age for TKR, at 65 or 70, but will demand an

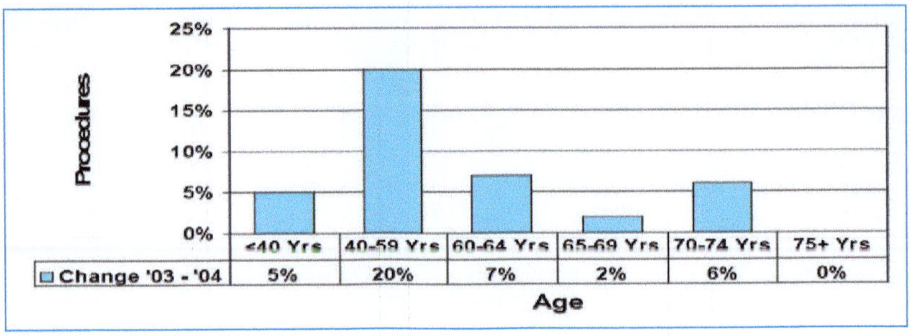

Fig. 4.5 Table showing projected percentage growth by age group in total knee replacement. 20% growth is predicted in the age group 40-59 years

immediate solution based on their significant symptoms, activity and quality of life. Thus, surgeons should be familiar with the more modern indications for each of these three solutions to knee joint pain.

4.3 Indications for Osteotomy

4.3.1 High Tibial Osteotomy

High tibial osteotomy (HTO) has become an established surgical procedure. Good to excellent results can be achieved with appropriate patient selection and correct surgical technique. HTO as a management option for medial knee osteoarthritis was first described in the 1960s [13] and popularised by Coventry [14]. The early technique was criticised by some as having high complication and failure rates, and its biomechanical validity was questioned [15]. These challenges and the success of knee arthroplasty were such that HTO fell into disuse during the 1980s and 1990s. However, with greater understanding of the basic science, refinements in surgical technique and the development of improved fixation technology there has been a resurgence of interest in HTO.

4.3.1.1 Indications

The principal indication for HTO is to treat established medial compartment osteoarthritis or overload of the medial compartment in the presence of menisectomy or osteochondral defects. This is achieved through offloading of the medial compartment by realigning the mechanical axis of the lower limb into valgus. A secondary indication for HTO is the management of knee instability [16].

The ideal candidate is a patient under 60 years of age who is a non-smoker, has a BMI <30 and presents with isolated medial joint line pain secondary to unicompartmental arthritis. There should be fixed flexion deformity of $< 5^{\circ}$, knee flexion of $> 120^{\circ}$ and, ideally, tibial metaphyseal varus of $> 5^{\circ}$ with normal ligament balance [16, 17].

HTO may also be undertaken in patients with cruciate ligament instability or patellofemoral arthritis but additional procedures and special attention to surgical technique are necessary. In the case of cruciate ligament insufficiency, the tibial slope can be adjusted accordingly (reduced for an ACL-deficient knee and increased in a PCL-deficient knee [16]), or the osteotomy can be combined with ligament reconstruction [18, 19]. A Fulkerson's osteotomy (or similar procedure) of the tibial tubercle may be performed in conjunction with HTO in the presence of patellofemoral disease. Obese patients or those with flexion contractures of up to 15° may also benefit, although they are less suited to the procedure.

4.3.1.2 Surgical Options

The most commonly used surgical options are medial opening wedge osteotomy and lateral closing wedge osteotomy. Dome osteotomy, chevron osteotomy, and progressive callus distraction using external fixation systems are alternative approaches [20].

Lateral closing wedge osteotomy was long considered the standard approach, but the technique involves either fibular osteotomy or disruption of the proximal tibiofibular joint, and the

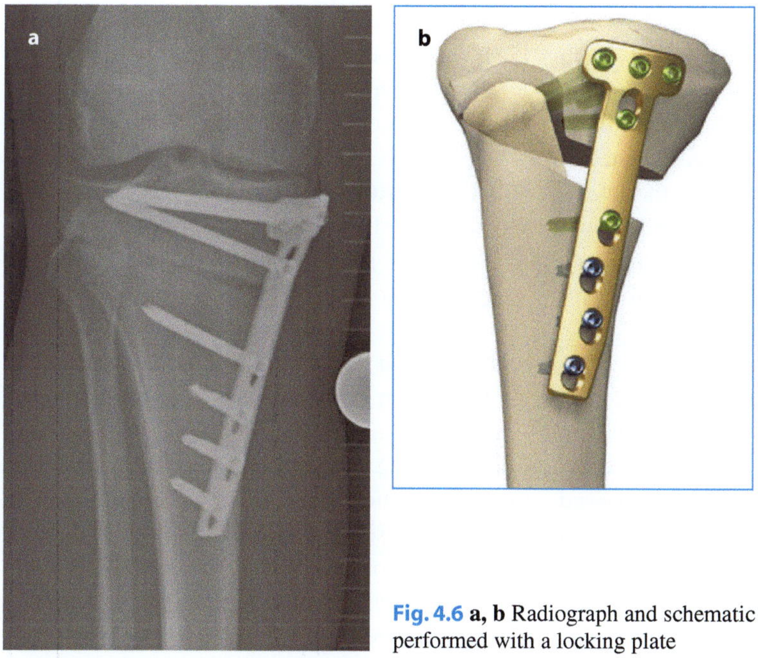

Fig. 4.6 a, b Radiograph and schematic of opening wedge osteotomy performed with a locking plate

exposure risks damage to the common peroneal nerve. Two saw cuts are necessary, causing bone loss and shortening that may compromise subsequent conversion to TKR.

Medial opening wedge HTO avoids extensive muscle detachment, involves only a single saw cut and allows more freedom to correct a deformity in both the coronal and sagittal planes [21]. Early problems with hardware failure and nonunion have been minimised with the recent introduction of better fixation systems. The TomoFix plate (Synthes, Switzerland), which is based on the principles of the locking compression plate, has been shown to yield a construct with enough stability to permit early weight-bearing and to allow osteotomy healing even in the presence of a lateral hinge fracture [22]. In a series of 262 patients, there was no loss of correction and only two nonunions using this plate [23]. Some authors routinely perform a bone graft to aid stability, but others have demonstrated that opening wedges of up to 20 mm can be safely left unsupported [16].

An additional important operative consideration in medial opening wedge HTO is the release of the superficial medial collateral ligament (MCL). Failure to do so results in increased medial compartment pressures rather than the desired reduction [24].

A modification of the opening wedge surgical technique has been proposed, with the use of a biplanar osteotomy combining the transverse cut with a second, vertically orientated cut running behind the tibial tubercle (Fig, 4.6a, b). This creates an anterior buttress improving torsional stability and allows more space proximally for fixation [21]. Osteotomies proximal to the tibial tubercle have been shown to reduce patellar height [25]. When large corrections, (>8-10° valgus) are required, it is therefore recommended that the second, vertically orientated cut is directed distally, which avoids this problem [16].

4.3.1.3 Workup

An adequate history must be taken, specifically noting sporting/recreational activities, smoking status and medical co-morbidities, including obesity. The examination must focus on the site of tenderness, the alignment of the limb, the range of motion at the knee and the integrity of the supporting ligaments. Weight-bearing anteroposterior, lateral, skyline and Rosenberg views (or tunnel views) must be obtained. Limb alignment is then assessed on full-length standing radiographs. Additional investigations, such as isotope-labelled bone scanning or magnetic resonance imaging (MRI) of the knee, may aid in establishing a failing or diseased medial compartment, along with the state of the lateral and patellofemoral compartments. Alternatively, knee arthroscopy may be undertaken, either as a separate procedure or immediately prior to committing to performing a HTO.

4.3.1.4 Preoperative Planning

The tibial metaphyseal varus angle should be determined and the principles of deformity correction, as set down by Paley, should be followed [26]. If a large correction is contemplated, a double osteotomy, involving the femur and tibia, may be required to avoid causing significant joint-line obliquity. The normal mechanical axis in the lower extremity passes through the medial compartment of the knee. In the coronal plane, overcorrection to the lateral compartment is generally desired. A number of different criteria exist for determining the mechanical axis, with early work stemming from Fujisawa et al. [27]. In fact, the 'Fujisawa point' is now generally accepted as 62% of the distance across the tibial plateau, measured from the medial side [16]. This typically translates to 3–5° of valgus relative to the native mechanical axis or 8–10° of valgus compared to the anatomical axis.

4.3.1.5 Postoperative Management

Cryotherapy and thromboprophylaxis using intermittent venous compression are recommended to reduce swelling. Some authors still insist on a period of non- or touch-weight-bearing depending on surgical technique and the fixation system. With the use of the TomoFix plate in medial opening wedge HTOs, early weight-bearing can be commenced even with large corrections. Typically, partial weight-bearing is started on the first postoperative day and then increased depending on the level of pain, with full-weight-bearing by no later than 6 weeks postoperatively [16]. Studies using radiostereophotogrammetric analysis support this schedule, showing that early weight-bearing causes no significant movement at the osteotomy site nor is there a loss of correction [28]. On occasion, the regime may need to be tailored according to any additional ligamentous or chondral procedures undertaken simultaneously.

4.3.1.6 Results

Good to excellent results have been reported by a number of groups worldwide using different surgical approaches, with recent published studies showing a 10-year survivorship of 74–97.6% and a 15-year survivorship of 65.5–90.4% [20]. At short-term (1-year) follow-up, a randomised controlled trial comparing medial opening with lateral closing wedge osteotomy found no difference in functional outcomes [29]. Additionally, a meta-analysis has demonstrated no difference in complication rate, conversion to TKR or functional scores in longer-term studies, although opening wedge HTO was associated with a greater angle of correction, increased posterior tibial slope and decreased patellar height [30].

4.3.1.7 Complications

The most common complications include nonunion (0.7–4.4%), psuedoarthrosis, infection (2.3–4%), injury to the peroneal nerve (2–16%), compartment syndrome, hardware failure and thromboembolic events [20]. Intraoperative fracture of the medial or lateral hinge (depending on approach) increases the chance of nonunion, as does smoking [31].

4.3.2 Conversion to TKR

Failed HTO requires conversion to TKR. A systematic review comparing primary TKR with conversion to TKR following closing wedge HTO showed longer operative time and less early range of motion but otherwise no significant differences between the groups at longer follow-up. Long-term results in patients undergoing bilateral TKR, having had unilateral conversion from HTO, do not significantly differ in terms of functional, radiographic and clinical outcomes or survivorship of the prosthesis at 15-year follow-up [7, 32]. Data regarding outcomes in TKR following opening wedge HTO are not yet available.

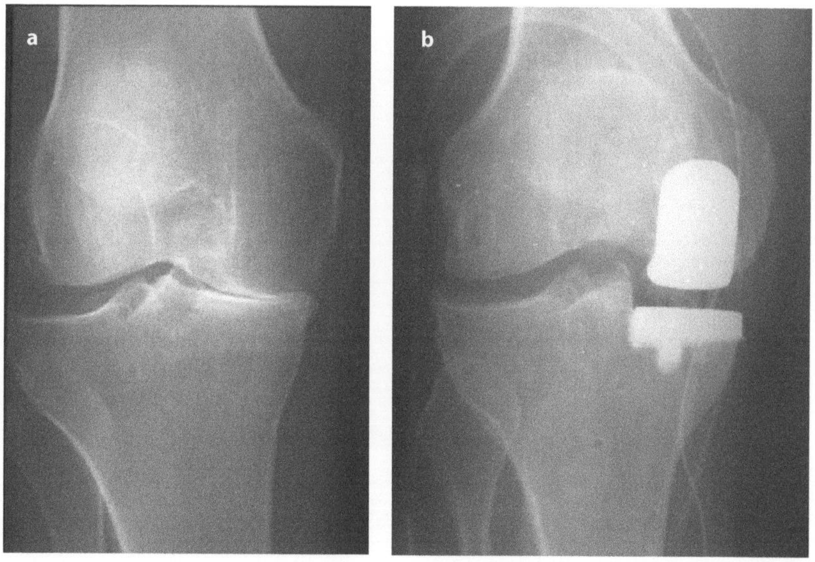

Fig. 4.7 Classical anteromedial arthritis seen on radiograph pre-op (**a**) and subsequently post-op after UKR (**b**)

Theoretically, medial opening wedge HTO allows easier conversion to TKR as there is no loss of bone stock, while the risk that the stem of the tibial component will impinge on the tibial cortex is less [17]. Therefore, although conversion to TKR may represent a technical challenge, the results of TKR following osteotomy are generally favourable.

4.4 Classical Indications for Unicompartmental Resurfacing

4.4.1 Preoperative Indications

The majority of UKR are carried out on the medial aspect. Thus, in the following the indications for the medial side are presented first, followed by a section on the indications for the lateral side.

Medial unicompartmental replacement is classically indicated for focal anteromedial arthritis limited to the medial aspect (Fig. 4.7a, b). Other compartments should not display radiographic signs of OA. Clinical examination should reveal a knee with less than 5° of fixed flexion deformity and less than 10° of varus malalignment that should be passively correctable [1]. History and examination should confirm the presence of a functional ACL as in particular for mobile-bearing designs the rate of failure, with ACL rupture, is reportedly higher [33]. The lack of an ACL gives rise to over-correction and early failure in addition to bearing dislocation, although this appears to be a problem related only to mobile-bearing prostheses. In addition to the clinical history and examination, the ACL rupture may be diagnosed radiologically based on the appearance of significant tibial lateral subluxation (Fig 4.8a) which may also indicate change or damage to the lateral compartment by tibial spine impingement (Fig 4.9). Lateral radiograph shows the particularly posterior position of the femur on the tibia as ACL rupture allows the contact point of the femur on the tibia to slide back from its normal anterior position (Fig. 4.8b)

Radiographically, some authorities recommend a valgus stress anteroposterior radiograph preoperatively to show a possible correction. A four-view series, AP standing, lateral, skyline view at 30° flexion, and a tunnel or intercondylar view at 45° flexion, should be obtained in all cases in order to assess the potential presence of arthritis elsewhere. MRI will reveal significant chondral defects if there is clinical concern regarding early changes in other compartments, but MRI is not part of the routine investigation when the clinical picture is well matched by the

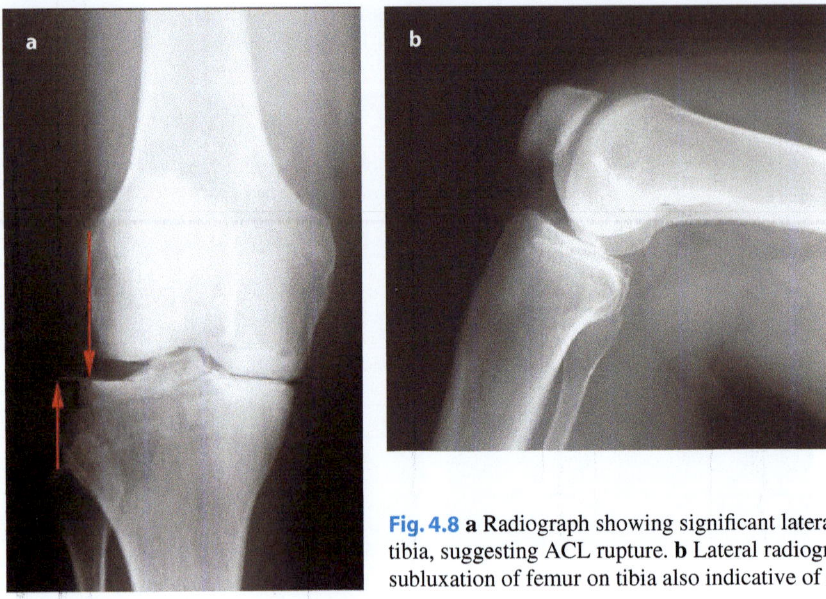

Fig. 4.8 a Radiograph showing significant lateral subluxation of the tibia, suggesting ACL rupture. **b** Lateral radiograph showing posterior subluxation of femur on tibia also indicative of ACL rupture

radiographic appearance. For similar reasons, the routine use of arthroscopy in knee assessment is not practiced, although many patients will have had arthoscopies in the past, details of which are useful in assessing disease progression. If the clinical position is in doubt and there is a possibility of ACL instability in addition to chondral damage as a cause of pain, arthroscopy and EUA are useful investigations prior to unicondylar replacement with or without ACL reconstruction.

Patients with varus medial arthritis may have either a degree of primary femoral valgus or lateral condylar hypoplasia (Fig. 4.10a). This is relevant when lateral condylar hypoplasia allows passive correction beyond neutral into a valgus malalignment. It may be of greater significance in mobile-bearing UKR, in which re-tensioning of the MCL is necessary to retain the mobile-bearing. In these cases fully re-tensioning the ligament pushes the knee into valgus alignment, with rapid acceleration of lateral OA and premature failure of the implant.

Previously, concern regarding tibial bone collapse under the prosthesis led surgeons to suggest a maximum weight limit of the patient (Fig. 4.10b). Suggestions vary in the absence of any detailed literature but an upper limit of 120 or 130 kg is considered appropriate.

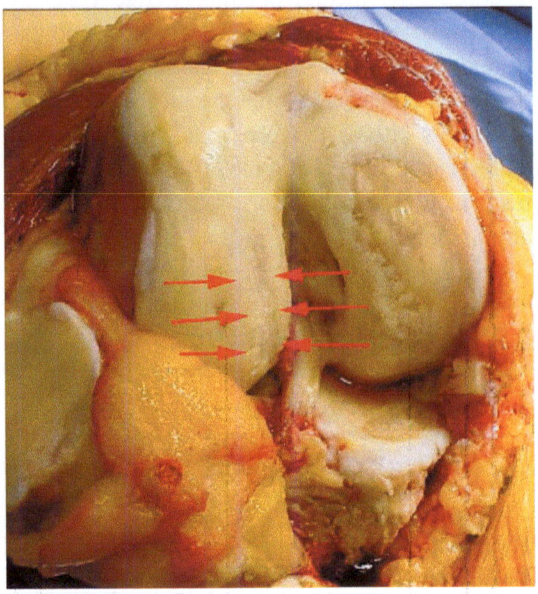

Fig. 4.9 Clinical picture showing tibial spine impingement on the inner aspect of the lateral femoral condyle, secondary to tibial subluxation

Poor bone density in elderly patients may preclude this group undergoing UKR due to concerns regarding tibial collapse. A second procedure, if the UKR fails or the OA progresses, is considered undesirable in the elderly. Therefore, many surgeons recommend the larger procedure of TKR in older patients.

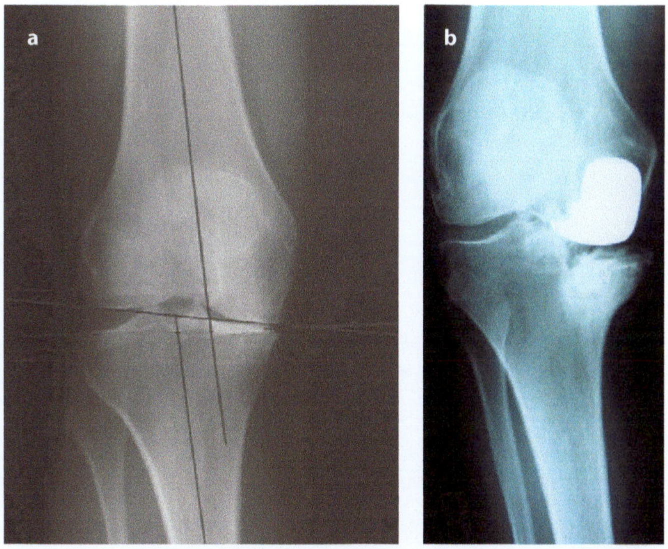

Fig. 4.10 **a** Radiograph showing significant lateral femoral condylar hypoplasia which may lead in to over correction into valgus. **b** Radiograph showing tibial bone collapse in an overweight patient

4.4.2 Intraoperative Indications

At surgery, inspection should be made of all other compartments. Grade II chondral changes (fibrillation of the chondral surface and partial-thickness chondral loss) are acceptable in the lateral compartment. Similar changes are also acceptable in the patellofemoral joint although in the view of some authors very significant changes in the patellofemoral joint may also be acceptable [34] (Fig. 4.11).

Surgeons should also check for the presence and function of the ACL, particularly if an unconstrained mobile-bearing model of UKR is used.

Many surgeons will determine the need for a UKR or TKR dependant on the intraoperative findings. Whilst this gives the surgeon maximum freedom, it is not the authors' practice, as in our opinion the combination of history, examination and radiographs should allow the surgeon to reach a definitive decision prior to surgery.

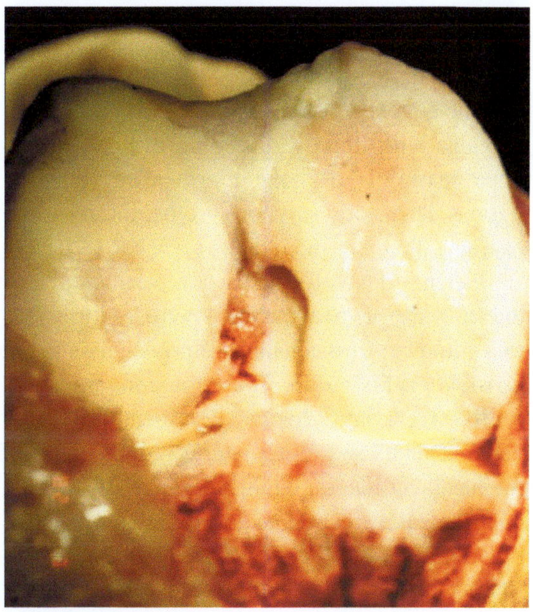

Fig. 4.11 Clinical photograph showing significant patellofemoral wear which may be acceptable in some circumstances for medial UKR surgery

4.4.3 Revised Indications

Currently, the indications for medial unicompartmental replacement are being revised, based on growing experience, developing designs and improved materials and techniques. Errors in surgical technique and prosthetic alignment coupled with older types of polyethylene led directly to many UKR failures. The resulting catastrophic polyethylene wear (Fig. 4.12a, b) caused significant bone loss and the requirement for a revision-type prosthesis rather than simple conversion to a primary TKR (Fig. 4.3a, b) [35]. Awareness of

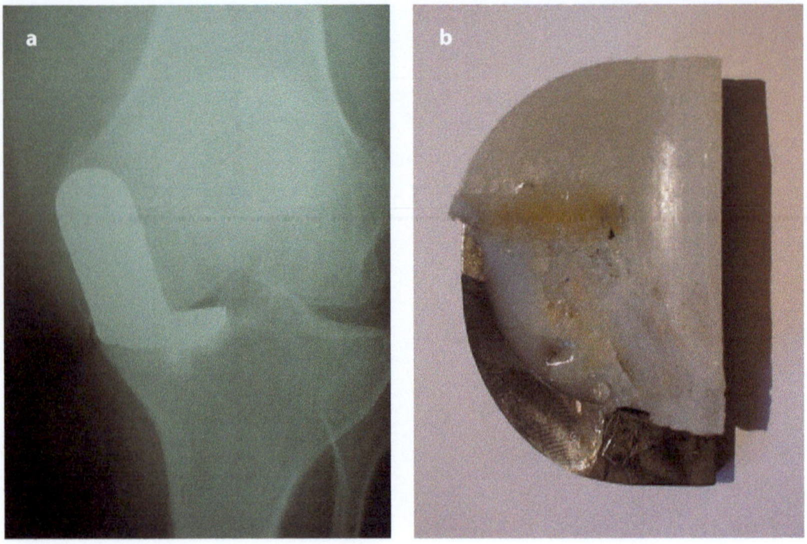

Fig. 4.12 **a** Radiograph showing significant malpositioning of UKR prosthesis leading to edge loading. **b** Explanted tibial prosthesis from the clinical case in 4.12 a. Accelerated polyethylene wear is shown as a direct result of malposition of the prosthesis and edge loading

the demands particular to UKR surgery, such as interprosthetic alignment to avoid edge loading and the advent of moderately cross-linked polyethylene with improved locking mechanisms in fixed-bearing UKR, have improved survivorship figures. Therefore, surgeons are beginning to re-examine the older indications for UKR [36].

Patients develop medial compartmental OA due to physiological habitual varus. Correction to a complete 0° mechanical hip-knee axis is not possible in this group. Thus, surgeons may prefer to leave a physiological alignment of 3° or 4° varus. This allows more natural re-tensioning of the medial collateral ligament, which is often lax due to medial wear. Changes in the nature of the polyethylene and the advent of moderate cross-linking have reduced polyethylene wear in the fixed-bearing UKR [37], allowing younger and more active patients to benefit from UKR. Thus, there has been a change in the balance between osteotomy and UKR, as more surgeons use the latter in a younger age group previously indicated for osteotomy [38].

Concerns regarding weight, BMI and the elderly patient also appear to be unconfirmed [39]. If appropriately performed, UKR does not have a higher failure rate, either in patients with elevated BMI or in the elderly; rather, UKR offers good symptom relief with a minimum of surgical intervention and much shorter rehabilitation [39]. Evidence from the Swedish Knee Registry [5] does not support the concern that this group suffers significantly more from disease progression and reoperation. Accordingly, it seems that UKR may be particularly beneficial in older patients.

Whilst the presence of a functional ACL is accepted as an important indication for mobile-bearing knees for the reasons outlined above, there is increasing evidence that a lax ACL in a functionally stable knee may not be a contraindication for a fixed-bearing UKR [33]. This is an important finding not only because of the persisting controversy but also because ACL-deficient patients make up a significant proportion of the younger patients presenting for consideration of UKR, due to the nature of the injury and associated meniscal tears leading to premature OA. Specifically, it appears there is no clinical difference in outcome between ACL-intact and ACL-deficient patients, providing that the knee is functionally stable prior to surgery. Theoretically, there will be a difference in the joint kinematics between these two groups [40] but with the newer, moderately cross-linked polyethylene resistant to cross-shear this difference may be only technical. In patients with symptomatic ACL instability, UKR can be satisfactorily combined with ACL reconstruction [41]. Occasionally, following UKR and the advent of a more mobile knee, a functional ACL instability is revealed. In

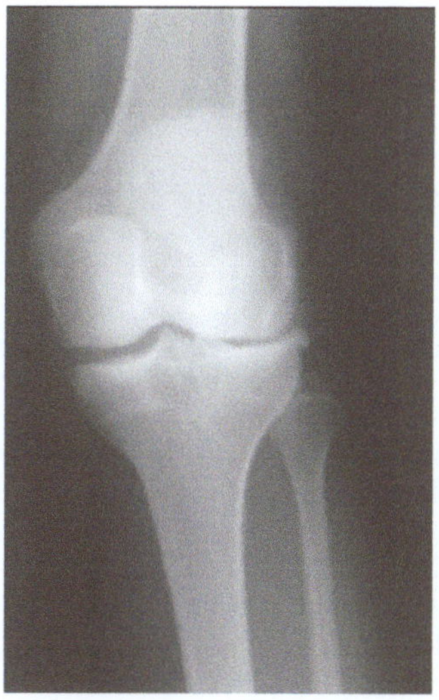

Fig. 4.13 Radiograph showing lateral osteo-arthritis suitable for lateral unicompartmental surgery

this case, ACL reconstruction is carried out as a secondary procedure.

There is increasing evidence that asymptomatic patellofemoral changes are not necessarily a contraindication to medial UKR [42]. This supports the view of Beard et al., who documented the results of a mobile-bearing practice [34]. Thus, patellofemoral change without clinical symptoms must no longer be included in the contraindications for mobile-bearing or fixed-bearing cases.

4.5 Lateral Unicondylar Resurfacing

Lateral resurfacing was previously rarely performed and it is contraindicated for an unconstrained mobile-bearing design. Recently, the number of patients undergoing lateral UKR with fixed-bearings has increased, with good results [43]. Suitable indications are isolated lateral OA, correctable valgus deformity and the absence of a fixed flexion deformity (Fig. 4.13). Valgus malalignment produces secondary lateral maltracking of the patella; therefore, surgeons should ensure that the patellofemoral joint is not involved before proceeding. Patients with obvious causes of lateral OA, such as post-total lateral menisectomy and lateral femoral hyperplasia, have good outcomes following lateral UKR. The tendency to over-correct a valgus malangulation at surgery should be avoided and the surgeon should be aware of the different positioning criteria of the prosthesis when used in the lateral compartment. Technically, lateral UKR is regarded as a more difficult procedure due to the challenges posed by exposure from the lateral side and prosthetic positioning. It is therefore advised that the surgeon become comfortably proficient in medial UKR before proceeding to lateral-type surgery.

4.6 Mobile- or Fixed-Bearing Unicondylar Surgery?

There are long-term outcome studies showing good results for both mobile-bearing and fixed-bearing UKR [3, 2]. In a paper comparing mobile-bearing with fixed-bearing for the medial side no significant difference was reported [44]; the choice is up to the surgeon, based on preference and training. Mobile-bearing UKR is contraindicated on the lateral side and therefore surgeons planning to offer UKR for patients with medial and /or lateral OA may wish to acquaint themselves with a fixed-bearing system that permits surgery on both compartments.

4.7 Total Knee Replacement

This procedure has a long history of development, good long-term survival figures [45] and well-established indications. For those patients with tricompartmental OA, significant deformity and fixed flexion, TKR offers both good relief of pain and functional improvement. TKR should always be the default option if the surgeon has doubts about the indications for osteotomy or UKR or is unfamiliar with the skills required for these procedures. However, in more active, younger patients, there are significant numbers of cases in which patients experience anterior knee pain, difficulty climbing stairs and pain or are unable to be involved in social sports [46]. Surgeons may feel the lower quoted revision rates for TKR are an important benefit in this group, but analysis of the data for young patients shows a significantly higher rate of revision (Fig. 4.4) [5], indicating unsatisfactory surgery or premature component failure under the higher activity of this group [12]. Early results indicate that preservation of the cruciate ligaments and the minimal intervention that are part of corrective osteotomy or UKR reward the patient with a greater functionality above that of TKR and similar to that of age-matched controls [9].

4.8 Revision Surgery

In this group, the surgeon must be mindful of subsequent revision surgery during the lifetime of the patient. Revision following TKR is increasingly successful when performed with a purpose-built revision prosthesis; however, eventual revision from osteotomy to TKR or UKR to TKR has more recently been shown to provide superior functional results [7]. This indicates that for the long-term outcome of these younger patients, who might require an arthroplasty after more than 50 years, the more minimal approach of osteotomy or UKR, with a higher initial functional performance, followed by eventual revision to a TKR, in which the performance is the same as following a primary TKR, may be the option of choice in suitable patients with the correct indications.

4.9 Conclusions

In UKR, as surgical skills have developed and both the materials and the designs have improved, the indications have changed, particularly with respect to a younger and more active population. Specialists have become more confident in performing UKR in these patients, thereby widening the previously strict indications. Lateral UKR can be expected increase in usage, with good results. Increasing accuracy with osteotomy techniques and fixation devices allows the earlier treatment of patients with OA, i.e. whilst chondral cartilage remains. TKR remains the treatment of choice in advancing tricompartmental disease, but given the increasing use of UKR and osteotomy it may be less commonly performed in the younger, more active OA population.

References

1. Price AJ, Rees JL, Beard D, Juszczak E, Carter S, White S, de Steiger R, Dodd CA, Gibbons M, McLardy-Smith P, Goodfellow JW, Murray DW (2003) A mobile-bearing total knee prosthesis compared with a fixed-bearing prosthesis. A multicentre single-blind randomised controlled trial. J Bone Joint Surg Br 85(1):62-7
2. Deshmukh RV, Scott RD (2001) Unicompartmental knee arthroplasty: long-term results. Clin Orthop Relat Res 392:272-8
3. Pandit H, Jenkins C, Gill HS, Barker K, Dodd CA, Murray DW (2011) Minimally invasive Oxford phase 3 unicompartmental knee replacement: results of 1000 cases. J Bone Joint Surg Br93(2):198-204
4. Schallberger A, Jacobi M, Wahl P, Maestretti G, Jakob RP (2011) High tibial valgus osteotomy in unicompartmental medial osteoarthritis of the knee: a retrospective follow-up study over 13-21 years. Knee Surg Sports Traumatol Arthrosc 19(1):122-7
5. Robertsson O, Ranstam J, Lidgren L (2006) Variation in outcome and ranking of hospitals: an analysis from the Swedish knee arthroplasty register. Acta Orthop 77(3):487-93
6. Coventry MB, Ilstrup DM, Wallrichs SL (1993) Proximal tibial osteotomy. A critical long-term study of eighty-seven cases. J Bone Joint Surg Am 75(2):196-201
7. Meding JB, Wing JT, Ritter MA (2011) Does high tibial osteotomy affect the success or survival of a total knee replacement? Clin Orthop Relat Res 469(7):1991-4
8. Gougoulias N, Khanna A, Maffulli N (2009) Sports activities after lower limb osteotomy. Br Med Bull 91:111-21
9. Willis-Owen CA, Brust K, Alsop H, Miraldo M, Cobb JP (2009) Unicondylar knee arthroplasty in the UK National Health Service: an analysis of candidacy, outcome and cost efficacy. Knee 16(6):473-8
10. Rajgopal V, Bourne RB, Chesworth BM, MacDonald SJ, McCalden RW, Rorabeck CH (2008) The impact of morbid obesity on patient outcomes after total knee arthroplasty. J Arthroplasty 23(6):795-800
11. Kurtz SM, Ong KL, Schmier J, Mowat F, Saleh K, Dybvik E, Kärrholm J, Garellick G, Havelin LI, Furnes O, Malchau H, Lau E (2007) Future clinical and economic impact of revision total hip and knee arthroplasty. J Bone Joint Surg Am 89 Suppl 3:144-51
12. Abdelgaied A, Liu F, Brockett C, Jennings L, Fisher J, Jin Z (2011) Computational wear prediction of artificial knee joints based on a new wear law and formulation. J Biomech 44(6):1108-16

13. Jackson JP, Waugh W (1961) Tibial osteotomy for osteoarthritis of the knee. J Bone Joint Surg Br 43-B:746-51
14. Coventry MB (1965) Osteotomy of the Upper Portion of the Tibia for Degenerative Arthritis of the Knee. A Preliminary Report. J Bone Joint Surg Am 47:984-90
15. Shaw JA, Moulton MJ (1996) High tibial osteotomy: an operation based on a spurious mechanical concept. A theoretic treatise. Am J Orthop (Belle Mead NJ) 25:429-36
16. Brinkman JM, Lobenhoffer P, Agneskirchner JD, Staubli AE, Wymenga AB, van Heerwaarden RJ (2008) Osteotomies around the knee: patient selection, stability of fixation and bone healing in high tibial osteotomies. J Bone Joint Surg Br 90:1548-57
17. Amendola A, Bonasia DE (2010) Results of high tibial osteotomy: review of the literature. Int Orthop 34:155-60
18. Noyes FR, Barber SD, Simon R (1993) High tibial osteotomy and ligament reconstruction in varus angulated, anterior cruciate ligament-deficient knees. A two- to seven-year follow-up study. Am J Sports Med 21:2-12
19. Aqueskirchner JD, Bernau A, Burkart AC, Imhoff AB (2002) Knee instability and varus malangulation - Simultaneous cruciate ligament reconstruction and osteotomy (Indication, planning and operative technique, results). Z Orthop Ihre Grenzgeb 140:185-93
20. Rossi R, Bonasia DE, Amendola A (2011) The role of high tibial osteotomy in the varus knee. J Am Acad Orthop Surg 19:590-9
21. Lobenhoffer P, Agneskirchner JD (2003) Improvements in surgical technique of valgus high tibial osteotomy. Knee Surg Sports Traumatol Arthrosc 11:132-8
22. Stoffel K, Stachowiak G, Kuster M (2004) Open wedge high tibial osteotomy: biomechanical investigation of the modified Arthrex osteotomy plate (Puddu Plate) and the TomoFix Plate. Clin Biomech (Bristol, Avon) 19:944-50
23. Lobenhoffer P, Agneskirchner J, Zoch W (2004) Open valgus alignment osteotomy of the proximal tibia with fixation by medial plate fixator. Orthopade 33:153-60
24. Agneskirchner JD, Hurschler C, Wrann CD, Lobenhoffer P (2007) The effects of valgus medial opening wedge high tibial osteotomy on articular cartilage pressure of the knee: a biomechanical study. Arthroscopy 23:852-61
25. Scuderi GR, Windsor RE, Insall JN (1989) Observations on patellar height after proximal tibial osteotomy. J Bone Joint Surg Am 71:245-8
26. Paley D (2002) Principles of deformity correction. Springer, New York
27. Fujisawa Y, Masuhara K, Shiomi S (1979) The effect of high tibial osteotomy on osteoarthritis of the knee. An arthroscopic study of 54 knee joints. Orthop Clin North Am 10:585-608
28. Brinkman JM, Luites JW, Wymenga AB, Van Heerwaarden RJ (2008) Early full weight-bearing in medial opening wedge HTO using an angle stable implant is safe using RSA analysis of stability. ESSKA Congress
29. Brouwer RW, Bierma-Zeinstra SM, van Raaij TM, Verhaar JA (2006) Osteotomy for medial compartment arthritis of the knee using a closing wedge or an opening wedge controlled by a Puddu plate. A one-year randomised, controlled study. J Bone Joint Surg Br 88:1454-9
30. Smith TO, Sexton D, Mitchell P, Hing CB (2011) Opening- or closing-wedged high tibial osteotomy: a meta-analysis of clinical and radiological outcomes. Knee 18:361-8
31. A WD, Toksvig-Larsen S (2004) Cigarette smoking delays bone healing: a prospective study of 200 patients operated on by the hemicallotasis technique. Acta Orthop Scand 75:347-51
32. Meding JB, Keating EM, Ritter MA, Faris PM (2000) Total knee arthroplasty after high tibial osteotomy. A comparison study in patients who had bilateral total knee replacement. J Bone Joint Surg Am 82:1252-9
33. Engh GA, Ammeen D (2004) Is an intact anterior cruciate ligament needed in order to have a well-functioning unicondylar knee replacement? Clin Orthop Relat Res. Nov (428):170-3
34. Beard DJ, Pandit H, Gill HS, Hollinghurst D, Dodd CA, Murray DW (2007) The influence of the presence and severity of pre-existing patellofemoral degenerative changes on the outcome of the Oxford medial unicompartmental knee replacement. J BoneJoint Surg Br. Dec 89(12):1597-601
35. Böhm I, Landsiedl F (2000) Revision surgery after failed unicompartmental knee arthroplasty: a study of 35 cases. J Arthroplasty 15(8):982-9
36. Pandit H, Jenkins C, Gill HS, Smith G, Price AJ, Dodd CA, Murray DW (2011) Unnecessary contraindications for mobile-bearing unicompartmental kneereplacement. J Bone Joint Surg Br 93(5):622-8
37. Collier MB, Engh CA Jr, McAuley JP, Engh GA (2007) Factors associated with the loss of thickness of polyethylene tibial bearings after knee arthroplasty. J Bone Joint Surg Am 89(6):1306-14
38. Engh GA, McAuley JP (1999) Unicondylar arthroplasty: an option for high-demand patients with gonarthrosis. Instr Course Lect 48:143-8
39. Fuchs S, Rolauffs B, Plaumann T, Tibesku CO, Rosenbaum D (2005) Clinical and functional results after the rehabilitation period in minimally-invasive unicondylar knee arthroplasty patients. Knee Surg Sports Traumatol Arthros 13(3):179-86
40. Banks SA, Fregly BJ, Boniforti F, Reinschmidt C, Romagnoli S. Comparing in vivo kinematics of unicondylar and bi-unicondylar knee replacements (2005) Knee Surg Sports Traumatol Arthrosc 13(7):551-6
41. Krishnan SR, Randle R (2009) ACL reconstruction with unicondylar replacement in knee with functional instability and osteoarthritis. J Orthop Surg Res 4:43
42. Berend KR, Lombardi AV Jr, Adams JB (2007) Obesity, young age, patellofemoral disease, and anterior knee pain: identifying the unicondylar arthroplasty

patient in the United States. Orthopedics 30(5 Suppl):19-23
43. Argenson JN, Parratte S, Bertani A, Flecher X, Aubaniac JM (2008) Long-term results with a lateral unicondylar replacement. Clin Orthop Relat Res 466(11):2686-93
44. Li MG, Yao F, Joss B, Ioppolo J, Nivbrant B, Wood D (2006) Mobile vs. fixed bearing unicondylar knee arthroplasty: A randomized study on short term clinical outcomes and knee kinematics. Knee 13(5):365-70
45. Bisschop R, Brouwer RW, Van Raay JJ (2010) Total knee arthroplasty in younger patients: a 13-year follow-up study. Orthopedics 33(12)
46. Diduch DR, Insall JN, Scott WN, Scuderi GR, Font-Rodriguez D (1997) Total knee replacement in young, active patients. Long-term follow-up and functional outcome. J Bone Joint Surg Am 79(4):575-82

UKR Surgical Technique: Pearls and Pitfalls

5

Norberto Confalonieri and Alfonso Manzotti

5.1 Introduction

Before beginning this chapter, perhaps a disclaimer is necessary: I'm not exclusively a knee surgeon, nor is knee surgery the most important and frequent part of my practice. I am neither a designer of the unicompartmental knee replacement (UKR) nor do I receive benefits for implanting them. I'm just saying this because the most frequent accusations, addressed to enthusiast knee surgeons using UKR, are that of expanding the indications and to obtain very positive but non-reproducible results by "normal" surgeons [1–3]. Likewise, there are surgeons inventors of new designs and models who exaggerate in their choices always with excellent results [4–8]. However, I believe, indeed, that almost all surgeons can obtain good results by just respecting the correct indications and following some basic rules of surgical technique.

I've been using the UKR prosthesis since 1988, with a series of over 1,400 patients [9]. I have implanted almost all models on the market and attempted both to understand the best way to improve my results, in a great majority of my cases, and to understand the errors of the few that were failures. Even when I dealt with computer-assisted surgery developing software, my first aim was to make the surgical procedure easy and reproducible [10]. Many of the things written on the pages of this book are still the subject of lively debate among us. There is no full agreement on all the rules, but I hope that the reader, looking at this book, can make up his or her own mind and act accordingly.

5.2 Principles of UKR Surgery

First of all, I believe the main rules to consider in UKR surgery are:

- Patient selection
- Implant design
- Operative technique

5.2.1 Patient Selection

Topics of this book are our patients with medial or lateral compartment osteoarthritis of different severity [11]. Often, this disease is the result of the congenital morphotype or traumatic events that have produced joint cartilage wear, with consequent mechanical axis deviation. First of all, it is mandatory to examine the patient and see if the problem is compartmental or general. For this, we use the "finger test": ask the patient to indicate with a finger where the knee is painful. If only one compartment is indicated and this corresponds to the pathological one, and the clinical examination is positive, the problem will probably be there and the Uni will be the correct solution. The main aim of our procedure is to remove the pain, and if, then, we get a better joint function and limb correction, then, why not even

N. Confalonieri (✉)
Orthopedic, Traumatology and Hand Surgery Department
CTO Hospital
Milan, Italy
E-mail: norberto.confalonieri@icp.mi.it

N. Confalonieri, S. Romagnoli (eds.), *Small Implants in Knee Reconstruction*,
DOI 10.1007/978-88-470-2655-1_5, © Springer-Verlag Italia 2013

aesthetics, which is so much the better [11]? But remember: no pain, no prosthesis!

5.2.2 Implant Design

To insert a prosthesis, you must create a joint space. You must know the thickness of the prosthesis (the wedge) and the model. In fact, the procedure of implanting the tibia is almost always the same, with a bone cut of varying dimensions [12, 13]. For the femoral component, there are two types of prosthesis: resurfacing, which provides a cartilage, and little bone fraction removal. The other prosthesis requires bone cuts in proportion to the thickness of the femoral component. It removes as much bone as the prosthesis thickness. This is important in determining the tibial cut. With resurfacing you can take into account the thickness of the femoral component: for example, for a thickness of 4.5 mm, you remove 2 mm of cartilage and bone, which leaves 2.5 mm of protrusion from the femur, and you can cut 2 mm less from the tibia. With the other, this is not possible, and the whole deformity correction should be taken into account during the tibial cut. Therefore, in severe axial deviations and using this last type of design, you need to know the maximum thickness of the tibial component because it may not be sufficient to correct the arthritis deformity. As an example: A 15° varus knee, 11 mm maximum thickness of the tibial component (minimum 7 mm): if you use a prosthesis with femoral cuts, even if you do not make any tibial cut, you will have a residual varus of 4° unless you use distal femoral cuts, but this is possible only with some prosthetic models.

It might be that a residual varus is plausible and physiological, but it is still a controversial topic, and there is no certain solution regarding whether this deformity should be totally corrected or not.

5.3 Operative Technique

The operative technique consists of five steps:

- Correction (planning).
- Minimal bone cut.
- Ligament balancing.
- Tibial cut.
- Femoral cut.

5.3.1 Correction

One indisputable fact is that the thickness of the prosthesis changes the axis of the knee according to the joint space that you have created. If the joint space is tight, the minimum wedge will also be tight and the mechanical axis will be overcorrected. If the joint space is abundant, the thickness of the tibial component chosen will decide the axis. A simple rule that we have developed is the "minimum tibia bone cut" (MBC), because it is important to cut the tibial plateau as little as possible in order to create good support for the prosthesis component. Our formula is: the minimum thickness of the prosthesis (TP) – the angular deformity (AD) = MBC.

Let's take an example: An 8° varus knee, and a resurfacing prosthesis with 4.5 mm of femoral and 7 mm of tibial thickness (total 11.5). Thus, you have 11.5 – 8 = 3.5 mm to remove. With resurfacing, you can also act on the femur. If you remove 2 mm of the femur, you have 2.5 mm of protrusion; you can cut only 1 mm of the tibia (3.5 – 2.5 = 1 mm) to provide a minimum joint space in which to introduce the minimal wedge in order to bring the axis to 0°. Obviously, if you want to undercorrect, you can increase the amount of femoral bone removal or increase the tibial cut. Using this concept, navigation is a useful tool to know the exact value of this procedure (Fig. 5.1).

If you use a prosthesis with femoral cuts, you need not consider the femoral component, because you have to remove all the bone exactly for the femoral component. That will leave you with only the thickness of the tibial component: 7 mm minimum, 11 mm maximum. It is evident that you must increase the thickness of the tibial component, because: 7 – 8 = –1. Even if you cut only 1 mm of bone, the joint space becomes 9 mm, so you can implant a tibial component of 9 mm (the rule becomes 9 mm – 8° = 1 mm). Here, if you

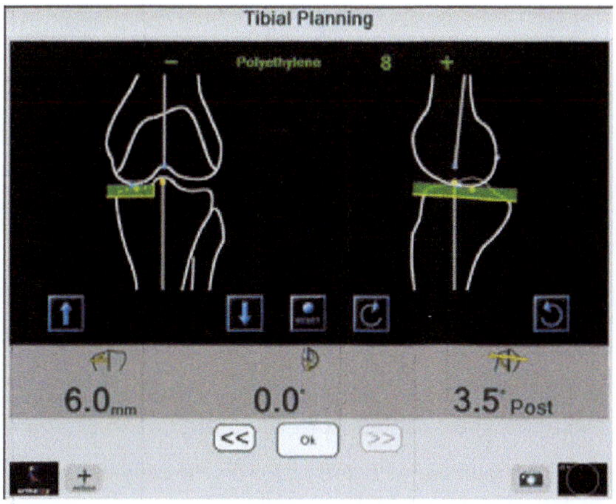

Fig. 5.1 Computer-guided determination of the minimal tibial cut yielding the perfect mechanical axis

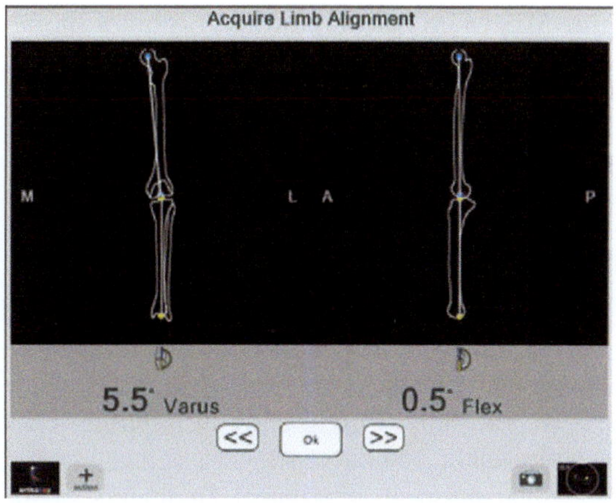

Fig. 5.2 Determination of the mechanical axis

want to undercorrect, keep the minimal thickness of the tibial and you'll have 2° of varus (9 mm – 7 mm = 2°). Sounds complicated, but it's only a matter of mental habit.

Another thing to be said is that sometimes the data do not match, either due to an incorrect orthostatic X-ray and resulting incorrect value of the deformity, or to an error in bone cuts, so you may find some problem with the introduction of the prosthesis. Experience and, for the person who uses it, the computer, will guide us to the best alternative choice of bone cuts (Fig. 5.2). But why would anyone want to undercorrect? And how much? And why in a high tibial osteotomy in a varus knee, is overcorrection of a few degrees recommended?

These questions are still without a definite answer. My experience with long-term follow-up leads me to say that it is better to have a mechanical axis close to 0° [14, 15]. UKR survivorship is close to that of TKR and, in the majority of cases, it fails either with a collapse of the bone under the tibial implant or, in rare cases, on the progression of osteoarthritis in other compartments [1–3, 14, 15]. Thus, it could be supposed that the more you keep the load on the prosthesis compartment, the more the bone suffers. Likewise, the more you transfer the load to the other compartment, and the more you free up the pathological compartment together with ligamentous stress, the better the joint works [16–18]. The rule to keep the morphotype constitutionally precise may be dangerous because the congenital deformity could be the cause of arthritic disease. We believe that an accurate examination of the contralateral knee, the clinical history, and the study of posture with a walking computerized platform (baropodometric test, gait analysis, etc.) should be taken in account together in order to decide the best correction [19–22].

5.3.2 Surgical Technique

Patient supine, knee flexed to 90°, thigh tourniquet inflated with limb at 90° to avoid the tension of the extensor apparatus when you flex the knee. Support for the foot to hold it steady when you flex it, lateral support to the thigh, freedom of motion: flexion–extension and intra and external rotation.

- Varus knee: skin incision less than 10 cm anterior–medial, starting at the upper pole of the patella to 2 cm below the tibial rim, near the anterior tibial tuberosity (ATT).
- Valgus knee: median skin incision, from the upper pole of the patella to the ATT. Lateral capsular arthrotomy. You have the possibility of lengthening the joint approach with the quadriceps tendon snip, using the effect of "sliding skin window."
  However, you should always take in account

that MIS (mini invasion surgery) is not a shorter incision, but respect the tissues under the skin, which are essential for joint function, and consider that the aesthetic scar effect depends sometimes on the suture!

For those who use the computer, please consider:

- Screws or pins for the rigid bodies supporting the sensors fixed outside the surgical incision, in the femur and tibia
- Registration of the centers of rotation of the hip, ankle, and knee
- Acquisition of anatomical landmarks of the tibial tuberosity, tibial plateau, femoral condyle, tibial slope, etc.
- Verification of the axial deformity and potential correction (ligament stress)

In all cases, it is necessary to consider:

5.3.2.1 Ligament Balancing

Consider even the ligament balance: a minirelease is possible to attain axial correction. In severe deformity >10°, the release also serves to free the compartment fixed by ligaments overstress.

5.3.2.2 Tibial Cut

We recommend that the frontal cut be perpendicular to the tibial mechanical axis. If the proximal tibial epiphysis is deformed >5° of varus, we recommend a valgus osteotomy in addition, associated with the UKR, in the same surgical step. But how much should we cut? Please follow the rule of the MBC, being ready to recut, if necessary. And how should we cut?

- Varus knee: The vertical cut; keeping the saw blade close to the anterior cruciate ligament (ACL), parallel to the femoral condyle. The horizontal cut: perpendicular to the mechanical axis.
- Valgus knee: The vertical cut: oblique medially starting just in front of the ACL and positioning the saw in contact with the posterior side of the femoral condyle, with an angle open anteriorly. This is to avoid prosthetic femoral impingement with the anterior tibial spine in extension during the "screw home mechanism" that produces a tibial extrarotation in extension. The horizontal cut: with an oscillating saw, perpendicular to the axis (Fig. 5.3).

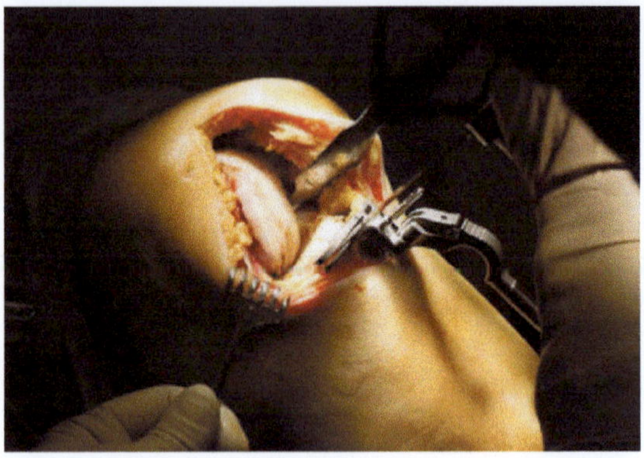

Fig. 5.3 Tibial cut with a retractor for the patella. The distal part of an intact ACL is visible

And the slope? Retaining the two ligaments, the joint space changes between flexion and extension. It usually drops down in flexion [12, 23, 24]. Our goal is to always get the same joint space in flexion and extension (Fig. 5.4). This can be achieved by adjusting the slope, or with the cuts of the femoral condyle, anterior and posterior. As you know, the two compartments are anatomically different and move differently [20–22, 25, 26]. The medial tibial plateau is concave with a degree of slope to allow the rolling of the femoral condyle in flexion, which has a radius of curvature that is larger posterior. This different offset has been stabilized and balanced in flexion by the meniscus. In contrast, the lateral tibial plateau is convex, to allow femoral roll back. Here, too, the meniscus has a fundamental role in the stabilization and containment of the excursion of the posterior condyle in flexion [19–22, 25, 26]. By removing the meniscus, we have to think about reducing the fall of the femur. On the other hand, we cannot cancel the slope, otherwise there will be a stress load on the posterior edge of the prosthesis, which tends to lift the front (anterior tilt) [24]. In addition, arthritic disease leads to wear of the femoral condyle, more frontal than posterior, increasing the problems of joint space. We must reach a compromise. In the medial compartment: you known the natural slope by means of the lateral X-ray or navigation, but we believe

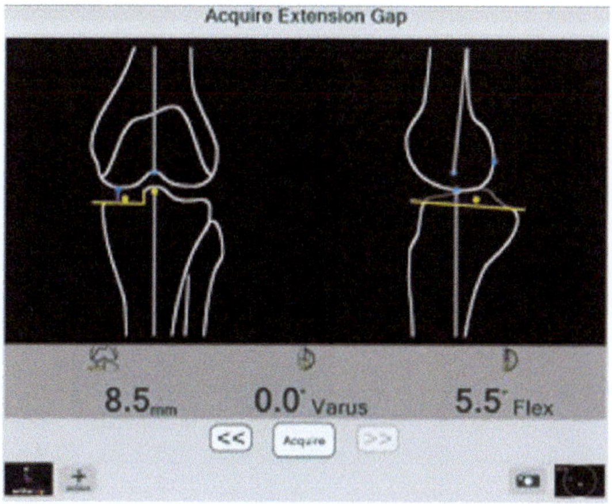

Fig. 5.4 Check of the joint spaces in flexion

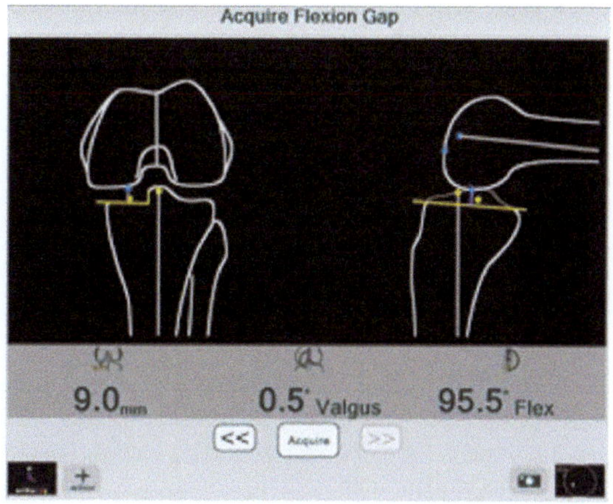

Fig. 5.5 Check of the joint spaces in extension

you should achieve a tibial slope ranging from 0° to 7°, which is proportional to the natural one, but no more than 7° to avoid ACL strain during flexion. At this point, you check the joint space in flexion and in extension by calibrated spacers or by the computer distractors. The spacer with the same extension/flexion thickness must enter and exit from the joint in both flexion and extension, without excessive difficulty, otherwise we have a conflict, usually in flexion, and it must be corrected [13, 27–29]. There are several solutions to increase the joint space. Cutting guides to increase the tibial slope, special inserts (shim, Fig. 5.5) on the distal femoral cutting guide in order to decrease the space in extension (less bone remotion), prosthetic models that have different thicknesses in front and posterior of the femoral component, etc. If you use femoral resurfacing, you can remove more bone posteriorly.

Of course, the computer helps you at this stage and gives you the exact measurements of the difference. In the lateral side, the hypoplastic femoral condyle, mainly responsible for valgus deformity, makes it hard to plan. If you adopt resurfacing, it is easier. You can use many millimeters of thickness of the component, removing only the cartilage, while for the posterior side, you cut the bone according to the thickness of the prosthesis. Be careful when you use a prosthesis with the femoral bone cuts. You may find it difficult to balance the spaces. Also, the slope on the lateral side must remain close to zero to allow the natural femoral condyle to roll back. Furthermore, you can adopt a thicker tibial component, trying to keep the morphotype without raising the joint line too much. If, however, you encounter osteoarthritis, the wear on the anterior condyle is greater than on the posterior, creating space in extension, which is not easy to fill. You must use implants that have distal anterior cuts (shims) that make it possible to resect less bone. However, you can only produce distal cuts up to 3 mm (maximum thickness of the shims). So, if you have a severe valgus knee (>15°, for instance), we recommend implanting a total replacement or performing uni resurfacing. A practical example: 18° valgus; if you use a prosthesis, with the cuts, with the possibility of 3-mm distally, the formula is: 14 mm (3 mm of femoral protrusion + 11 mm of the maximum tibial thickness) – 18°= –4 mm. Also, you resect only 1 mm of the tibial plateau, leaving 5° of valgus (4 + 1).

5.3.2.3 Femoral Cut

The cutting tools and techniques for the femoral component are divided into two groups: one involves the femoral cut joined to the tibia, the other is independent of the tibia. Our aim, however, is always the same: to implant the femoral component perpendicular to the tibia cut to pro-

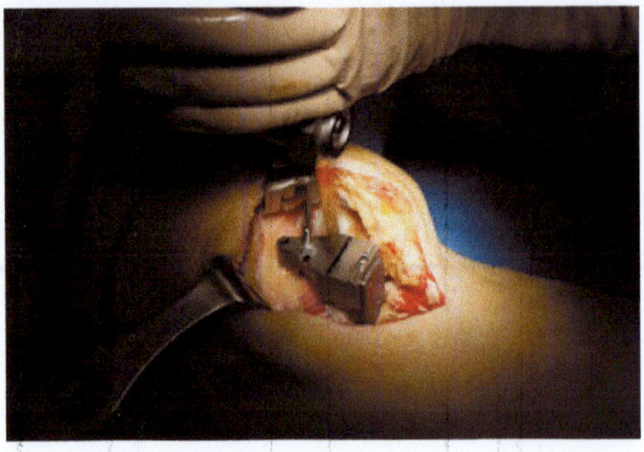

Fig. 5.6 Distal femoral cut with the cutting guide joined to the tibial cut in extension

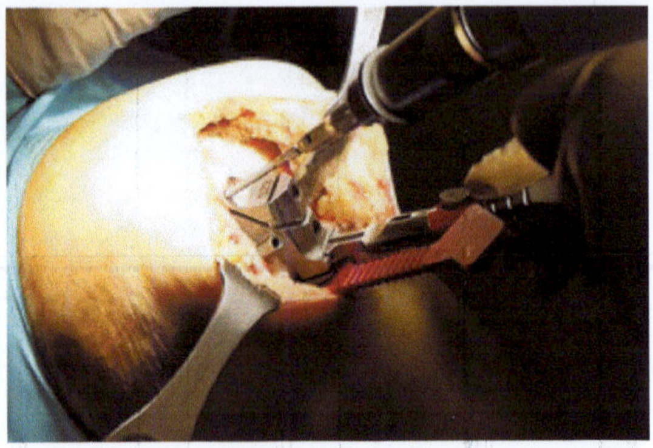

Fig. 5.7 Chamfers with a spacer supporting the femoral cutting guide in flexion

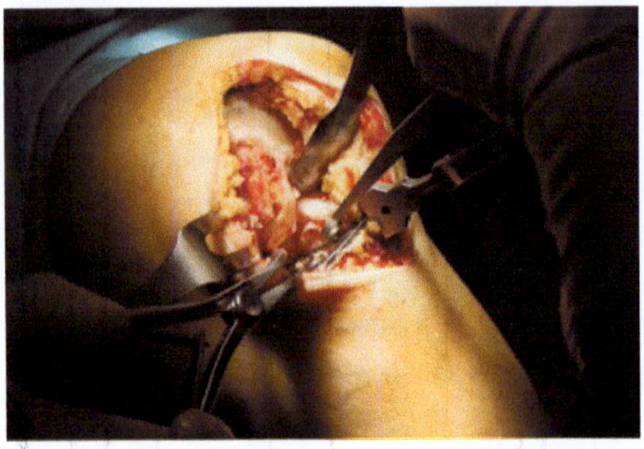

Fig. 5.8 Tibial preparation

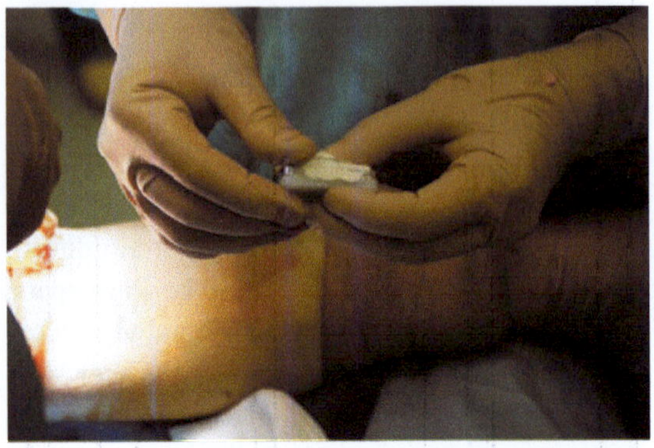

Fig. 5.9 Cemented implant: the polyethylene and metal back can be assembled in order to avoid cement cracks or dislocation of the metal back

vide more surface contact and avoid pick wear [19, 20]. If you use cutting guides joined (laying beside) to the tibial cut, the procedure is pretty forced (Fig. 5.6). The only option will be to cut anteriorly and posteriorly with the guide inserted to correct the arthritis deformity both in extension and flexion; otherwise, it will be difficult to implant the prosthesis perpendicular to the mechanical axis of the lower limb (Figs. 5.7, 5.8). This is to obtain the maximum area of the prosthesis supporting the load bearing.

If you use free guides, you need intramedullary femoral instrumentation, or a computer, to be able to implant the femoral component perpendicular to the mechanical axis. But it is not necessarily perpendicular to the tibial component. Therefore the design of the implant will have more tolerance to curves, or guides (milling), that transform the femoral condyle with a single radius of curvature using mobile bearing congruent. Everything is correct when the components are perpendicular to each other and to the mechanical axis, and the limb is correct and well balanced in flexion and extension (Fig. 5.9 and 5.10).

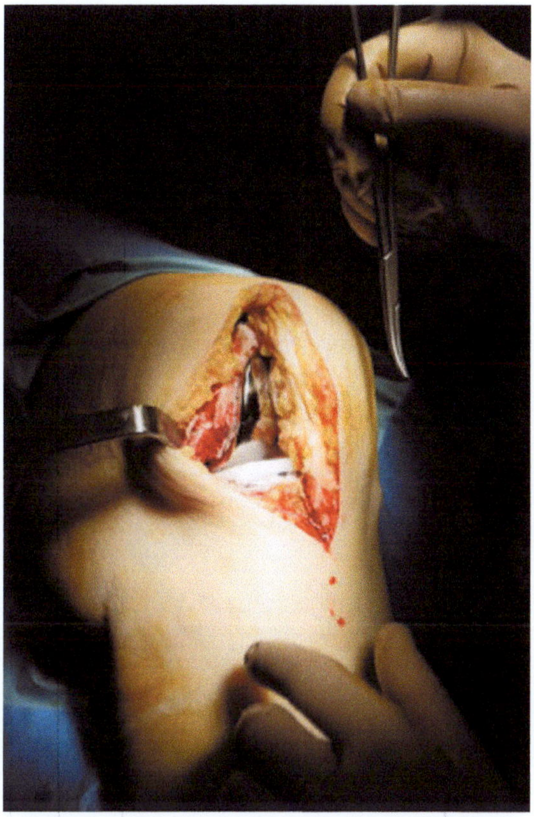

Fig. 5.10 Final check with the implanted components

References

1. Newman JH, Ackroyd CE, Shah NA (2001) Unicompartmental or total knee replacement? J Bone Joint Surg 80-B:862-865
2. Newman J, Pydisetty RV, Ackroyd C (2009) Unicompartmental or total knee replacement: the 15-year results of a prospective randomised controlled trial. J Bone Joint Surg Br 91(1):52-7
3. Swienckowski JJ, Pennington DW (2004) Unicompartmental knee arthroplasty in patients sixty years of age or younger. J Bone Joint Surg 86-A Suppl 1(Pt 2):131-42
4. Hanssen AD, Dorr LD, Kurosaka M, Maloney WJ, Romagnoli S, Ranawat CS (2002) Case challenges in knee surgery: what would you do? J Arthroplasty 17(4 Suppl 1):83-9
5. Pandit H, Van Duren BH, Gallagher JA, Beard DJ, Dodd CA, Gill HS, Murray DW (2008) Combined anterior cruciate reconstruction and Oxford unicompartmental knee arthroplasty: in vivo kinematics. Knee 15(2):101-6
6. Heyse TJ, Khefacha A, Peersman G, Cartier P (2011) Survivorship of UKA in the middle-aged. Knee 29 [Epub ahead of print]
7. Heyse TJ, Khefacha A, Fuchs-Winkelmann S, Cartier P (2011) UKA after spontaneous osteonecrosis of the knee: a retrospective analysis. Arch Orthop Trauma Surg 131(5):613-7
8. Repicci JA (2003) Mini-invasive knee unicompartmental arthroplasty: bone-sparing technique. Surg Technol Int 11:282
9. Confalonieri N, Manzotti A, Pullen C (2007) Navigated shorter incision or smaller implant in knee arthritis? Clin Orthop Relat Res 463:63-7
10. Confalonieri N, Manzotti A, Montironi F, Pullen C (2008) Tissue sparing surgery in knee reconstruction: unicompartmental (UKA), patellofemoral (PFA), UKA + PFA, bi-unicompartmental (Bi-UKA) arthroplasties. J Orthop Traumatol 9(3):171-7
11. Kozinn SC, Scott R (1989) Unicondylar knee arthroplasty. J Bone Joint Surg 71A(1):145-50
12. Assor M, Aubaniac JM (2006) Influence of rotatory malposition of femoral implant in failure of unicompartmental medial knee prosthesis. Rev Chir Orthop Reparatrice Appar Mot 92(5):473-84
13. Hopkins AR, New AM, Rodriguez-y-Baena F, Taylor M (2010) Finite element analysis of unicompartmental knee arthroplasty. Med Eng Phys 32(1):14-2
14. Jeffery RS, Morris RW, Denham RA (1991) Coronal alignment after total knee replacement. J Bone Joint Surg Br 73(5):709-14
15. Fehring TK, Odum S, Griffin WL, Mason JB, Nadaud M (2001) Early failures in total knee arthroplasty. Clin Orthop Relat Res (392):315-8
16. Choong PF, Dowsey MM (2011)Update in surgery for osteoarthritis of the knee. Int J Rheum Dis 14(2):167-74
17. Dieppe P, Lim K, Lohmander S (2011) Who should have knee joint replacement surgery for osteoarthritis? Int J Rheum Dis 14(2):175-80
18. Chapple CM, Nicholson H, Baxter GD, Abbott JH (2011) Patient characteristics that predict progression of knee osteoarthritis: a systematic review of prognostic studies. Arthritis Care Res 63(8):1115-25
19. Telli S, Pinskerova V (2002) The shapes of the tibial and femoral articular surfaces in relation to tibiofemoral movement. J Bone Joint Surg Br 84(4):607-13
20. Lankester BJ, Cottam HL, Pinskerova V, Eldridge JD, Freeman MA (2008) Variation in the anatomy of the tibial plateau: a possible factor in the development of anteromedial osteoarthritis of the knee. J Bone Joint Surg Br 90(3):330-3
21. Pinskerova V, Samuelson KM, Stammers J, Maruthainar K, Sosna A, Freeman MA (2009) The knee in full flexion: an anatomical study. J Bone Joint Surg Br 91(6):830-4
22. Freeman MA, Pinskerova V (2005) The movement of the normal tibio-femoral joint. J Biomech 38(2):197-208
23. Amis AA, Senavongse W, Darcy P (2005) Biomechanics of patellofemoral joint prostheses. Clin Orthop Relat Res (436):20-9

24. Hernigou P, Deschamps G (2004) Posterior slope of the tibial implant and the outcome of unicompartmental knee arthroplasty. J Bone Joint Surg Am 86-A(3):506-11
25. Iwaki H, Pinskerova V, Freeman MA (2000) Tibiofemoral movement 1: the shapes and relative movements of the femur and tibia in the unloaded cadaver knee. J Bone Joint Surg Br 82(8):1189-95
26. Hill PF, Vedi V, Williams A, Iwaki H, Pinskerova V, Freeman MA (2000) Tibiofemoral movement 2: the loaded and unloaded living knee studied by MRI. J Bone Joint Surg Br 82(8):1196-8
27. Møller JT, Weeth RE, Keller JO, Nielsen S (1985) Unicompartmental arthroplasty of the knee. Cadaver study of the importance of the anterior cruciate ligament. Acta Orthop Scand 56(2):120-3
28. Dennis D, Komistek R, Scuderi G, Argenson JN, Insall J, Mahfouz M, Aubaniac JM, Haas B (2001) In vivo three-dimensional determination of kinematics for subjects with a normal knee or a unicompartmental or total knee replacement. J Bone Joint Surg Am 83-A Suppl 2 Pt 2:104-15
29. Argenson JN, Komistek RD, Aubaniac JM, Dennis DA, Northcut EJ, Anderson DT, Agostini S (2002) In vivo determination of knee kinematics for subjects implanted with a unicompartmental arthroplasty. J Arthroplasty 17(8):1049-54

6 Unicompartmental Knee Arthroplasty with a Mobile-Bearing Prosthesis: Long-Term Results

Hemant G. Pandit, David W. Murray, and Christopher A. F. Dodd

6.1 Introduction

Anteromedial osteoarthritis (OA) of the knee, a distinct pathological condition described by White et al. in 1991 [1], is an ideal indication for unicompartmental knee arthroplasty (UKA). In this condition, the cartilage erosion in the medial compartment begins typically in the anterior half of the tibial plateau, the cartilage being preserved over the posterior third (Fig. 6.1).

There is a corresponding lesion on the distal femoral condyle. The femoral condyle sits within this tibial defect in extension, producing a varus deformity that is corrected on flexing the knee as the preserved cartilage over the posterior condyle of the distal femur rides over the intact cartilage of the posterior tibial plateau. In these cases, the medial collateral ligament is not shortened (Fig. 6.2) and the varus deformity remains correctible in near extension by application of a valgus stress.

The anterior cruciate ligament (ACL) is also usually preserved and the retention of these structures tend to prevent OA from progressing to other compartments of the knee. This pattern of OA accounts for one in three cases of osteoarthritic knees undergoing arthroplasty in some centres.

UKA is a well-accepted treatment option for anteromedial OA as it has many advantages over total knee arthroplasty (TKA). These include less perioperative blood loss, reduced risk of infection, a shorter recovery period, better range of movement and lower morbidity and mortality.

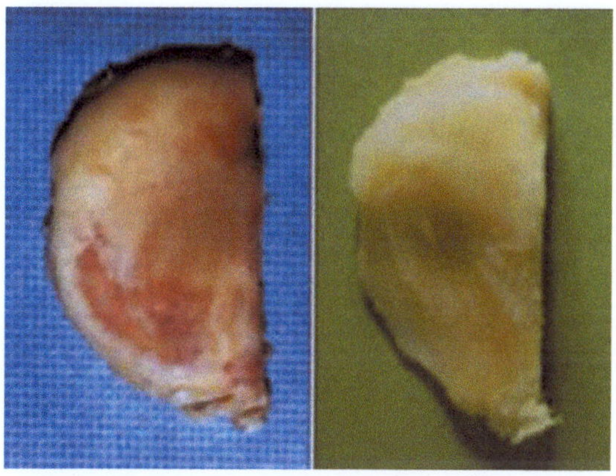

Fig. 6.1 Typical tibial plateau specimen confirming the presence of cartilage erosion in the anterior half

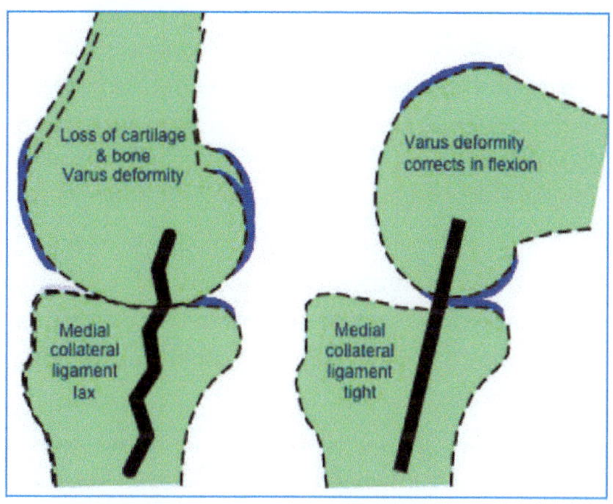

Fig. 6.2 Femoral movement in extension and flexion. The intact posterior tibial cartilage allows the femur to move out of the defect each time the patient flexes the knee

C. A. F. Dodd (✉)
Nuffield Department of Orthopaedics, Rheumatology and Musculoskeletal Sciences (NDORMS), University of Oxford, Nuffield Orthopaedic Centre, Headington, Oxford, UK
E-mail: cafdodd@aol.com

N. Confalonieri, S. Romagnoli (eds.), *Small Implants in Knee Reconstruction*,
DOI 10.1007/978-88-470-2655-1_6, © Springer-Verlag Italia 2013

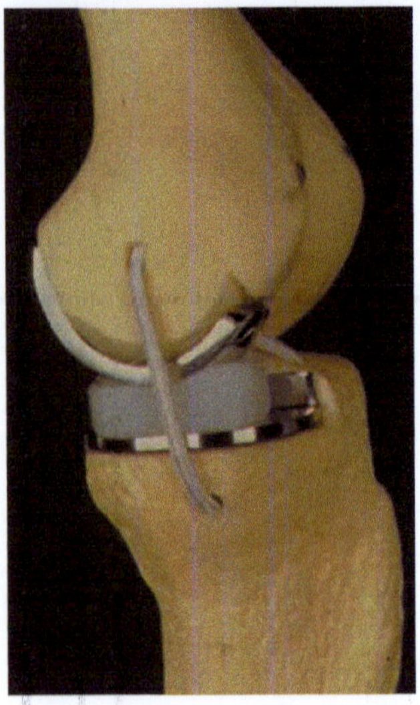

Fig. 6.3 The Oxford Knee

As the cruciate ligaments are preserved, the procedure has the ability to restore knee function to near normal. The knee feels more natural and pain relief is as good or better than following a TKA.

This chapter describes the long-term outcome of patients undergoing UKA, with particular reference to the Oxford Knee (Biomet Europe). Its unique design features are outlined below followed by the methods used to describe the long-term outcome and the outcome data for these patients.

6.2 Implant Design

The Oxford Knee (Fig. 6.3) is the only mobile-bearing fully congruous UKA design approved by the FDA. It has a spherical femoral and a flat tibial component, both made of cobalt chrome. Between the two lies an unconstrained mobile-bearing, the upper surface of which is spherically concave and congruent with the femur while the lower surface is flat and congruent with the tibia. The bearing is congruent in all positions of knee flexion.

Therefore the contact area is large (around 6 cm^2) and the contact pressure is low. This form of articulation, while imposing no constraints upon movements, diminishes polyethylene wear to very low values. Both in vivo and in vitro measurements have confirmed the same.

In vitro measurement of retrieved bearings has shown a mean linear wear rate (combining both articular surfaces, including backside wear) of 0.03 mm per year, and even less (0.01 mm per year) if the knee had been functioning normally without any impingement. Furthermore, the rate of wear is no more rapid when thinner (3.5 mm) rather than thicker components are implanted. The use of the thin polyethylene bearing is advantageous, especially in young and active patients, as the bone stock is preserved.

In vivo measurements by Kendrick et al. [2] used model-based radiostereometric analysis to measure the combined wear of the upper and lower bearing surfaces in 13 Oxford Knees at a mean of 20.9 years (17.2–25.9) postoperatively. The mean linear penetration of the polyethylene bearing was 1.04 mm (0.307–2.15), with a mean annual wear rate of 0.045 mm/year (0.016–0.099).

6.3 Phases in the Development of the Oxford Knee

In phase 1 (1976), the femoral surface was prepared with cutting blocks and saw blades to remove the angular cuts of bone to fit the non-articular surface of the metallic femoral component. This did not, however, allow accurate ligament balancing (flexion/extension gap) and bearing dislocation was an occasional problem.

Phase 2 (1986) saw the introduction of a spherical mill to address this problem. The femoral component was changed to a spherical concave inner surface and the femoral bone surface was thus prepared with a rotating mill around a central spigot. This allowed accurate soft-tissue balancing by incremental 1-mm milling of the distal femoral surface.

The phase 3 design, introduced in 1998, provided new instrumentation and an increased range of components to facilitate the implantation through a short incision (minimally invasive surgical approach). Although the Oxford Knee was the first of its kind, there are currently several other mobile-bearing implants based on a similar philosophy. The AMC knee (Uniglide) differs from the Ocford Knee with respect to the shape of the femoral component. The radius of the femoral component is constant in the AMC design up to 45° of flexion but decreases towards the posterior position of the condyle, which can affect knee kinematics. This is not the case with the Oxford Knee, in which the radius of curvature is constant throughout. Various studies have demonstrated the restoration of near-normal knee kinematics following Oxford Knee implantation [3, 4] There are very few series reporting the results of the AMC Uniglide implant.

The other category of mobile UKA relates to the LCS mobile-bearing. This device employs a polyradial femoral component articulating with a dished polyethylene bearing that runs back and forth in a track on a metal tibial tray. Again, the polyradial nature of the articulation means that the congruency is lost after 30°; beyond this flexion the device acts as a fixed-bearing implant. More damaging, however, is the conflict between the bearing movement and the track; indeed, many devices jammed and failed. The mobile iteration of the LCS UKA is therefore no longer used.

6.4 Long-Term Outcome

Ideally, the long-term outcome should reflect the results and outcome of all the patients who have undergone a particular procedure for the entire lifespan of that implant; that is, the end-point should be either that the patient has died or that the implant has been revised. This approach is, obviously, not realistic; instead, the next best assessment is a prediction of the real long-term outcome. This is best achieved by survivorship analysis, which is widely used in reporting the results of joint arthroplasty. The method allows the failure rate of an implant to be predicted based on the results of a series of operations that may have different lengths of follow-up but are assumed, for the purposes of the analysis, to have all been performed at the same time. The method calculates a cumulative survival rate from the failures occurring at differing time periods. It is commonly used to determine the results obtained with in a population with a single series of prosthesis or to study and compare the results from a larger populations in which different prostheses were used, as in National Joint Registries. In most survivorship studies, all-cause revision is reported as the primary end-point. This can be further modified to differentiate revisions performed for various reasons, for example, aseptic loosening (as is commom in the American literature), from failures secondary to infection, type of revision implant used, etc. Survival analysis may be performed using either the life table method or the Kaplan-Meier method.

Whichever method is employed, there are a number of features that must be understood about the reported data. Survival figures are cumulative, which allows a prediction of the expected failure rate in the long term, reducing the need for a large number of prostheses to have reached the long-term follow-up end-point. However, the number at risk at each time point must be known since if the number reduces to less than 15 it becomes difficult to interpret the data. Loss to follow-up is also important, and studies should present worst- as well as best-case scenarios.

The long term results of mobile-bearing UKA are available from three main sources: cohort studies, prospective trials and arthroplasty registries (regional or national).

6.5 Cohort Studies

Khanna and Levy outlined and compared 17 published clinical studies, comprising 2,847 patients. Follow-up ranged from 2 to 22 years during which there were 77 (2.7%) device-related failures [5]. The survivorship ranged from 84.0% (at 10 years) to 100% (at 10 years), with the majority of studies quoting survivorship > 94%.

Cohort studies are usually based around the observed results of cases treated by a single surgeon or a small group of surgeons (usually from a single unit). Their advantage is that groups of patients are followed in detail and with often near-complete follow-up. The indications for surgery, operative technique and postoperative

Table 6.1 Summary of 10-year survival studies

Year	Author	Phase	Number	Mean age (years)	Mean follow-up (range)	Survival % (95% CI)
1998	Murray et al. [6]	1 and 2	144	71 (35–91)	7.6 (6–14)	97 (93–100)
1999	Kumar and Fiddian [12]	2	100	71	5.6 (1–11)	85 (78–92)
2001	Svard and Price [10]	1 and 2	124	70 (51–86)	12.5 (10.1–15.6)	95
2002	Emerson et al. [14]	2	50	64	6.8 (2–13)	92
2004	Keys et al. [9]	2	40	68 (40–80)	7.5 (6–10)	100
2004	Rajasekhar et al. [8]	2	135	72 (53–88)	5.8 (2–12)	94 (84–97)
2006	Vorlat et al. [13]	2	141	66 (46–89)	5.5 (1–10)	82 (SE 6.9)
2009	Mercier et al. [11]	3	43	69 (47–86)	14.9	75
2011	Pandit et al. [7]	3	1000	66 (32–87)	5.6 (1–11)	96

rehabilitation tend to be standardised. However the total number of patients is often small and may include non-continuous series, with exclusions. Additionally, these studies are open to bias as they are often reported by the designer(s) or the enthusiasts such that the results may not be representative of the implant outcome in general orthopedic practice. Nonetheless, these cohort studies provide important information as to the success or failure of the intervention and can usually be treated as the best-case scenarios.

A 10-year follow-up of the Oxford Knee was reported in nine studies, with a wide range in the reported survival (Table 6.1). In six of the nine studies cumulative survival at ten years was 94% or greater. In three series, however, the cumulative survival was 85% or less. The designer series by Murray et al. [6] for phases 1 and 2 of the Oxford Knee reported a 10-year cumulative worst-case survival rate of 97% (confidence interval (CI): 93–100%). In that series 44 knees were at risk at 10 years and no failures were due to polythene wear or aseptic loosening of the tibial component. Pandit et al. [7] reported the designer series of the phase 3 Oxford Knee, with 1000 knees; the survivorship at 10 years was 96% (number at risk at 10 years: 121) (Fig. 6.4).

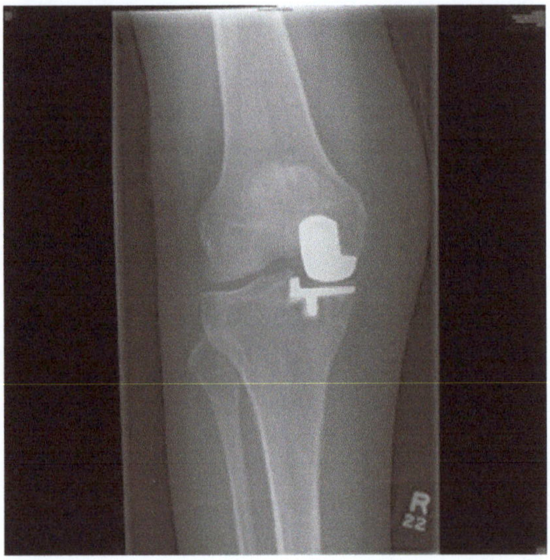

Fig. 6.4 X-ray showing a phase 3 Oxford Knee in situ at 12 years

Rajasekhar et al. [8] obtained similar results, with a 94% cumulative survival of phase 2 Oxford Knees at 10 years while Keyes et al. [9] reported excellent results with their first 40 phase 3 Oxford knees. The latter study had an average follow-up of 7.5 years, with a survivorship at 10 years of 100%, without any patients lost to follow-up. In another independent series of phase 1 and 2 knees, Svard and Price [10] showed a cumulative survival of 95% for 124 patients at 10 years.

Mercier et al. [11] reported an overall survival of 74.7%. They specifically drew attention to their broad selection criteria, including ACL-deficient knees and inflammatory arthropathy, neither of which are ideal indications for UKA. If these cases are excluded from this series, the 10-year survival is >85%. In a similar fashion, Kumar and Fiddian reported a 10-year survival of 85% (CI: 78–92%) at a mean follow-up of 5.6 years [12]. They also drew attention to inflam-

Table 6.2 Summary of 20-year survival studies

Year	Author	Phase	Number	Mean age (years)	Survival (95% CI)	Survival (95% CI)
2010	Price and Svard [16]	1, 2 and 3	683	69.7	92.1 (+ 33.2)	97 (93–100)
2010	Barrington and Emerson [17]	2	54	64	94 (-)	85 (78–92)

matory arthropathy as an inappropriate indication for patient selection. Vorlat et al. showed the effect of previous high tibial osteotomy (HTO) on the outcome of Oxford Knee [13]. The overall cumulative survival at 10 years in their series was 82%; however, four of the failures were in eight patients who had previously undergone HTO.

In 2002 Emerson et al., compared 51 fixed-bearing UKA with 50 mobile-bearing UKA. Survivorship analysis based on component loosening and revision showed a 93% survival for the fixed-bearing UKA and a 99% survival for the mobile-bearing UKA (Oxford knee) at 11 years. The latter implants had no tibial component failure, in contrast to the fixed-bearing implant (six of the eight failed UKA were due to tibial component failure). This study cohort was part of a study in which the Oxford knee was introduced into the USA [14]. The surgical technique used in that study included subtle release of the medial collateral ligament (MCL), which could have predisposed to the failures in the mobile-bearing group secondary to progression of arthritis in the retained lateral compartment (n = 4).

These last four papers show the importance of indications and technique on outcome and that extending the indications outside the recommended ones has an adverse effect on the results.

6.6 Twenty-Year Studies

Price and Svard reported the continuation of their 10-year study, which was also reported at 15 years (Table 6.2) [15, 16]. Their report included all cases in which there was no loss to follow-up. Among the 683 consecutive knees that were assessed the overall cumulative survival was 92% at 20 years. The most common cause for revision was the progression of arthritis in the retained lateral compartment although over the 20-year period this occurred in only ten patients (1.5%). This study also reinforces the importance of adhering to the present indication of excluding patients with previous HTO or ACL deficiency, as the inclusion of these cases reduced survival to 71%. Another interesting feature of this 20-year series is the number of relatively few failures that occurred in the second decade. There is a consistent trend across all the series in that infection and dislocation tended to present as early complication after UKA, with lateral compartment arthritis and loosening accounting for the majority of mid-term failures. None of the failures in the second decade, as reported by Price and Svard, were due to polyethylene wear, suggesting that the design features of reducing contact stress successfully prevent catastrophic wear for at least 20 years. Barrington and Emerson also reported 20-year results with the Oxford Knee (Table 6.2) [17], with a survivorship of 94% and no revisions for bearing dislocation, tibial subsidence or polyethylene wear. They also reported excellent functional scores: the mean American Knee Society Score improved from 47 (preoperative) to 94 (postoperative).

In assessing the few available studies that reported on long-term clinical outcome, it is clear that no consistent clinical outcome assessment tools were used, making generalised interpretation rather difficult. The common theme, however, seems to be that clinical scores improve significantly from the postoperative period within the first year and remain almost unchanged over the subsequent follow-up period. The long-term data of Price and Svard and of Pandit et al. suggest that the significant increase in clinical scores does not decrease with time. The patients' function is as good 10 years postoperatively as it is at one year.

6.7 Randomised Controlled Trials

Prospective randomised controlled trials of a prosthesis or surgical technique allow many of the flaws of cohort studies to be overcome, but they are much less common and more difficult to conduct. This is, in general, a reflection of the cost and complexity of the organisation and execution of such studies. When available, however, they provide better qualitative data than cohort studies, although they have yet to include cumulative revision rates at 10 years from a randomised controlled trial for a mobile-bearing UKA.

6.8 Joint Registries

The primary function of national joint registries is to assess the success of treatment in large population-based cohorts. The data provided represent clinical practice without the inherent bias in cohort studies and can be used to compare the outcome of implant designs. Consequently, registers have always taken revision as the marker of failure and cumulative revision rate as the comparator between implants. While revision is a definite end point and therefore can be easily measured, there are some difficulties with the interpretation of revision rates. Unfortunately, arthroplasty registers collect limited data and exert no control over patient selection, surgical expertise and indications for revision.

Analysis of the data from every national register shows that the failure rate of UKA is between four and six times higher than that of TKA. This suggests either a higher proportion of unhappy patients or other factors, such as ease of revision, acting to distort the results. The evidence as to the cause of this higher failure rate is found in the New Zealand Joint Register. The New Zealand Joint Registry publishes not only the revision rates but also the equally relevant clinical outcomes (Oxford Knee Scores), allowing comparison of these two measurements. UKA patients consistently had a better knee score than TKA patients; however, the revision rate of the former was nearly three times higher than that of the latter because the sensitivity of the revision rate to clinical failure differs for the two implant types. For example, of knees with a very poor outcome (Oxford Knee Score < 20), only about 12% of TKAs were revised compared with about 63% of UKAs with similar scores. This confirms the limitations of joint registries. While they do provide information on the various types of implants, their usage and survival, the data should be interpreted with caution. There are many factors that contribute to the success (or failure) of an implant; of course, registries should not be used to compare a unicompartmental implant with a total knee replacement implant. Another interesting (obvious but easily ignored) fact about an implant is that its success is decided by the surgeon who implants it, as demonstrated by the Swedish Registry. In 1995, the registry data suggested that Oxford Knee was not performing well in Sweden; therefore, the registry wrote to all surgeons in Sweden advising them to stop the procedure. However, surgeons who always had good results with the Oxford Knee continued to use it. The 2005 data from the same registry showed Oxford Knee to be the best performing UKA, presumably in great part due to instructional courses and the effect of education. This shows that the registries should be used with caution when comparing UKAs with one another and should not be used to predict how well a particular UKA will perform over time.

Registries are, nonetheless, helpful in identifying individual surgeons who are not performing as well as their colleagues. The National Joint Registry of England and Wales provides funnel plots for individual surgeons; those with failure rates outside two standard deviations of the average are identified and contacted by the registry (in confidence) to help them (and, in turn, their patients) by highlighting the high failure rates. These surgeons can be further trained or be urged to stop UKA surgery altogether.

Three national registries have reported specific data for the Oxford Knee at approximately the 10-year time point. Other national registries (for example the New Zealand and the Norwegian registries) do not report separate outcomes for fixed- vs. mobile-bearing UKA and in some cases do not differentiate between medial and

Table 6.3 Breakdown of causes of revision and its incidence as percentage at 10 and 20 years

	10-year studies (4116 patients)	20-year studies (736 patients)
Bearing	0.9	0.4
Bearing dislocation	0.7	0.3
Bearing fracture	0.1	0.0
Bearing impingement	0.1	0.1
Wear	0.4	0.0
Polyethylene wear with major osteolysis	0.0	0.0
Loosening (total)	1.1	1.4
Loosening (not specified)	0.2	0.1
Loosening (both)	0.1	0.3
Femoral loosening	0.2	1.0
Tibial loosening	0.6	0.0
Pain	0.3	0.4
Progression	1.1	2.2
Patellofemoral joint progression	0.0	0.0
Lateral progression	1.1	2.2
Infection	0.4	0.7
Prosthesis fracture	0.1	0.0
ACL rupture	0.2	0.0
Plateau fracture	0.1	0.0
Recurrent haemarthrosis	0.1	0.0
Instability	0.1	0.0
Total revisions	4.6	5.0

lateral UKA. The England and Wales National Joint Registry presently reports revision rates for specific implants but results are only available for the last three years. Therefore, these registries have not been included in this analysis. In the 2009 Annual Report of the Swedish Knee Arthroplasty Register, the cumulative 8-year survival for the Oxford Knee was >91% [18]. The Australian Orthopedic Association Joint Registry data from 2009 [19] reported a cumulative survival of 87.1% at 8 years while the Finnish Arthroplasty Register reported a 10-year survival of 81% for the Oxford Knee, slightly better than for the fixed-bearing device (79%, Miller Galante). There is no further detailed information in these reports for mobile-bearing UKA.

6.9 Reasons for Revision

As stated earlier, the revision rates are low in various large cohort studies and the majority of the revisions tend to occur early. The main reasons for failure of a TKA in the second decade tend to be wear and / or component loosening. Unlike TKA, there are very few revisions in the second decade after implantation of the Oxford Knee. The reasons for revision are summarised in Table 6.3. Not only is the incidence very low but in the majority of cases the UKA can be revised to a primary TKA without the need for augments or stems.

The excellent survival, low morbidity and mortality along with the ease of revision to primary TKA make UKA an ideal treatment option in patients with anteromedial osteoarthritis.

References

1. White SH, Ludkowski PF, Goodfellow JW (1991) Anteromedial osteoarthritis of the knee. J Bone Joint Surg Br 73:582-6
2. Kendrick BJL, Simpson DJ, Bottomley NJ, Kaptein BL, Garling EH, Gill HS, Dodd CAF, Murray DW,

Price AJ (2010) An in vivo study of linear penetration in the Oxford unicompartmental knee arthroplasty at twenty years. BASK, Oxford
3. Pandit HG (2009) Sagittal plane kinematics after knee arthroplasty. medical sciences. Oxford: DPhil, University of Oxford
4. Price AJ, Rees JL, Beard DJ, Gill HS, Dodd CAF, Murray DW (2004) Sagittal plane kinematics of a mobile-bearing unicompartmental knee arthroplasty at 10 years: a comparative in vivo fluoroscopic analysis. J Arthroplasty 19:590-7
5. Khanna G, Levy BA (2007) Oxford unicompartmental knee replacement: literature review. Orthopedics 30 Suppl:11-4
6. Murray DW, Goodfellow JW, O'Connor JJ (1998) The Oxford medial unicompartmental arthroplasty: a ten-year survival study. J Bone Joint Surg Br 80:983-9
7. Pandit H, Jenkins C, Gill HS, Barker K, Dodd CA, Murray DW (2010) Minimally invasive Oxford phase 3 unicompartmental knee replacement: results of 1000 cases. J Bone Joint Surg Br 93:198-204
8. Rajasekhar C, Das S, Smith A (2004) Unicompartmental knee arthroplasty. 2- to 12-year results in a community hospital. J Bone Joint Surg Br 86:983-5
9. Keys GW, Ul-Abiddin Z, Toh EM (2004) Analysis of first forty Oxford medial unicompartmental knee replacement from a small district hospital in UK. Knee 11:375-7
10. Svard UC, Price AJ (2001) Oxford medial unicompartmental knee arthroplasty. A survival analysis of an independent series. J Bone Joint Surg Br 83:191-4
11. Mercier N, Wimsey S, Saragaglia D (2010) Long-term clinical results of the Oxford medial unicompartmental knee arthroplasty. Int Orthop 34:1137-43
12. Kumar A, Fiddian NJ (1999) Medial unicompartmental arthroplasty of the knee. The Knee 6:21-3
13. Vorlat P, Putzeys G, Cottenie D, Van Isacker T, Pouliart N, Handelberg F, Casteleyn PP, Gheysen F, Verdonk R (2006) The Oxford unicompartmental knee prosthesis: an independent 10-year survival analysis. Knee Surg Sports Traumatol Arthrosc 14:40-5
14. Emerson RH, Jr., Hansborough T, Reitman RD, Rosenfeldt W, Higgins LL (2002) Comparison of a mobile with a fixed-bearing unicompartmental knee implant. Clin Orthop Relat Res 404:62-70
15. Price AJ, Svard U (2006) 20-year survival & 10 year clinical results of the Oxford medial UKA. The Annual Meeting of the American Academy of Orthopaedic Surgeons. Chicago, USA
16. Price AJ, Svard U (2010) A second decade lifetable survival analysis of the oxford unicompartmental knee arthroplasty. Clin Orthop Relat Res 469:174-179
17. Barrington JW, Emerson RH Jr (2010) The Oxford Knee: First Report of 20-year Follow-up in the U.S. Annual Meeting of the American Academy of Orthopaedic Surgeons, New Orleans, podium no 422
18. Swedish Knee Arthroplasty Register (2009) Annual Report 2009
19. Australian Orthopaedic Association National Joint Replacement Registry (2009) Annual Report

7 Lateral Unicompartmental Knee Replacement: Long-Term Survival Study

Sergio Romagnoli, Francesco Verde,
and Sara Zacchetti

7.1 Introduction

Unicompartmental knee replacement (UKR) has well known advantages over total knee replacement (TKR), such as less invasiveness, respect of both cruciate ligaments, better function, and less morbidity. However, the survival rates of UKR are typically inferior to those obtained with TKR. The higher failure rate of the former has been ascribed to the effects of degeneration in other compartments and to polyethylene wear. Despite this history, recent surveys have documented an evident improvement in the survivorship rate probably based on the large diffusion of the UKR and in a consequent improvement in the indications, surgical technique, and prostheses. However, long-term clinical results, which are the hardest to obtain, are needed to confirm the positive short-term experience (Fig. 7.1) [1-3] (unpublished data).

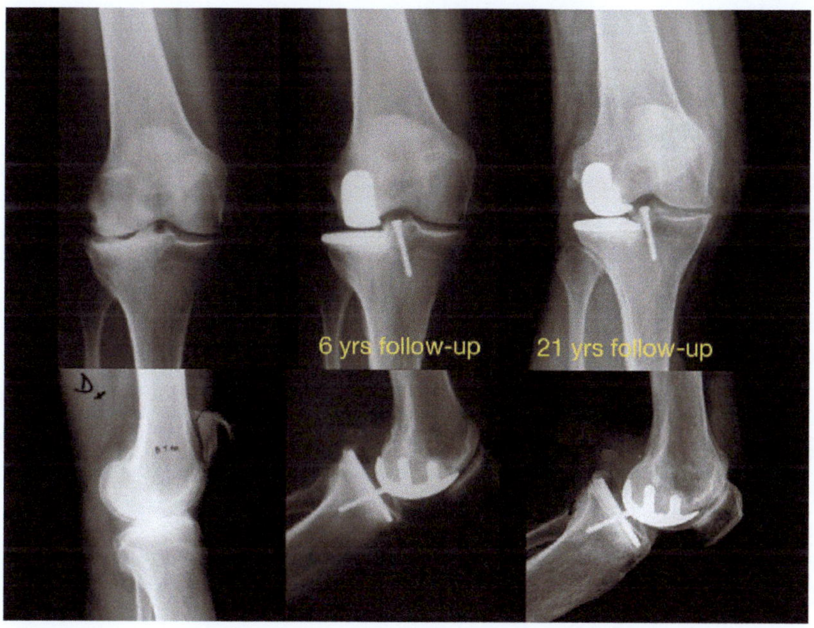

Fig. 7.1 Lateral unicompartmental implant: long-term follow-up

S. Romagnoli (✉)
Galeazzi Orthopedic Institute
Milan, Italy
E-mail: sergio.romagnoli@libero.it

N. Confalonieri, S. Romagnoli (eds.), *Small Implants in Knee Reconstruction*,
DOI 10.1007/978-88-470-2655-1_7, © Springer-Verlag Italia 2013

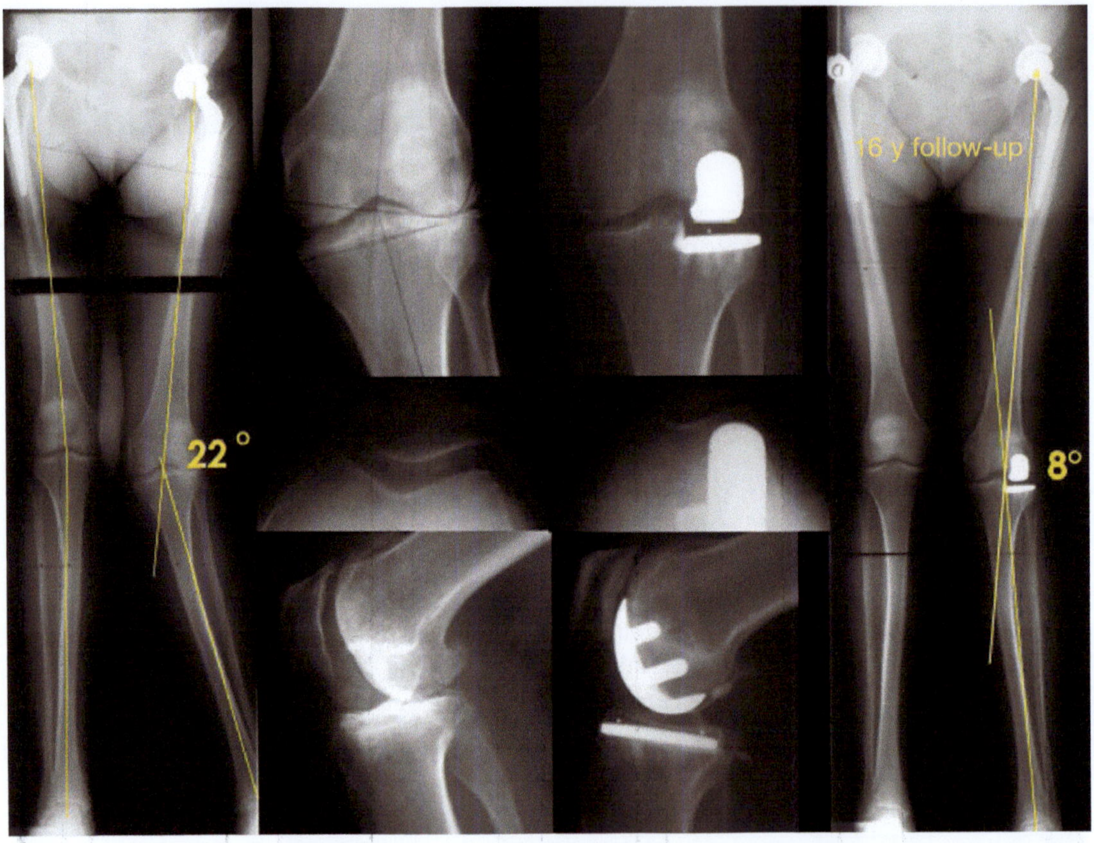

Fig. 7.2 Severe valgus in hip dysplasia sequelae: wide mechanical axis correction with lateral UKR

7.2 Pathomechanics of Unicompartmental Knee Arthritis

The arthritic joint modifications in the frontal, sagittal, and coronal planes are the basis of the triplanar deformity of the knee referred to as "rotatory arthritis of the knee" (RAK) [3-5]. RAK is proportional to the degree of changes in all three planar dimensions and it leads to progressive changes in the joint due to alterations in the static and dynamic loads. Intra-articular and/or extra-articular factors underlie RAK. It involves one of the two femorotibial compartments through cartilage, bone, and meniscus wear, with ligament, joint capsule and soft-tissue lesions as a cascade of events compromising joint kinematics.

Patients with RAK present with typical clinical and radiological signs, which allow it to be distinguished from intra- or extra-articular unicompartmental knee arthritis and related prognostic factors. The extra-articular elements influence the adductor movement of the knee (Fig. 7.2). They consist of: (a) the femoral and tibial axes (mechanical, anatomic) and their relationship, (b) the morphology of the tibia and the femur (diaphyseal, metaphyseal axis), (c) the overall limb alignment, (d) the pelvic width, (e) the patient's height and body status.

Intra-articular elements relate to cartilage, meniscal, and ligamentous defects. Cartilage wear leads to augmentation of the contact stresses between the femoral condyle and tibial plateau. Consequently, osteophytes develop, increasing bony contacts, reducing rotation, and resulting in abnormal femorotibial movements. Treatment is aimed at correction of the defect, while maintaining most of the joint structure to gain nearly normal kinematics of the knee. UKR offers tech-

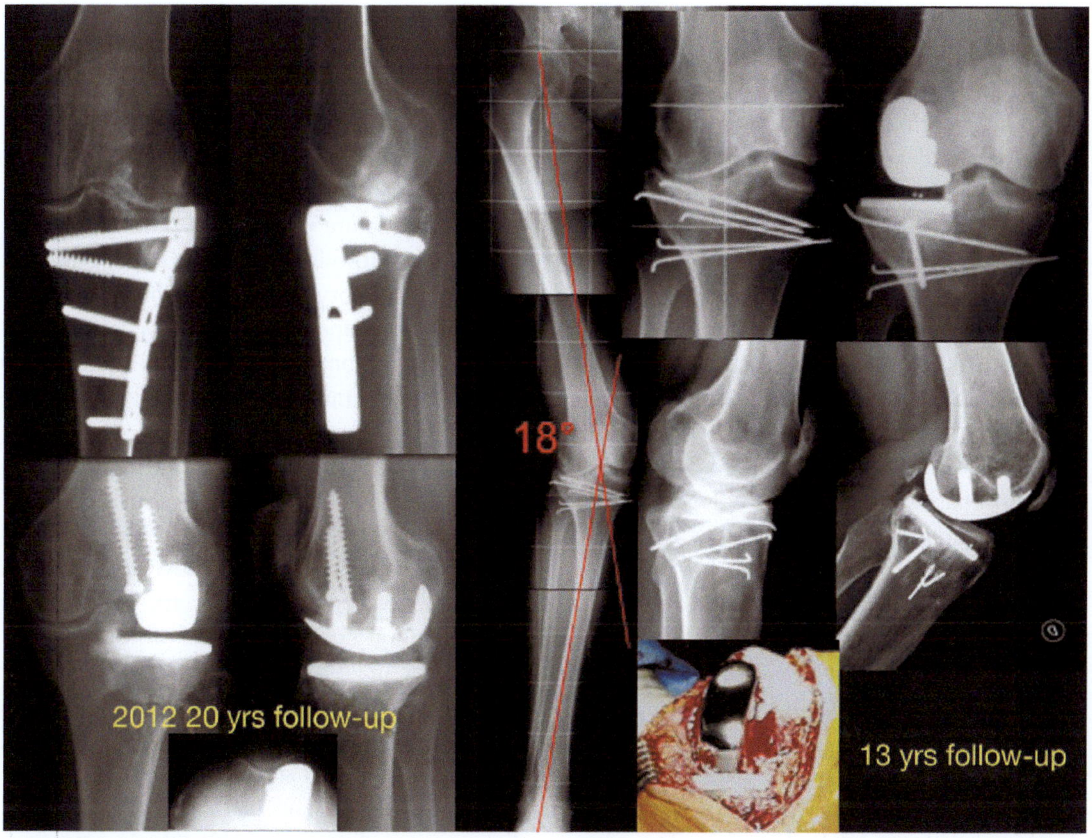

Fig.7.3 Two cases of post-traumatic valgus knee arthritis: in the first, there has been a contemporary complete removal of the plate, in the second, only partial pins have been removed

niques for defect correction while preserving the bone, cartilage, and ligaments not involved in the degenerative arthritis of the knee.

7.2.1 Valgus Knee and Lateral Compartment Disease

In the valgus knee, deformity is more acceptable than in the varus knee because of the specific adaptive capabilities of the subtalar joint. However, the femoral lateral condyle increases movement toward the center of the knee, causing wear of the central lateral tibial plateau. On the horizontal plane, loads and forces are directed toward the knee center. The lateral meniscus and joint soft tissues are not directly stressed. Recently, the large diffusion of arthroscopic meniscectomy in the treatment of meniscal tears has led to more frequent observations of chondropathies of the lateral femoral condyle and tibial plateau and thus of consequent progressive arthrotic degeneration in the lateral compartment.

7.2.2 Postraumatic Valgus Disease

Another very important issue is post-traumatic lateral compartment degeneration due to isolated lateral tibial plateau fracture. Indeed, fracture of the tibial plateau, even if surgically treated, is frequently the cause of an acquired varus or valgus deformity. These cases typically occur in young patients. A UKR procedure becomes mandatory to treat both the pain and the limited function due to degeneration of the single compartment affected, even if the bony defect requires a component thickness of >12 mm in the medial or lateral compartment as a secure limit for this indication [6].

Special consideration must be given in these cases to the type of arthritic degeneration, the patient's characteristics, and possibly the presence of internal fixation, such as screws or plates, from previous surgical treatment.

Arthritic degeneration can occur as a consequence of an extra-articular diaphyseal fracture with a >10° valgus mechanical axis, either acquired or because of an intra-articular trauma. In the first case, a preceding osteotomy may be indicated to correct the mechanical axis before the UKR. In the second case, the limit is the bony defect.

The age of the patient is a controversial issue. Most patients with this pathology are young such that mini-invasive treatment is mandatory; however, in elderly patients the low quality of bone at the implant site could be problematic. If a previous scar is present, it should, if possible, be used. In addition, internal fixation that does not invade the compartment should be preserved, if possible.

As an alternative to a previous scar, internal fixation removal, whether partial or total, can be combined with the UKR (Fig. 7.3). The advantage of this surgical strategy compared to TKR is less morbidity.

Based on our experience between 1991 and 2010, comprising 305 post-traumatic cases, 3.9% were knee implants, 37 were UKR, 14 were bilateral/unilateral knee replacements, 131 were standard TKRs, and 123 involved a semi-constrained prosthesis. Among the 37 post-traumatic UKRs, 35 were lateral and two were medial, with an average follow-up of 6.3 years (2–19 years). There was only one revision, corresponding to a failure rate of 2.7%.

7.3 Patients and Methods

7.3.1 Patients

From February 1991 to January 2010, the senior surgeon in our institution performed 184 consecutive lateral UKRs in 176 patients for lateral unicompartmental arthritis of the knee. The patients were followed-up prospectively and then evaluated at the last follow-up, in January–February 2012. The average follow-up was 13.2 years (2–20 years). Patients were selected based on clinical and radiological symptoms and signs. Clinically, the indications for surgery were: knee pain, absence of femoropatellar joint symptoms, fix flexion contracture < 10°, range of motion > 80°, and valgus deformity < 15°. The patients did not have inflammatory arthritis, hemochromatosis, hemophilia, parapatellar tenderness, patellofemoral joint symptoms, or joint instability. The 145 women and 31 men had an average age at surgery of 67 years (40–89); their average height was 168.2 cm (158–177 cm) and their average weight was 75 kg (54–91 kg). Arthritis involved the lateral compartment of the knee in all 184 cases. Two knees were previously treated with high tibial osteotomy (HTO), six had necrosis of the femoral condyle, and 35 were post-tibial plateau fractures; none had a lesion of the ACL. Primary arthritis was diagnosed in 141 knees. Five patients underwent simultaneous bilateral UKRs and three had staged bilateral procedures. At surgery, the patients had no more than type I disease (according to the Ahlback classification) in the other compartments [7, 8].

Patients were followed-up yearly for a period of 3 years and then every 2 years. Fourteen patients (14 knees) died from causes unrelated to the arthroplasty, three with < 10 years of follow-up, three with 10 years, and eight with > 10 years. At the most recent follow-up of 170 knees in 162 patients, 29 men and 133 women were evaluated. Follow-up of 112 patients (118 knees) consisted of clinical and radiological evaluation, while 45 patients (47 knees) were interviewed only by phone because they were not able to attend the clinic. Five knees were lost at follow-up. All patients were interviewed regarding the level of personal satisfaction. Postoperative knee function was evaluated using the Hospital for Special Surgery Knee Score before surgery and at last follow-up. Radiological imaging consisted of anteroposterior weight-bearing and lateral and patellar skyline views of the knee. Radiographic measurements of the mechanical and anatomical axis, cement interface, and the prosthesis-cement interfaces were evaluated in 11 zones for the pres-

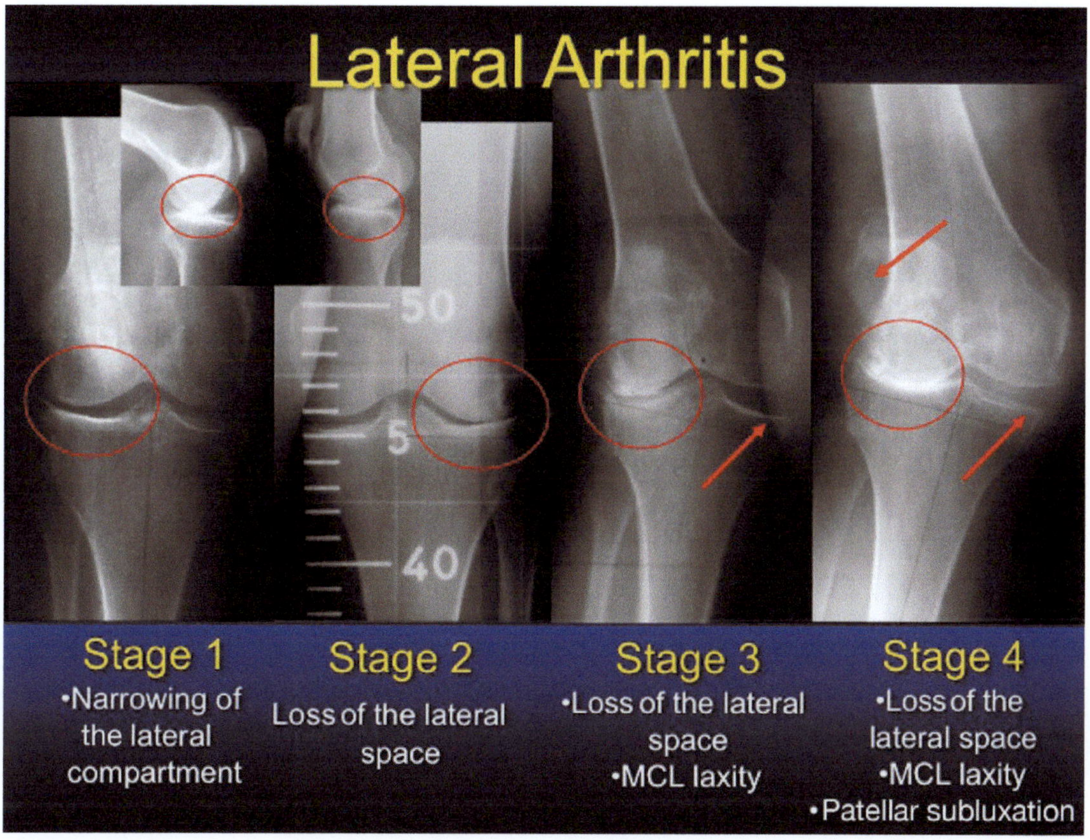

Fig. 7.4 Classification of valgus knee arthritis according to Romagnoli [9]. *MCL* medial collateral ligament

ence and extent of radiolucencies. The latter were reported to be progressive if there was an increase in size from one zone to an adjacent zone over time. Arthritis was graded in four stages according to the method of Romagnoli (Fig. 7.4) [9].

Stage 1 consists of narrowing of the lateral joint space and grade 1–3 chondromalacia, in stage 2, there is closure of the lateral joint space and grade 4 chondromalacia. Stage 3 is characterized by closure of the lateral joint space and MCL laxity, while in stage 4 there is closure of the lateral joint space, MCL laxity, and patellar dislocation (Fig. 7.4).

In addition, the opposite compartment and the patellofemoral joint were radiographically evaluated in all followed patients using the preoperative radiographs as the baseline. Radiographic progression of the opposite compartment and the patellofemoral joint was determined. These changes, if present, were graded on a four-point scale. Grade 1 radiographic change was defined as not-measurable joint-space loss but with radiographic changes such as osteophytes. Grade 2 radiographic changes consisted of joint space loss up to 25%. In grade 3 radiographic changes, joint space loss increases to 50%, while in grade 4 the loss exceeds 50% [10]. Kaplan survival analysis was used to evaluate the long-term results, with revision as the end point [11, 12].

7.3.2 Surgical Technique

The skin incision is 6- to 9-cm long and parapatellar lateral for valgus disease [13]. The lateral approach relies on the advantage of preservation of the quadriceps (Fig. 7.5).

In fact, the articular exposition is obtained by passing through the lateral intermuscular septum, thereby reducing muscular invasiveness. After

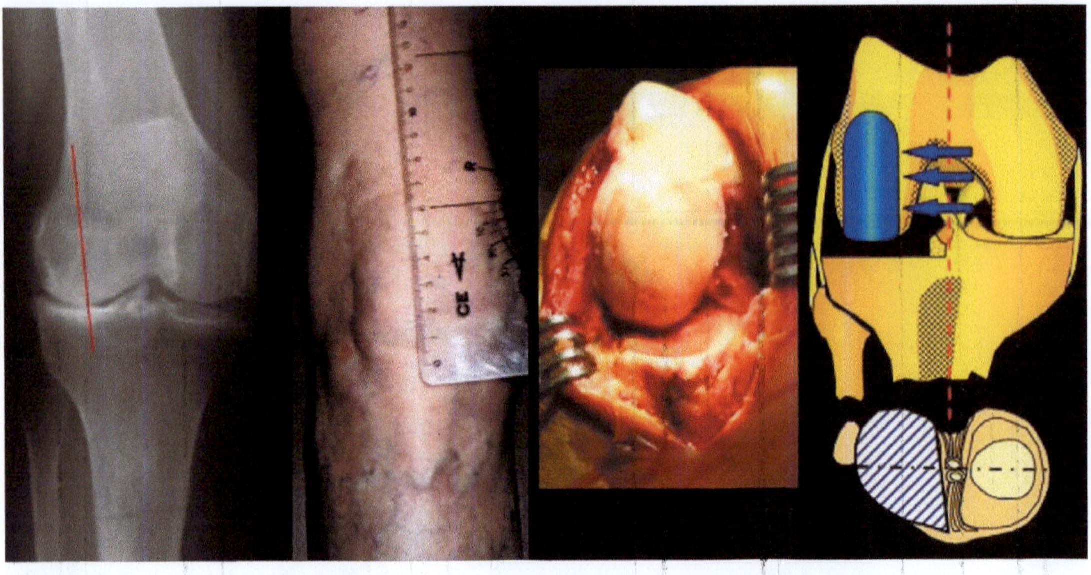

Fig. 7.5 A lateral approach, avoiding quadriceps damage and femoral component lateralization

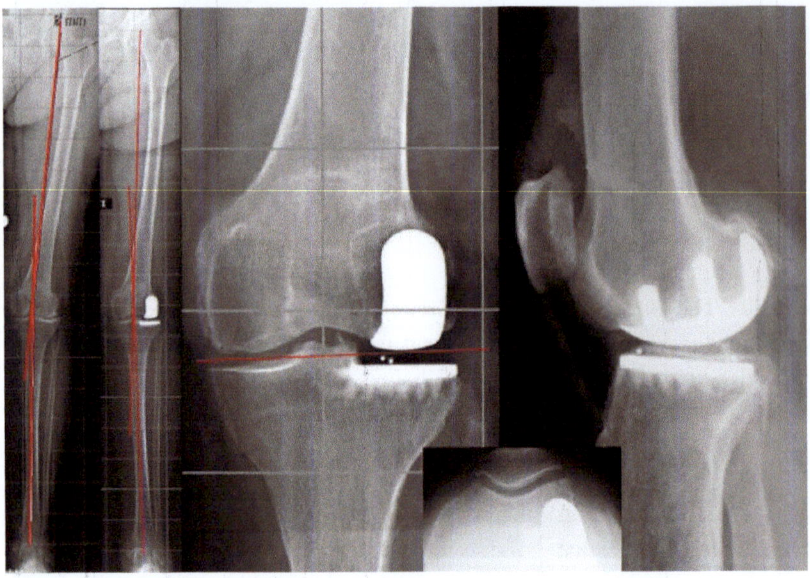

Fig. 7.6 Correct joint line reproduction with a lateral UKR implant

the capsulotomy, the patella is subluxed, never everted, and the knee is thoroughly inspected. The anterior horn of the meniscus is removed while Hoffa's fat pad and the ACL are protected. Once the tibial cuts have been made, the operation proceeds with positioning of the tibial guide, followed by a sagittal cut 10–15° oblique to the anteroposterior axis. The horizontal tibial cut is perpendicular to the mechanical axis in the lateral compartment, thereby ensuring correct joint line reproduction (Fig. 7.6). In the sagittal plane, the inclination of the tibial cut should be between 0° and 3° (slope).

Once it has been cut, the lateral tibial plateau takes on a more symmetric, semicircular shape than the medial one (Fig. 7.7).

Furthermore in case of fracture, a medio-lateral deformation with consequent enlargement is

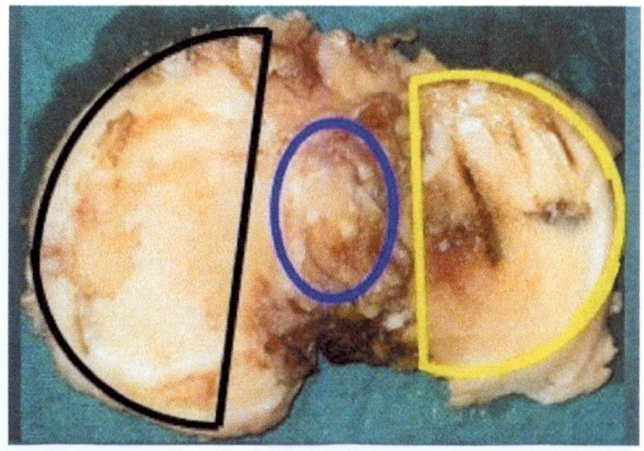

Fig. 7.7 Differences in the shape of the medial vs. the lateral tibial compartment

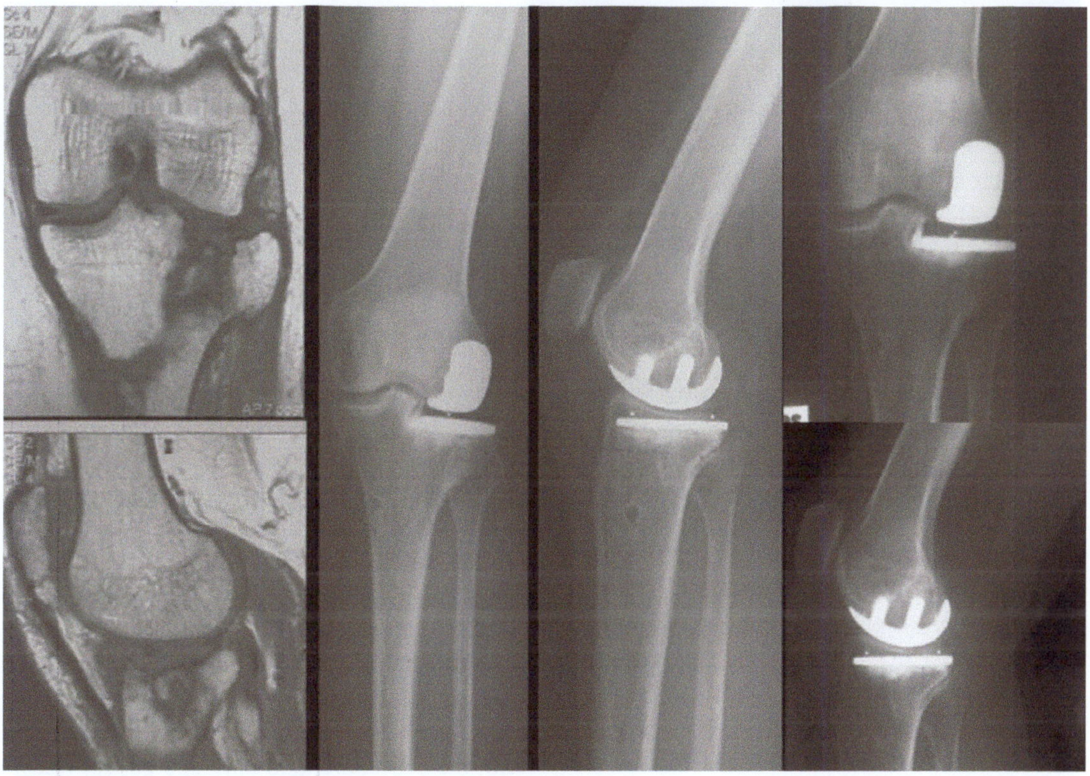

Fig. 7.8 Mediolateral enlargement of the lateral tibial plateau as a fracture sequela. X-ray control at 6 and 18 years of follow-up

possible (Fig. 7.8). In such cases, it is better to utilize a specific prosthesis with a more semicircular shape that is much more adaptable in uniformly covering the tibial surface.

The femoral component has to be positioned perpendicular to the center of the tibial component during both bending and extension. This is accomplished by lateralizing the femoral component (translating it closer to the outer border of the condyle). Also, the femoral cut must be very conservative in the lateral compartment because of the condylar hypoplasia of the valgus deformity, which is such that normally a thicker femoral component is needed to obtain joint line and axial limb correction. Finally, the mechanical axis should be under-corrected to remain within 3–6° in valgus.

The joint surfaces are prepared, drilled, and

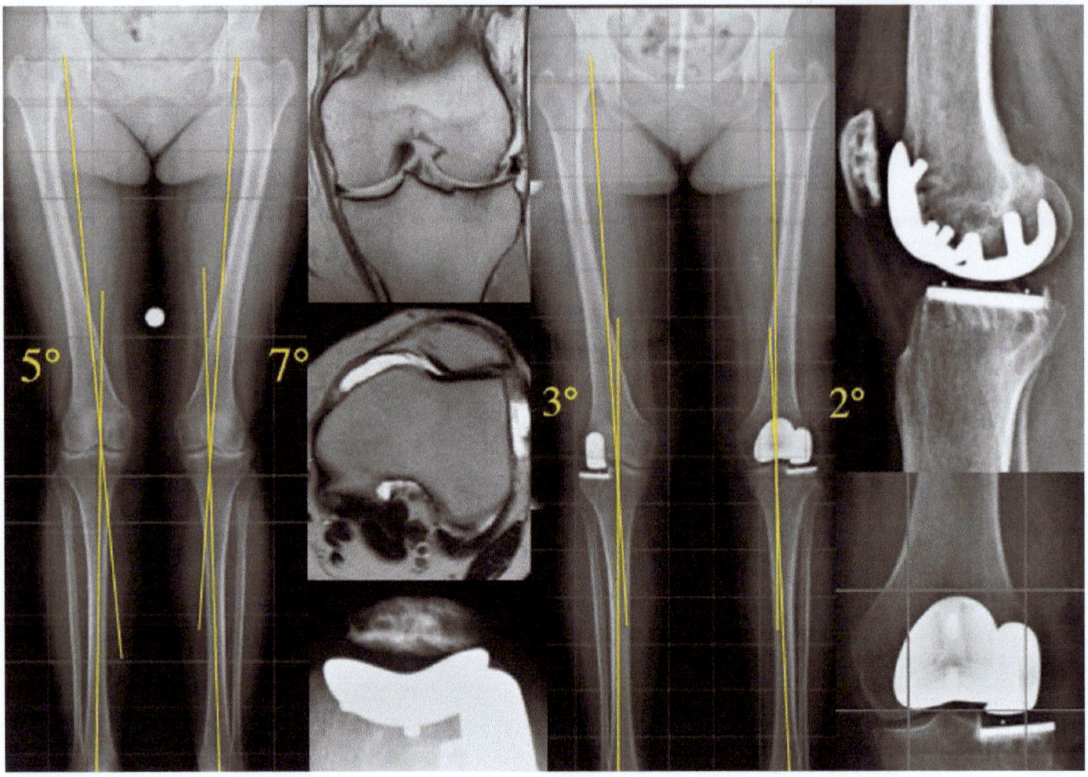

Fig. 7.9 Bilateral simultaneous implant: lateral UKR in the right knee and a bicompartmental implant in the left knee

freed of sclerotic areas by drilling. A standard cementing technique is used to fix the prosthesis. In case of bilateral pathology, we perform a bilateral simultaneous one-stage implant. In other cases, when there is associated patellofemoral arthritis, a patellofemoral prosthesis can be added, i.e., a bicompartmental implant (Fig. 7.9).

Passive movements are started very early in the post-operative period. Weight-bearing is allowed during the first post-operative day.

7.4 Results

Clinically, the average preoperative Hospital for Special Surgery Knee Score was 59 points (range: 48–69) but improved postoperatively to 94 (60–100). The average preoperative range of movement (ROM) was 105.4° (80–130°) At the final follow-up, the average ROM was 124.8° (103–140°). Eighty-one knees (64.8%) had a ROM > 120°; 139 patients had no pain (88.5%) while 17 patients had slight or occasional pain (10.8%) and one had persistent pain (0.6%).

At the time of the latest follow-up, 129 patients (82.4%) were enthusiastic regarding the procedure, 27 patients (17.6%) were satisfied with the procedure, and only one patient (0.6%) was not satisfied.

Radiographically, no component showed evidence of loosening, defined as no change in the position of the components as determined on sequential radiographs. There was no radiographic evidence of osteolysis. In eight patients, radiolucencies < 2 mm thick and non-progressive were demonstrated. In some cases these involved more than one zone but, in general, all of them occurred at the tibial component, near the cement-bone interface.

The average preoperative deformity was 9.7° of mechanical axis valgus (range: 4–22°). The

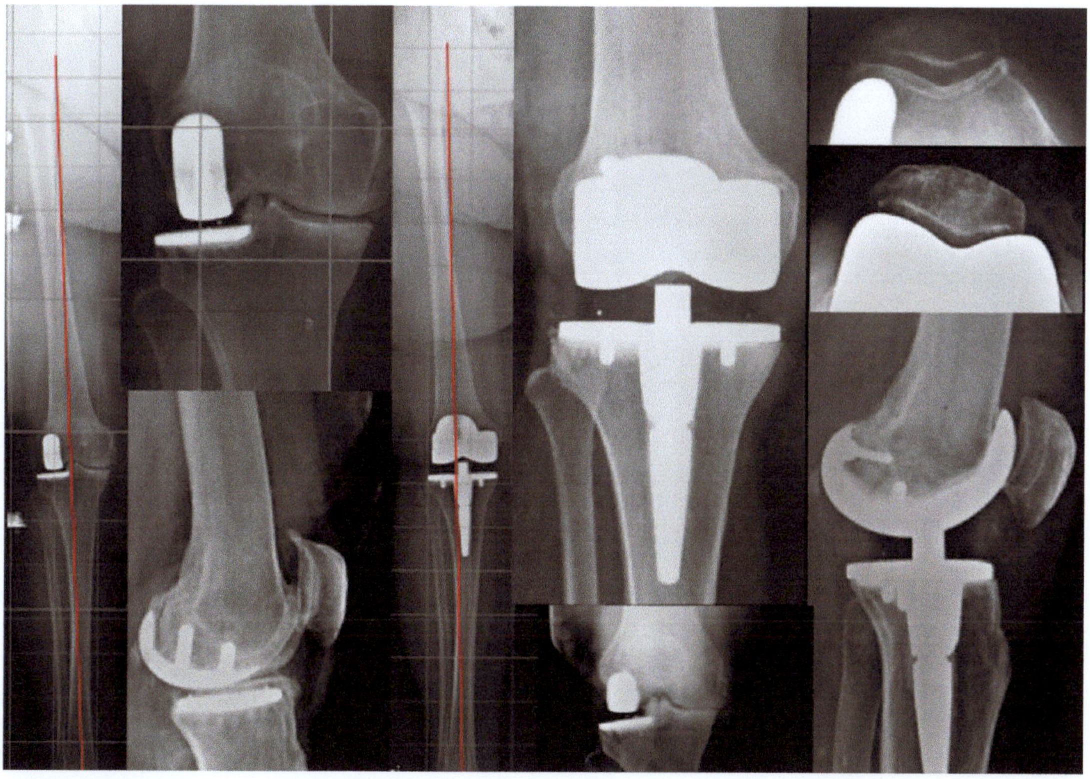

Fig. 7.10 Lateral UKR revision with a TKR due to an ACL deficiency and medial compartment degeneration, as seen at the 10-year follow-up

average postoperative alignment was 3.3° (0–8°) of mechanical axis valgus for an average correction of 6.4°.

Among the 118 X-ray evaluations, there was no radiographic progression of the opposite compartment in 93 knees (78.8%) whereas 27 knees (22.8%) had grade 2 progression and five knees (4.2%) had grade 3. There was no radiographic progression in the patellofemoral joint in 76 knees (64.8%), but 48 knees (40.7%) had a grade 2 progression and one knee had a progression of grade 3 (0.8%).

There were 11 revisions [14]: one occurred 5 years after surgery, due to capsulo-ligament instability and femoropatellar joint degeneration. In two others, 5.5 and 3 years after implantation, capsuloligament instability and ACl deficiency were documented. In the first case, the patient underwent revision surgery because of continuous anterior knee pain. Capsuloligament instability, due to laxity in the lateral collateral ligament, and femoropatellar joint degeneration, as confirmed during surgery even if in another orthopedic center, were clinically evident. In the second case, the capsulo-ligament instability had caused problems during gait and stairs, even if without pain. Both patients underwent revision surgery, during which a secondarily acquired ACL deficiency was demonstrated. There were no cases of component instability or polyethylene wear. One patient, 10 years after surgery for ACL deficiency and medial compartment degeneration, underwent revision with a TKR (Fig. 7.10). No failure was registered in the HTO group, nor was there necrosis of the femoral condyle. One case was due to under-correction of a valgus deformity, which is one of the more common causes of failure in that procedure. There were two cases of medial femoral condyle necrosis revised with TKR. Four patients had a medial UKR because of medial compartment degeneration, resulting in bi-UKRs (Fig. 7.11).

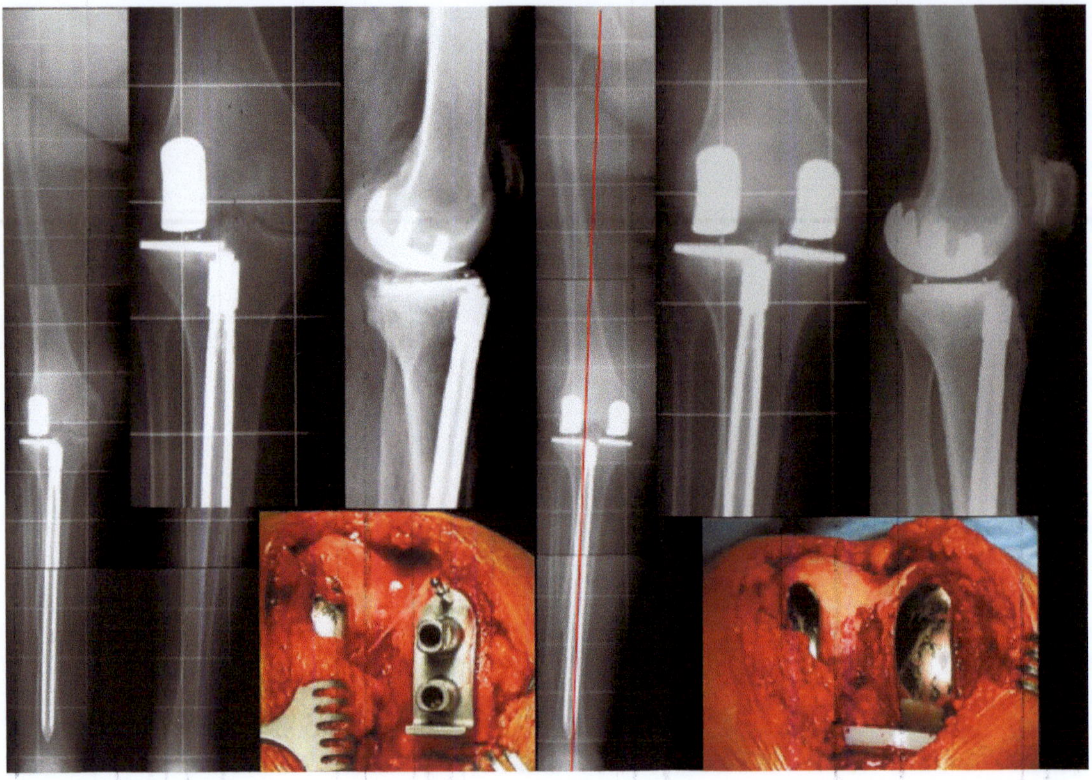

Fig. 7.11 Lateral UKR revision with a medial UKR in a patient with medial compartment degeneration due to tibial fracture sequelae

The cumulative survival rates at 10 and 20 years were 92.47% and 90.00%, respectively (Table 7.I) (Fig. 7.12).

7.5 Discussion

The indications for UKR have been defined. The procedure is recommended for osteoarthritis in either of the femorotibial compartments, medial or lateral.

The axial deformities, whether varus or valgus, should be correctable and there should be full-thickness cartilage in the not-involved compartment. The femoropatellar joint has always been a major concern in knee replacement, and the controversy has yet to be resolved. Some authors argue that it is a secure limit even for a single damage site. Others feel that realignment of the limb due to the femorotibial substitution weakens the patella and decreases its loading capacity, consequently causing anterior pain. We approach such patients considering the clinical data (symptoms and lifestyle) and the radiological grade even if there has been no direct surgical inspection. Age and weight are no longer a restriction for UKR, as no differences have been described between slim and overweight patients. On clinical examination, anterior subluxation and tibial external rotation have to be considered [10]. On anteroposterior and lateral weight-bearing X-ray views, anterior and external tibial translation is evaluated. Cartilage defects, such as femoral condyle-tibial intercondylar notch contacts, are located. Erosions of the patellofemoral joint are common; if they involve the medial patellar facet and the medial flange of the patellar groove of the femur, surgery unloads the damaged areas and relieves symptoms. When all the criteria for UKR are respected, the procedure is indicated. Even if

Table 7.1 Survival of 184 lateral UKRs

Years since surgery	N. at start	Failure	Width	Lost to FU	N. at risk	Failure %	Success %	Surv rate	%var	% SE
0-1	184	2	14	0	177	1.13	98.87	98.87	0.62	0.79
1-2	168	3	17	0	159.5	1.88	98.12	96.99	1.78	1.33
2-3	148	0	5	0	145.5	0.00	100.00	96.99	1.95	1.40
3-4	143	0	11	0	137.5	0.00	100.00	96.99	2.06	1.44
4-5	132	1	11	0	126.5	0.79	99.21	96.20	2.78	1.67
5-6	120	2	5	0	117.5	1.70	98.30	94.50	4.18	2.05
6-7	113	0	11	0	107.5	0.00	100.00	94.50	4.57	2.14
7-8	102	2	7	0	98.5	2.03	97.97	92.47	6.54	2.56
8-9	93	0	15	0	85.5	0.00	100.00	92.47	7.53	2.74
9-10	78	0	6	0	75	0.00	100.00	92.47	8.59	2.93
10-11	72	0	8	0	68	0.00	100.00	92.47	9.47	3.08
11-12	64	0	12	0	58	0.00	100.00	92.47	11.11	3.33
12-13	52	0	10	0	47	0.00	100.00	92.47	13.71	3.70
13-14	42	1	3	0	40.5	2.47	97.53	90.00	20.00	4.47
14-15	38	0	7	0	34.5	0.00	100.00	90.00	23.48	4.85
15-16	31	0	6	0	28	0.00	100.00	90.00	28.94	5.38
16-17	25	0	4	0	23	0.00	100.00	90.00	35.23	5.94
17-18	21	0	10	0	16	0.00	100.00	90.00	50.64	7.12
18-19	11	0	4	0	9	0.00	100.00	90.00	90.02	9.49
19-20	7	0	3	0	5.5	0.00	100.00	90.00	147.31	12.14
20-21	4	0	4	0	2	0.00	100.00	90.00	405.10	20.13
Total		11	173	0						

FU follow-up

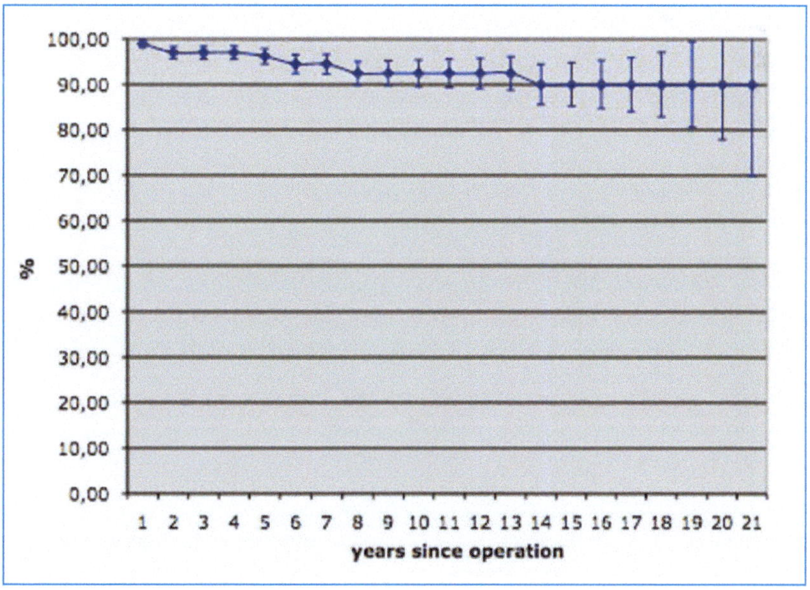

Fig. 7.12 Survival curve for the Allegretto (Centerpulse, Baar, Switzerland). See Table 7.1 for details

not well reported in the literature, treatment of the lateral isolated tibial plateau fracture is, in our opinion, an underestimated problem especially in young patients. We assume that the use of UKR in these cases reduces the risk of complications such as infections and postoperative stiffness compared to the rates seen in TKR.

Based on the correct indications, appropriate surgical expertise, and appropriate instruments, UKR is a safe and reliable choice for the treatment of unicompartmental arthritis of the knee.

References

1. Cartier P, Sanouiller J-L, Greisamer RP (1996) Unicompartmental knee arthroplasty surgery: 10- year minimum follow-up period. J Arthroplasty 11:782-8
2. Marmor L (1993) Unicompartmental arthroplasty of the knee with a minimum ten-year follow-up period. Clin Orthop 286:154-9
3. Romagnoli S, Verde F, Eberle RW (2006) 10 year minimum follow-up of medial unicompartmental knee arthroplasty with the allegretto prosthesis. JBJS-BR 88-B Supp_I, 100
4. Romagnoli S, Morasso V, Bibbiani E (1994) La gonartrosi rotatoria e le protesi monocompartimentali. Minerva Ortop Traumatol 45(10):485-8
5. Romagnoli S (1996) The unicompartmental knee prosthesis and the rotatory gonarthrosis kinematic. current concept in primary and revision total knee arthroplasty. Lippincott-Raven, Philadelphia, pp 69-83
6. Romagnoli S, Verde F (2011) Le protesi "mono" in esiti di frattura; La protesi monocompartimentale con ricostruzione del LCA. In: Confalonieri N (ed) La protesi monocompartimentale del ginocchio. Cic Editore
7. White SH, Ludkowski PF, Goodfellow JW (1991) Anteromedial osteoarthritis of the knee. J Bone Joint Surg (Br) 73-B:582-6
8. Ahlback S (1968) Osteoarthrosis of the knee: a radiographic investigation. Acta Radiol Suppl 277:7-72
9. Romagnoli S, Grappiolo G, Camera A (1998) Indicazioni e limiti delle protesi monocompartimentali. Il ginocchio-Anno XIV-Vol.1
10. Romagnoli S, Grappiolo G, Ursino N, Broch C (2000) Dexa evaluation of bone remodeling in the proximal tibia after unicompartmental prosthesis. Traumalinc 2:2 Pabst Science Publishers
11. Murray DW, Carr AJ, Bulstrode CJK (1993) Survival analysis of joint replacement. J Bone Joint Surg (Br)75-B:697-704
12. Peto R, Pike MC, Armitage P et al (1977) Design and analysis of randomised clinical trials requiring prolonged observation of each patient. Br J Cancer 35:1-40
13. Romagnoli S (2001) The Mini-Incision: More Hype than Help! In Opposition. Current Concepts in Joint Replacement. Presented by Current Concepts Institute, Cleveland, Ohio
14. Romagnoli S, Bibbiani E, Castelnuovo N, Cusmà G, Verde F (2008) The problem of UKR revisions. J Bone Joint Surg Br 90-B (Supp. I) 182

Computer-Assisted Unicompartmental Knee Replacement: Technique and Results

8

Jean Yves Jenny and Dominique Saragaglia

8.1 Introduction

Unicompartmental knee replacement (UKR) has become increasingly popular after the development of minimally invasive techniques [1]. The question of adequate indications for UKR has been extensively debated, although a consensus has yet to be accepted in the literature. Furthermore, this procedure was previously considered as more demanding than total knee replacement (TKR), especially because the instrumentation was not as accurate as that for TKR.

In the early 1970s, Marmor [2] developed a UKR implantation (medial femoral condyle and medial tibia plateau) procedure with very simple instrumentation. However, this was virtually a free-hand technique and it resulted in a high rate of inaccurate implantation. Specifically, the expected orientation of the tibial resection in the coronal and sagittal planes was very difficult to achieve. In the early 1980s, Cartier and Cheaib [3] introduced a tibial guiding system, aimed at achieving a higher accuracy of the proximal tibial resection. They also developed a trial femoral implant with spikes, allowing testing for the most appropriate positioning of the femoral component and for the most appropriate ligament tension. In the early 1990s, more sophisticated instruments were developed, similar to those for TKR, and mostly using intramedullary guiding rods. These instruments improved the accuracy of the procedure [4] but also increased its invasiveness, with a longer skin incision, the need for muscle incision, and violation of the medullary canal.

At the same time, it was extensively demonstrated that the accuracy of implantation, and especially restoration of the coronal mechanical femoro-tibial angle, was the most significant prognostic factor in the long-term survival of a UKR [1, 5-7]. Over-correction may rapidly lead to progression of the degenerative changes in the opposite femorotibial joint, while under-correction may induce accelerated polyethylene wear and early tibial loosening. Inappropriate reconstruction of the sagittal tibial slope may cause excessive anterior or posterior positioning of the femoral component on the tibial polyethylene component, with excessive wear and risk of tilting. Inappropriate ligament tension may lead to excessive wear (if overly tightened), or the risk of luxation of a mobile-bearing component (if too loose) [8, 9]. Conventional technique relies mainly on the surgeon's skill, which is known to be variable.

In the late 1990s, computer-assisted TKR was developed to overcome the inaccuracy of conventional implantation [10, 11]. Such devices were shown to allow a substantially more accurate reconstruction of the coronal femorotibial mechanical axis and a more accurate assessment of ligamentous balancing [7]. Computer navigation was then adapted to UKR, with encouraging results [12-18]. In the following we report our experience with a computer-assisted UKR using the OrthoPilot navigation system.

J.Y. Jenny (✉)
Hôpitaux Universitaires de Strasbourg, Centre de Chirurgie Orthopédique et de la Main, Illkirch, France
E-mail: jean-yves.jenny@chru-strasbourg.fr

N. Confalonieri, S. Romagnoli (eds.), *Small Implants in Knee Reconstruction*,
DOI 10.1007/978-88-470-2655-1_8, © Springer-Verlag Italia 2013

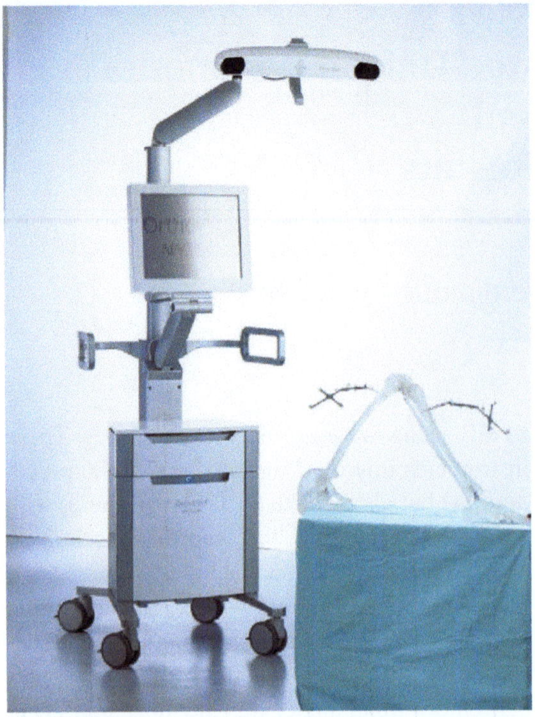

Fig. 8.1 The navigation system

8.2 Computer-Assisted Technique

The standard navigated operative technique for UKR has been described in detail elsewhere [19]. Briefly, OrthoPilot (AESCULAP, Tuttlingen, Germany) is an intra-operative non-image based system (Fig. 8.1). Three infrared localizers are implanted on screws in the distal femur and in the proximal tibia and then strapped on the dorsal part of the foot. The relative motion of two adjacent localizers is tracked by an infrared camera (Polaris, Northern Digital, Toronto, Canada). The dedicated software calculates the center of rotation of this movement, and so defines the respective centers of rotation of the hip, knee, and ankle joints. These centers are then used to calculate the mechanical axes of the femur and tibia in the coronal and sagittal planes. A localizer is then fixed on the tibial or femoral resection blocks, and the software displays on line the orientation of this block with respect to the mechanical axes of the bone. The surgeon can fix the block with the desired orientation before performing the bony resection, with a classical motorized saw blade. The trial implants are tested and, if satisfactory, the definitive prosthesis is implanted.

8.3 Navigation of a Tibial Resection Only (DS)

8.3.1 Surgical Technique

Preoperative planning is performed on standard anteroposterior and lateral X-rays obtained with the patient in standing position, bilateral Merchant view, and standing long-leg X-rays to measure the hip-knee-ankle (HKA) angle and the varus deformation of the proximal tibia. The posterior tibial slope is measured on the standard lateral X-ray

The patient lies supine, a tourniquet is applied at the proximal part of the thigh. The navigation system is set at the level of the patient's head, on the opposite side, at a distance of 1.80–2.20 m from the operated knee.

The navigation trackers are inserted first: the femoral tracker is fixed on the anteromedial part of the distal femur, 10 cm proximal to the patella; the tibial tracker is fixed on the anteromedial part of the proximal tibia, 10 cm below the joint line (Fig. 8.2).

A 7- to 9-cm medial parapatellar skin incision is used, according to the patient's body weight and the elasticity of the involved soft tissue. The joint approach may be performed by a subvastus incision; alternatively, a parapatellar approach with a 3–4 cm incision of the vastus medialis is possible.

The standard navigation technique is performed: (1) kinematic registration of the hip joint (circumduction), the knee joint (flexion-extension and rotation), and the ankle joint (flexion-extension); (2) anatomic registration of the specific landmarks: center of the intercondylar notch, center of the tibial plateau (Fig. 8.3), most distal point of the medial femoral condyle, most posterior point of the femoral condyle, medial and lateral epicondyles, medial and lateral malleoli, center of the ankle joint.

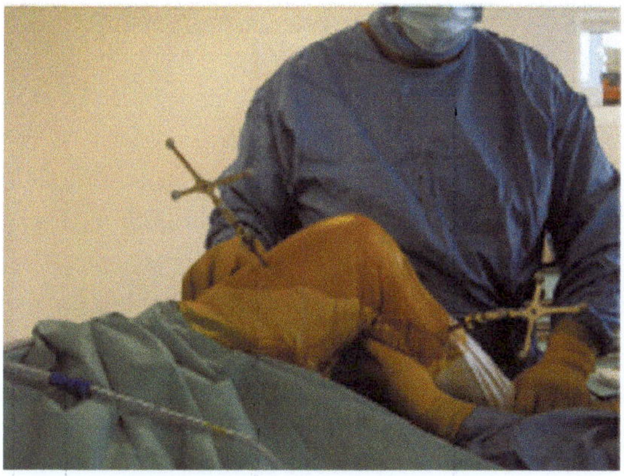

Fig. 8.2 Implantation of the trackers

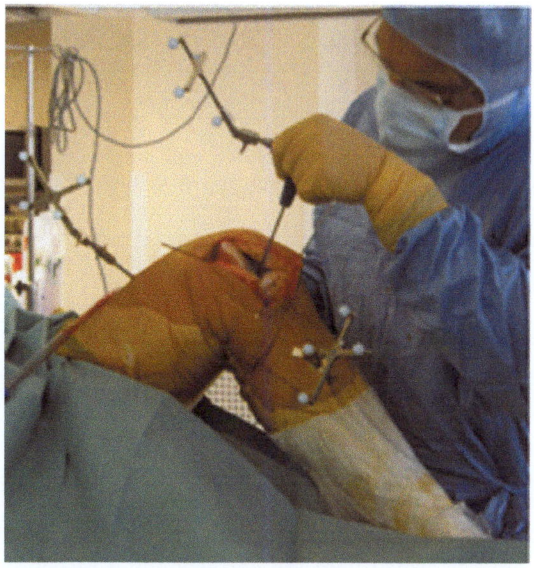

Fig. 8.3 Palpation of the anatomical landmarks

The navigation system displays the HKA in real time. A plausibility check is performed by comparison of this angle to the radiologic HKA. The reducibility of the deformation is assessed. If an over-correction is detected, it is considered as a contraindication for a mobile-bearing UKR because of the risk of overcorrection of the HKA. In such cases, a standard varus under-correction involves a laxity of the medial collateral ligament, with a high risk of bearing dislocation.

The tibial resection bloc is oriented with a free-hand technique according to the indication of the software (Fig. 8.4). We routinely choose a varus orientation of 2–3°, a posterior slope of 3–5°, and a resection height of 4–6 mm to avoid a cancellous bone support with a risk of later subsidence. However, the height of the resection should be adapted to the varus deformation: the greater the varus deformation, the shorter the resection [5, 7]. When the expected orientation is achieved, the resection block is secured with three threaded pins.

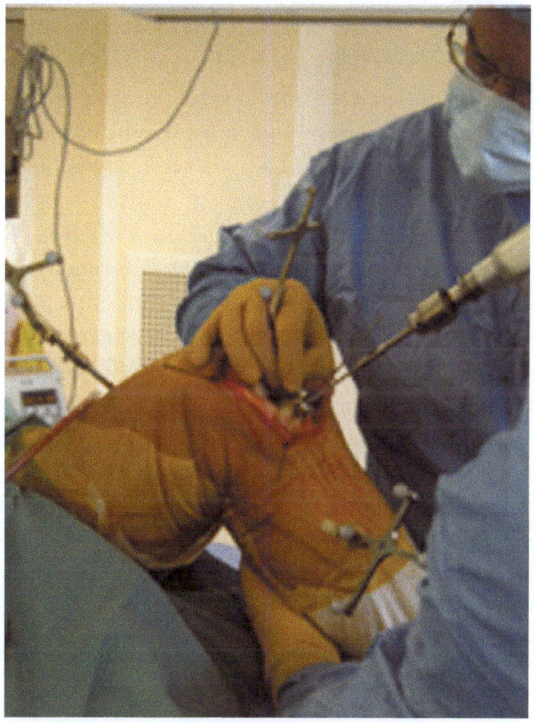

Fig. 8.4 Tibial navigation only: tibial resection

The proximal tibial resection is performed with an oscillating saw. The femoral resection is not navigated. A metallic spacer is inserted between the tibial resection and the distal part of the medial femoral condyle in full extension. The medial collateral ligament should be tightened. Knee recurvatum must be avoided because of the risk of excessive anterior condyle resection with a subsequent patellar impingement. The distal femoral guide is fixed on the spacer (Fig. 8.5) and then secured to the femur with three threaded pins. The distal femoral resection is performed with an oscillating saw. The size of the femoral component is determined with a template. The posterior femoral resection and the chamfer cut

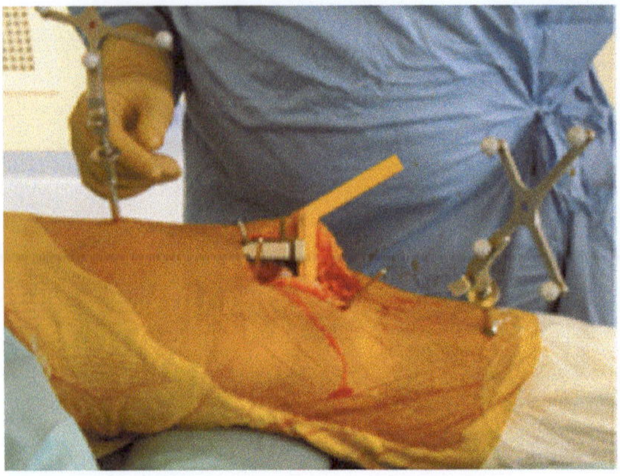

Fig. 8.5 Tibial navigation only: femoral resection

are performed with the corresponding resection guide.

The trial implants are placed on the resected bones, and the accurate limb axis correction (HKA = 177° ± 2°) and the ligamentous balance are controlled with the navigation system. We look for a 1° laxity with a mobile-bearing implant. When a greater laxity is needed to achieve a 3° varus HKA, we implant a fixed-bearing prosthesis. The classical indication of UKR is respected; if the preoperative varus deformation is < 10°, there is typically no under-correction > 5°. In other cases, a medial release may be performed or the indication may be changed to a TKR.

When the values are correct, the final implants are cemented. The final axis correction is again controlled by the navigation system.

8.3.2 Results

Our first experience was published in 2009 [12], with a case-control comparison of 20 navigated vs. 20 conventional implantations. The expected HKA (178° ± 1°) was achieved in 85% of the cases in the navigated group and in only 60% without navigation. In a second study, based on 21 implantations by one senior surgeon (DS), the expected HKA was achieved in 94%, the expected tibial mechanical axis (3° ± 1° varus) in 90.1%, and the expected tibial slope (3° ± 2°) in 95.2% of the cases.

8.4 Mini-Invasive Complete Navigation (JYJ)

8.4.1 Surgical Technique

The standard instruments were initially designed for a conventional 15–20 cm approach. Minimally invasive instruments were adapted for use with a typical 10-cm skin incision. We developed a new implant dedicated to this navigated technique (Univation, Aesculap, Tuttlingen, Germany), based on the concept of extra-articular fixation of the resection guides to further decrease the invasiveness of the procedure. The implantation side of the metallic femoral component is cylindrically shaped whereas the articular surface is spherical. The implant was designed to obtain full contact between the articular surface and the meniscal bearing throughout the entire range of motion. The meniscal polyethylene bearing has a proximal surface perfectly congruent with the femoral component and a fully flat inferior surface completely congruent with the metallic tibial tray. Both metallic components are designed for cemented implantation.

The software was modified because the minimally invasive approach does not allow direct palpation of the lateral femorotibial joint. The positions of the lateral articular points were calculated using the software and through radiographic preoperative planning.

Preoperative planning involves coronal long-leg X-rays with unipodal support and standard standing anteroposterior and lateral views. Two specific measurements are obtained prior to surgery: (1) coronal orientation of the distal femur (angle between the mechanical femoral axis and the distal bicondylar line); (2) the expected size of the femoral component (with appropriate templates).

The procedure begins with a quadriceps-sparing medial arthrotomy, typically 6 cm in length (Fig. 8.6). The navigation references are positioned: First. one bicortical screw is fixed to the anteromedial femoral cortex, 10–15 cm proximal to the joint line; a special device is secured on this screw to fix the femoral tracker (and later the femoral guiding system). Second, two pins are fixed to the anteromedial tibia cortex, 15 cm distal to the joint line; a special device is secured on this screw to fix the tibial tracker.

Kinematic registration is performed by moving the hip, knee, and ankle joints. Anatomic registration is limited to the medial femorotibial joint. A forced valgus maneuver is used to test the reducibility of the deformity extension, without movement of the ligament, obtaining the angle of reduction needed to achieve the proper correction for the patient in question.

The tibial resection guide is oriented with a free-hand technique (Fig. 8.7). The typical orientation is as follows:

- varus orientation of 50% of the expected postoperative varus deformation;
- posterior tibial slope of 3°;
- height of resection between 3 and 6 mm according to the reducibility of the deformation (the greater the reducibility, the lower the resection).

Horizontal resection of the medial tibial plateau is performed with an oscillating saw, and the vertical resection with a dedicated chisel of right-angle design in order to preserve the tibial attachment of the anterior cruciate ligament and to control the orientation of this resection to the proximal one. The medial tibial plateau and the medial meniscus are removed. The accuracy of the resection is controlled with a navigated plate. Any correction may be made at this moment.

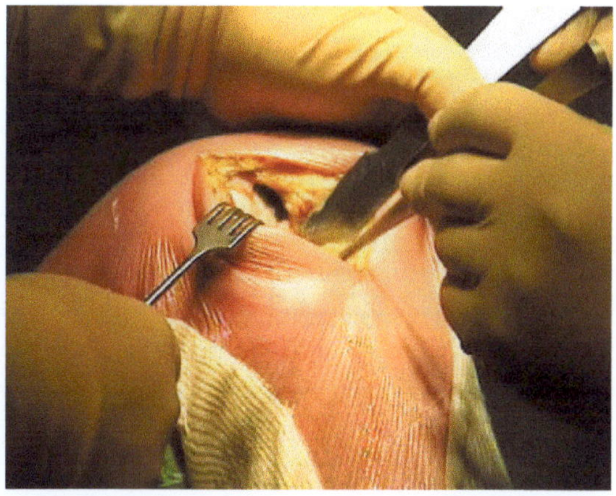

Fig. 8.6 Full navigation: skin incision

The medial femorotibial gap is measured at 0° and 90° of knee flexion with a laminar spreader (Fig. 8.8). The results are displayed on a planning screen in order to choose the appropriate femoral resection: coronal and sagittal orientation, height of the distal and posterior resections, thickness of the tibial component, and residual laxity in extension and in flexion (Fig. 8.9). These data may be virtually adapted to fit the surgeon's preferred

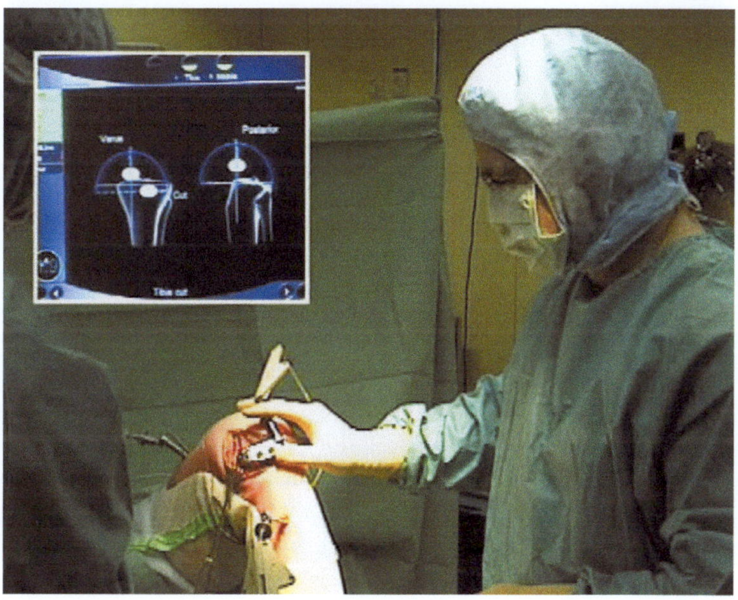

Fig. 8.7 Proximal tibial resection

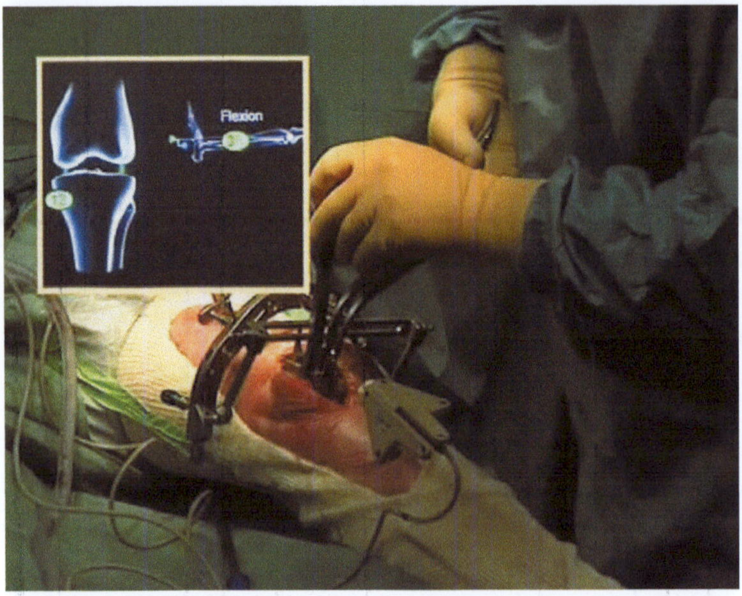

Fig. 8.8 Gap measurement

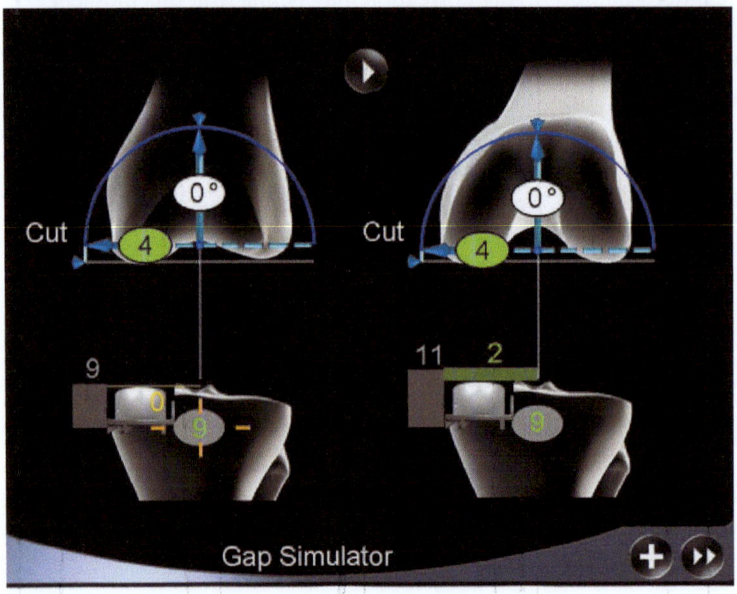

Fig. 8.9 Planning screen

approach and the patient's anatomy. The typical goal is as follows:

- varus orientation of 50% of the expected postoperative varus deformation;
- sagittal orientation of the posterior resection with a 10° flexion angle with respect to the sagittal mechanical femoral axis;
- adaptation of the heights of the distal and posterior resections to leave a 2-mm laxity.

A navigated bow is fixed by two bicortical screws on the distal femur and oriented along the knee flexion-extension axis. The distal and posterior resection guides are fixed to this bow and finely oriented according to the indication of the navigation system to achieve the planned goal. No instrument is fixed directly within the joint (Fig. 8.10).

A template is fixed to the mobile part of the

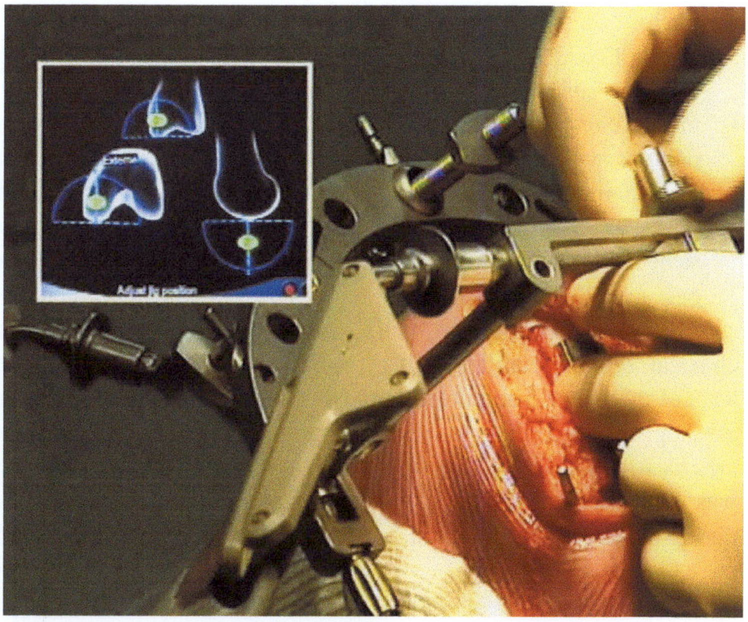

Fig. 8.10 Bow fixation

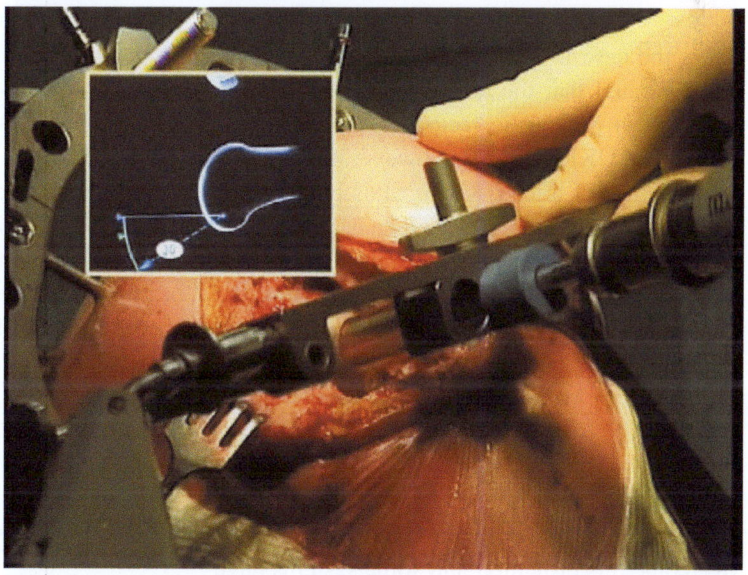

Fig. 8.11 Femoral resection

bow, and the posterior femoral resection is performed with an oscillating saw according to plan. A second template is fixed to the mobile part of the bow, and the cylindrical distal femoral resection is performed with a burr (Fig. 8.11). The position of the trial femoral implant may be controlled by the navigation system, with control of the axis correction and testing of the ligamentous balance. Finally, the implants are cemented. The thickness of the mobile bearing is finally defined to obtain a 2° residual laxity in flexion and in extension.

8.4.2 Results

More than 250 knees have been operated on with this technique in our department. The first 81 knees, with more than 2 years of follow-up, have been re-examined [20]. The functional result was satisfactory according to the following criteria:

- mean clinical Knee Society Score (KSS) of 91 points (on a scale from 0 to 100 points);
- mean functional KSS of 94 points (0–100 points);
- mean pain KSS of 42 points (0–50 points);
- mean Oxford Knee Score of 20 points (on a scale from 12 to 60 points, 12 points being the best score).

The expected correction of the coronal mechanical femorotibial angle was achieved for 94% of the knees. The implantation was considered optimal according to all five radiological criteria for 77% of the knees. The survival rate was 97% after 2 years. Most revisions occurred during the development period.

8.5 Discussion

As is the case in TKR, it has been extensively demonstrated that the accuracy of implantation is a critical prognostic factor for the long-term survival of UKRs [1, 5-7]. However, the optimal limb alignment after UKR remains unclear [4], although there is general agreement that poor alignment increases the risk of early polyethylene wear and early loosening [21, 22]. Thus, the need to promote more accurate and more precise implantation techniques is clear.

Also as in TKR, conventional, manual instrumentation, relying mainly on the surgeon's intraoperative assessment of the position of the resection guides, may result in a poor accuracy [4]. Therefore, navigation systems were developed to overcome this difficulty, and some systems have been validated in the early phase of navigation era [14, 17]. Since the pioneer period of navigation, several studies have demonstrated that its use in UKR provides a higher accuracy of implantation [16, 18, 23], while the opposite results were obtained in only a single study [24]. One might even assume that the efficacy of navigation is higher for UKR than for TKR, as the former is a more demanding procedure.

Nonetheless, navigation systems are only a tool and as such must be adapted to the surgeon's needs-explaining the efforts at tailored systems allowing the surgeon to choose the particular steps to be navigated vs. those to be performed conventionally.

Minimally invasive procedures have been primarily developed for UKR [25, 26]. These techniques may decrease surgical damage to the joint, with an easier and faster rehabilitation [27-29]. However, there may be a higher risk of prosthetic misplacement because of the narrower joint approach, with less visualization of the relevant anatomic landmarks [30, 31]. These techniques must not compromise the accuracy of implantation, which obviously remains the primary goal. Navigation systems can offer the possibility to achieve a high degree of accuracy with a less invasive approach [19]. Our results confirm that the use of a navigation system can provide the same accuracy of implantation with a minimally invasive approach as navigated implantation with a conventional approach.

8.6 Conclusions

Computer navigation in UKR allows greater accuracy of implantation than conventional techniques. Given the increased technical difficulty of this procedure compared to TKR, it may even be the most useful and powerful indication for navigation.

References

1. Borus T, Thornhill T (2007) Unicompartmental knee arthroplasty. J Am Acad Orthop Surg 15:9-18
2. Marmor L (1982) The Marmor knee replacement. Orthop Clin North Am 13:55-64
3. Cartier P, Cheaib S (1987) Unicondylar knee arthroplasty. J Arthroplasty 2:157-162
4. Jenny JY, Boeri C (2002) Accuracy of implantation of a unicompartmental knee arthroplasty with 2 different instrumentations: a case-controlled comparative study. J Arthroplasty 17:1016-1020
5. Hernigou P, Deschamps G (1996) Prothèses unicompartimentales du genou. Rev Chir Orthop 82 Suppl 1:23-60
6. Hernigou P, Deschamps G (2004) Alignment influences wear in the knee after medial unicompartmental arthroplasty. Clin Orthop Relat Res 423:161-165
7. Scott RD (2006) Three decades of experience with unicompartmental arthroplasty: mistakes made and les-

sons learned. Orthopaedics 29:829-831
8. Mercier N, Wimsey S, Saragaglia D (2010) Long-term clinical results of the Oxford medial unicompartmental knee arthroplasty. Int Orthop 34:1137-1143
9. Neyret P, Chatain F, Deschamps G (1996) Matériel et options dans les prothèses unicompartimentales du genou. Rev Chir Orthop 82 Suppl 1:48-52
10. Jenny JY, Boeri C (2001) Implantation d'une prothèse totale de genou assistée par ordinateur. Etude comparative cas-témoin avec une instrumentation traditionnelle. Rev Chir Orthop 87:645-652
11. Saragaglia D, Picard F, Chaussard C, Montbarbon E, Leitner F, Cinquin P (2001) Mise en place des prothèses totale du genou assistée par ordinateur : comparaison avec la technique conventionnelle. A propos d'une étude prospective randomisée de 50 cas. Rev Chir Orthop 87:18-28
12. Ayach A, Plaweski S, Saragaglia D (2009) Computer-assisted uni knee arthroplasty for genu varum deformity. Results of axial correction in a case-control study of 40 cases. 9th annual meeting of CAOS-International proceedings. WingSpan, Livermore, CA, pp 4-7
13. Cossey AJ, Spriggins J (2005) The use of computer-assisted surgical navigation to prevent malalignment in unicompartmental knee arthroplasty. J Arthroplasty 20:29-34
14. Jenny JY, Boeri C (2003) Unicompartmental knee prosthesis implantation with a non-imaged-based navigation system : rationale, technique, case-control comparative study with a conventional instrumented implantation. Knee Surg Sports Traumatol Arthrosc 11:40-45
15. Jenny JY (2008) Navigated unicompartmental knee replacement. Sports Med Arthrosc rev 16:103-107
16. Jung KA, Kim SJ, Lee SC, Hwang SH, Ahn NK (2010) Accuracy of implantation during computer-assisted minimally invasive Oxford unicompartmental knee arthroplasty: a comparison with a conventional instrumented technique. Knee 17:387-391
17. Perlick L, Bäthis H, Tingart M, Perlick C, Lüring C, Grifka J (2004) Minimally invasive unicompartmental knee replacement with a nonimage-based navigation system. Int Orthop 28:193-197
18. Rosenberger RE, Fink C, Quirbach S, Attal R, Tecklenburg K, Hoser C (2008) The immediate effect of navigation on implant accuracy in primary mini-invasive unicompartmental knee arthroplasty. Knee Surg Sports Traumatol Arthrosc 16:1133-1140
19. Jenny JY, Ciobanu E, Boeri C (2007) The rationale for navigated minimally invasive unicompartmental knee replacement. Clin Orthop Relat Res 463:58-62
20. Jenny JY, Saussac F, Louis P (2011) Navigated, minimal invasive, mobile bearing unicompartmental knee prosthesis. A 2-year follow-up study. Paper presented at the 12th EFORT Meeting (European Federation of Orthopedic and Traumatology Societies), Copenhagen
21. Larsson SE, Larsson S, Lundkvist S (1988) Unicompartmental knee arthroplasty. Clin Orthop Relat Res 232:174-181
22. Ridgeway SR, McAuley JP, Ammeen DJ, Engh GA (2002) The effect of alignment of the knee on the outcome of unicompartmental knee replacement. J Bone Joint Surg Br 84:351-355
23. Seon JK, Song EK, Park SJ, Yoon TR, Lee KB, Jung ST (2009) Comparison of minimally invasive unicompartmental knee arthroplasty with or without a navigation system. J Arthroplasty 24:351-357
24. Lim MH, Tallay A, Bartlett J (2009) Comparative study of the use of computer-assisted navigation system for axial correction in medial unicompartmental knee arthroplasty. Knee Surg Sports Traumatol Arthrosc 17:341-346
25. Price AJ, Webb J, Topf H, Dodd CAF, Goodfellow JW, Murray DW (2001) Rapid recovery after Oxford unicompartmental arthroplasty through a short incision. J Arthroplasty 16:970-976
26. Romanowski MR, Repicci JA (2002) Minimally invasive unicondylar arthroplasty: eight-year follow-up. J Knee Surg 15:17-22
27. Haas SB, Cook S, Beksac B (2004) Minimally invasive total knee replacement through a mini midvastus approach: a comparative study. Clin Orthop Relat Res 428:68-73
28. Muller PE, Pellengahr C, Witt M, Kircher J, Refior HJ, Jansson V (2004) Influence of minimally invasive surgery on implant positioning and the functional outcome for medial unicompartmental knee arthroplasty. J Arthroplasty 19:296-301
29. Reilly KA, Beard DJ, Barker KL, Dodd CA, Price AJ, Murray DW (2005) Efficacy of an accelerated recovery protocol for Oxford unicompartmental knee arthroplasty. A randomised controlled trial. Knee 12:351-357
30. Berend KR, Lombardi AV Jr, Mallory TH, Adams JB, Groseth KL (2005) Early failure of minimally invasive unicompartmental knee arthroplasty is associated with obesity. Clin Orthop Relat Res 440:60-66
31. Hamilton WG, Collier MB, Tarabee E, McAuley JP, Engh CA Jr, Engh GA (2006) Incidence and reasons for reoperation after minimally invasive unicompartmental knee arthroplasty. J Arthroplasty 21:98-107

9 The Bi-Unicompartmental Knee Prosthesis

Sergio Romagnoli, Francesco Verde, Michele Corbella, and Sara Zacchetti

9.1 Introduction

The bi-unicompartmental knee prosthesis [1-5] is a system that uses two independent components, femoral and tibial, to preserve the tibial eminentia with the anterior cruciate ligament (ACL). Although in the majority of prosthetic knee systems the cruciate ligaments are sacrificed or only the posterior cruciate ligament (PCL) is preserved, a long-term research objective has been to reproduce the normal articular kinematics of the knee, replacing only the worn areas while respecting the capsule and ligaments (Fig. 9.1).

The recent development of tissue-sparing surgery has given new impetus to the utilization of prosthetic systems that respect the undamaged capsuloligamentous structures of the knee. This type of implant, while not an entirely novel knee prosthesis, represents the evolution of the first experiences of Marmor, Gunston, and Lubinus, whose principles remain valid in many aspects of biomechanical and gait analyses.

9.2 Epidemiology

The presence of the ACL in the treatment of bicompartmental arthritis limits the surgical options. Of course, the link between the ACL and its mechanical function must eventually be established. We have carried out survivorship studies of a bicompartmental prosthesis and the unicompartmental Allegretto (Zimmer), with 10-15 years of follow-up [6]. In addition, we have evaluated many other long-term unicompartmental survivorship studies reported in the literature (Goodfellow, Berger, etc.). The results are consistent, confirming the long-term stability on anteroposterior (AP) views. This shows that the ACL is able to maintain the same mechanical function over a period of years. In fact, in our study, in which 124 patients received a unicompartmental prosthesis, there was only one case of failure due to ACL deficiency. With patient age as a criterion, among 500 cases of total knee arthroplasty (TKA), 7.6% of the patients were < 55 years of age, 25.8% were 55–65 years of age, 39.5% were between 65 and 75 years of age, and 27.1% were over the age of 75. This means that 33.4% were below 65 years of age and thus had a high functional demand. Within this group, 29.8% had an intact ACL and were therefore candidates for cruciates-preserving prostheses.

9.3 Indications

Our indications are: patients with femorotibial degeneration but asymptomatic with respect to the patella, cruciate ligaments integrity, flexion deformity < 10°, varus-valgus deformity < 15°, range of active movement (ROM) > 90°, and tibial bone defect < 12 mm [1-4]. Radiographic evaluation is based on standard AP, lateral, and skyline projections demonstrating femorotibial degeneration higher than grade I and femoropa-

S. Romagnoli (✉)
Galeazzi Orthopedic Institute
Milan, Italy
E-mail: sergio.romagnoli@libero.it

N. Confalonieri, S. Romagnoli (eds.), *Small Implants in Knee Reconstruction*,
DOI 10.1007/978-88-470-2655-1_9, © Springer-Verlag Italia 2013

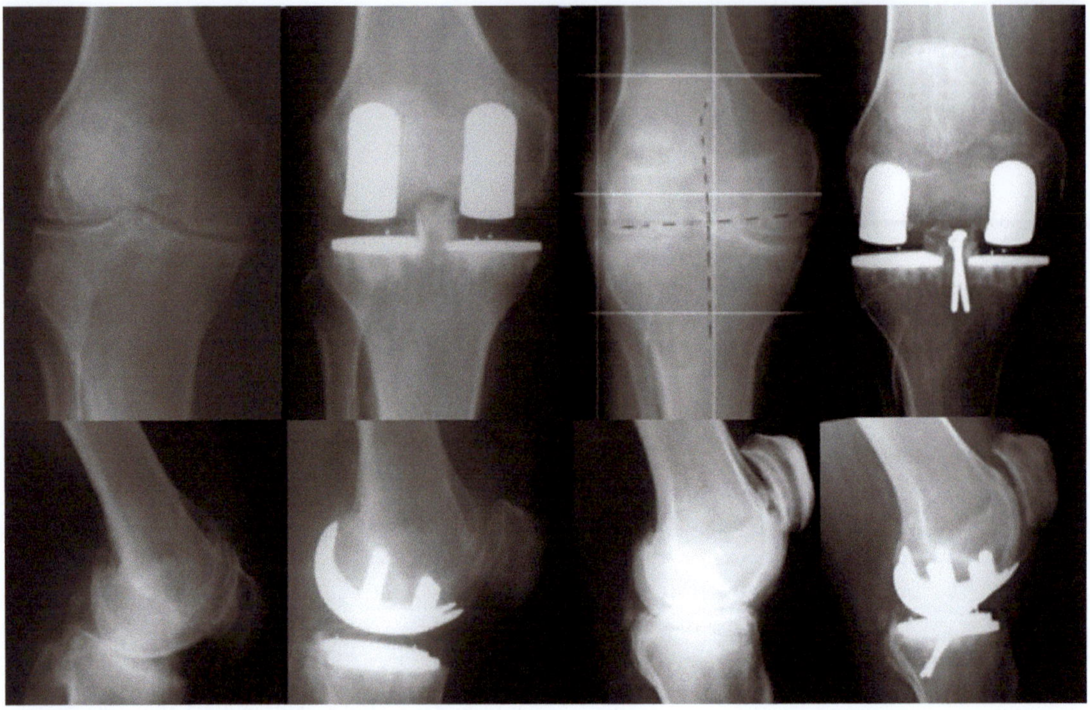

Fig. 9.1 Two bi-unicompartmental implants: *left* at 17 years of follow-up of a 63-year-old male patient; *right* at 15 years of follow-up of a male patient with spina bifida

tellar involvement lower than grade II according to the Ahlback scale. Also, on a weight-bearing long AP X-ray view the mechanical axis can be calculated, showing the correct range of deformity. In some cases magnetic resonance imaging shows features of instability such as ACL deficiency and patellofemoral status. Clinically, the knee must be quite stable and only a mild laxity due to cartilage wear is tolerated. Femorotibial signs of disease are generally present, such as pain while walking and doing stairs or effusion. Patient age and weight are not limits, but this procedure is particularly recommended for young patients (< 65 years) with a good level of activity and a BMI < 32. In fact, a bi-unicompartmental knee replacement (UKR) prosthesis is an option when a high performance of the knee is requested by young patients. In some well selected cases, when bi-femorotibial compartment degeneration is a correct bi-UKR indication but ACL deficiency represents a clear limit, an ACL reconstruction procedure is possible in men under the age of 60 years. Secondary patellofemoral joint degeneration with anterior pain should be kept in mind in patient selection. The standard of evaluations are: symptomatology, X-ray evaluation of the alignment and possible overload, and the intraoperative observation of third or fourth degree chondromalacia. Symptomatology, only if associated with a second parameter, such as X-ray or intra-

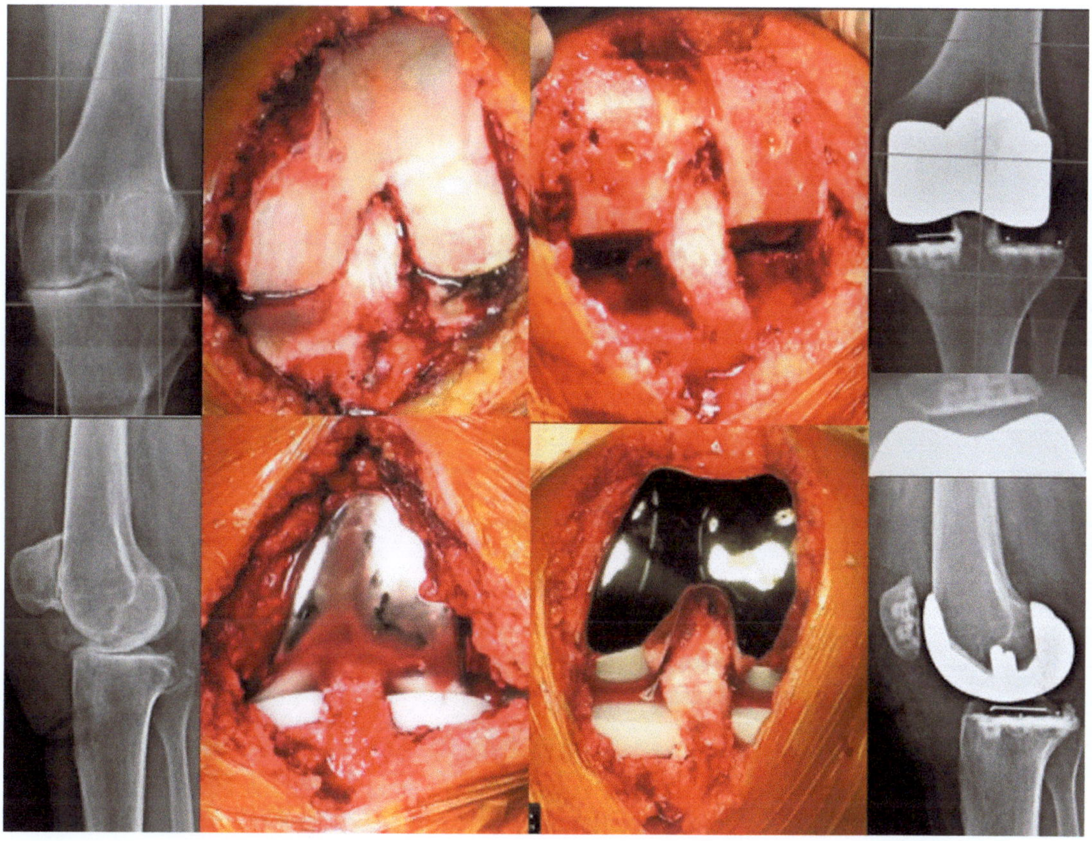

Fig. 9.2 Bi-unicompartmental implant with a bicondylar femoral component in a 61-year-old female

operative findings, is a clear limit to the use of independent unicondylar femoral components. In these cases the alternative is a bicondylar femoral component that also covers the trochlear surface or the inclusion of a patellofemoral prosthesis (Fig. 9.2).

Sometimes bi-UKR can be the result of a UKR revision due to late degeneration and pain in the not treated femorotibial compartment [3, 4]. Obviously, in this kind of prosthesis, performed over the course of years, the previous implant must be stable and the only contraindications are polyethylene wear and ACL deficiency (Fig. 9.3).

Contraindications are active inflammatory arthritis, ligament instability, severe deformity, and fractures if the bone defect is > 12 mm.

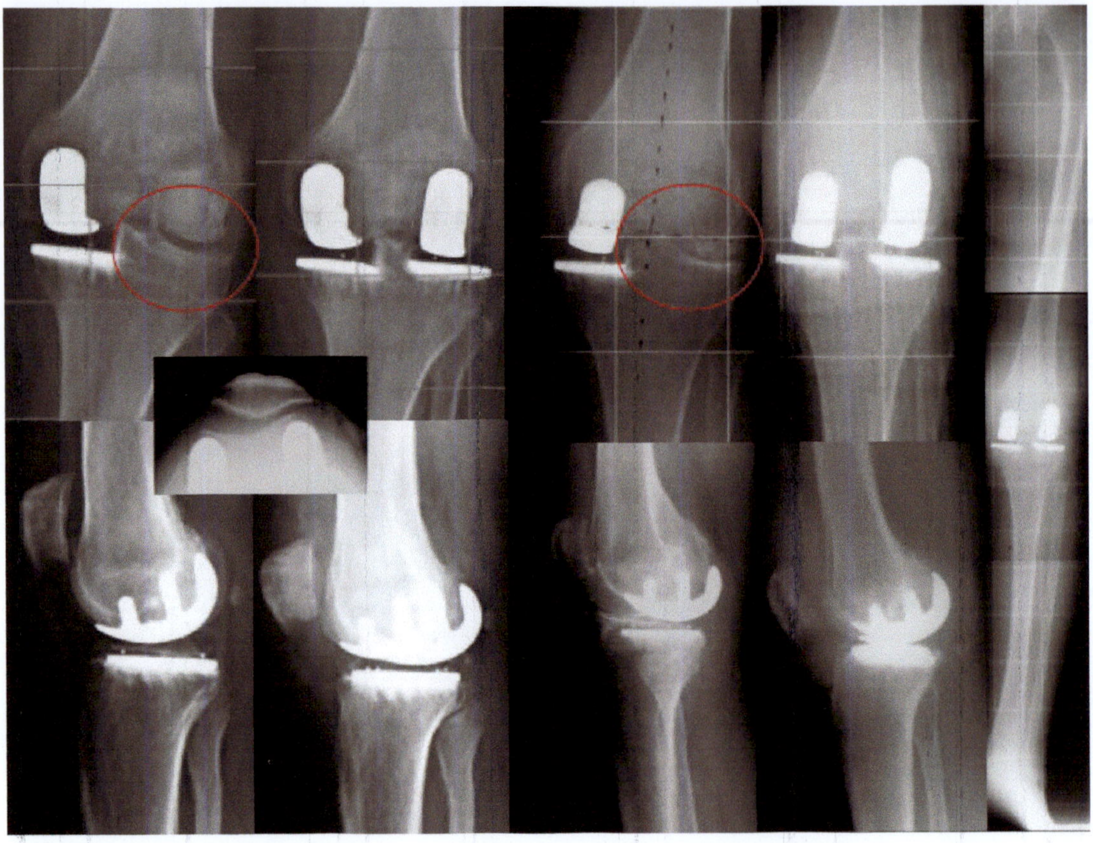

Fig. 9.3 Two cases of a bi-unicompartmental implant as a result of UKR revision: *left* at 20 years of follow-up an 84-year-old male patient; *right* at 15 years of follow-up of a 74-year-old female patient

9.4 Surgical Technique

Bi-UKR uses the same surgical technique as UKR but it is applied to the medial and lateral compartments. Two different approaches are possible: a double mini-skin incision or an isolated medial parapatellar mini-invasive approach.

In the first option, the procedure begins in the compartment of the deformity; once it has been corrected with the implant trials, the other side is addressed. An advantage of this solution is the possibility to further reduce the quadriceps aggression. Thus, essentially, there are two independent implants. The patellar vascularization, in this case, is guaranteed by respecting the superomedial area (Fig. 9.4).

The second choice relies on a mini-invasive parapatellar medial incision of 8–10 cm. In this case, a mini mid-vastus incision allows patellar subluxation, well-exposing the medial and lateral compartments and avoiding patellar eversion (Fig. 9.5). Once the compartments are exposed, surface bone cuts are performed with the tibia first technique.

Tibial cuts are performed, with an oblique cut 15–20° along the AP axis in the medial compartment and 10–15° along the lateral axis. The horizontal cut must be perpendicular to the epiphyseal axis, in order to respect the height and obliquity of the joint line while avoiding any consequent release. In the majority of cases, the tibial cut in the sagittal plane (slope) must differ between the two compartments, lateral 0–3° and medial 3–6°, in order to reproduce the anatomical preoperative slope and respect PCL stability. Once the tibial resection has been completed, the asymmetric features of the tibial plateau must be considered. The lateral compartment is more symmetric than the medial and semicircular compartments regarding

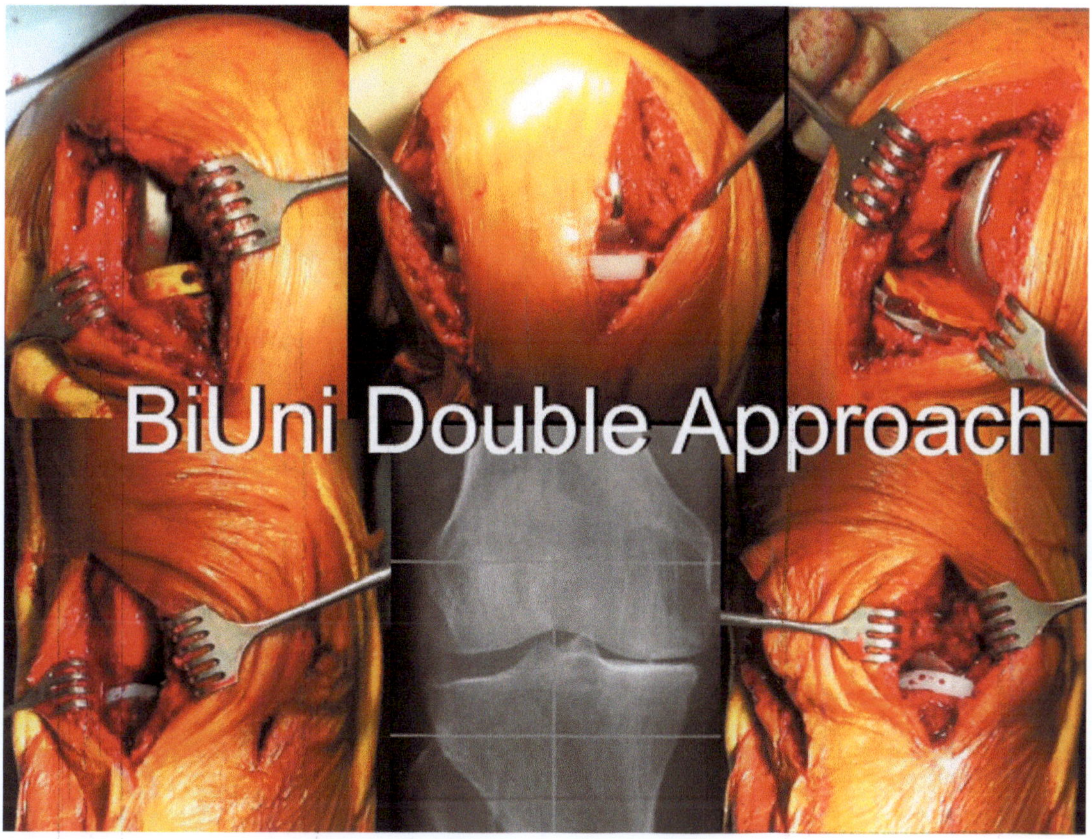

Fig. 9.4 Double mini-invasive approaches: parapatellar, medial, and lateral

their shape. It is thus better to utilize a dedicated prosthesis with a more semicircular shape as it is much more adaptable, allowing uniform coverage of the lateral tibial surface (Fig. 9.6).

The next step involves checking the stability in extension with trials and marking the anterior limits on the femoral condyles to fit the limit of the right anterior position for the femoral cutting guide. We perform the distal cut in extension and the posterior cut in flexion using two different tensor-guides that calibrate the same amount of resection, obtaining a balanced flexion-extension gap. First, the distal cut in extension indicates the desired degree of stability; the tensor is adjusted to avoid overcorrection and release. Subsequently, with the knee in flexion, the same calibrated amount of tension and resection is performed on the posterior condyle. Only 2–3 mm are removed from the femoral condyles, corresponding to the same thickness of the prosthesis to be implanted. From the tibial surface, an amount generally between 3 and 7 mm for each compartment is removed, with less removal on the deformity side. This approach explains why the implant can be considered a resurfacing prosthesis. Furthermore, there is no need for further resection because, if the indications are followed, a morphotype correction is not needed. Regarding the position, a component lateralization is necessary.

The components of the prosthesis will be lateralized to maintain perpendicularity on the tibial components in extension and in flexion. Finally, femoral components with different sizes and flexion degrees are implanted, which create two different radii of curvature. This achieves motion and stability with respect to the rotational axis of each compartment [3, 4]. Once the stability has been checked with trials, the sclerotic bone is removed from the surfaces, followed by drilling and component cementation. The lateral tibial component is cemented first, proceeding to the medial and, finally, to the femoral components.

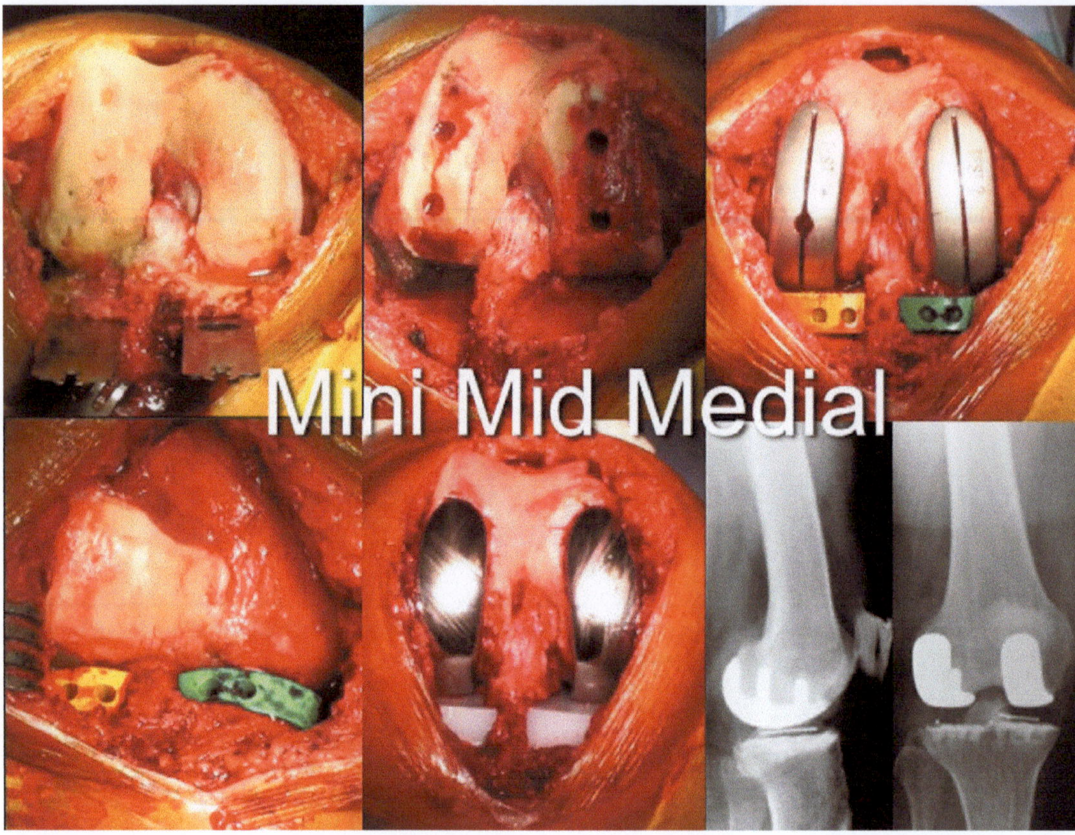

Fig. 9.5 Mini-mid-medial approaches: complete bicompartmental exposure, trials in situ and X-ray control

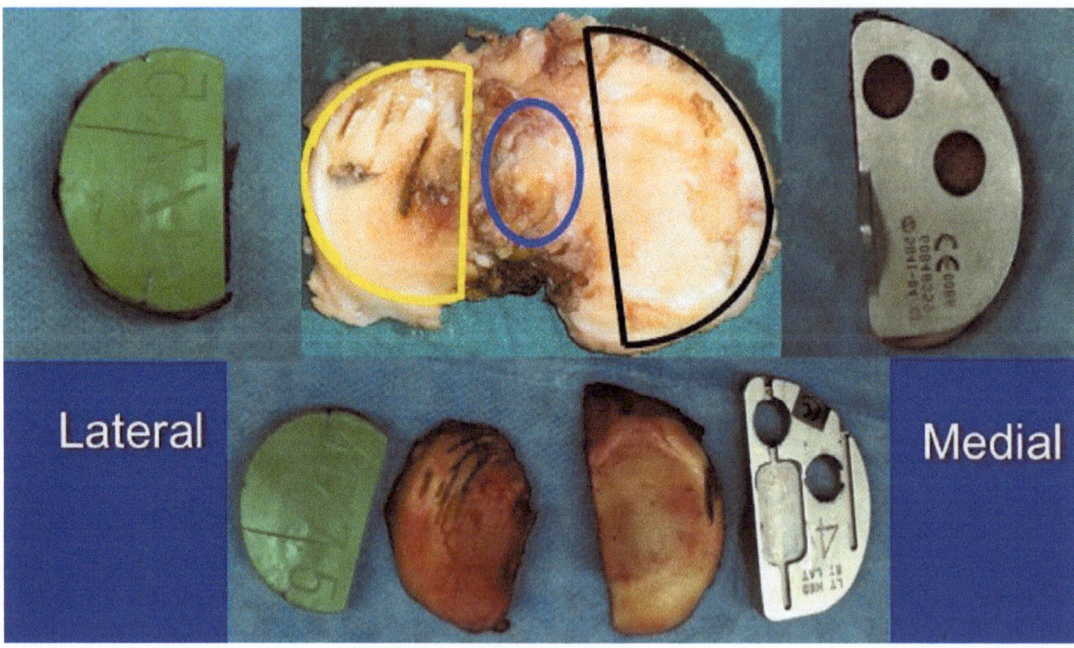

Fig. 9.6 Comparison between the shape of tibial plateau and prosthetic trials

Reconstruction also can be performed in well-selected young patients in whom the only contraindication is ACL deficiency. Our first such patient was operated on in 1996 (Fig. 9.7) [5]. ACL reconstruction was done in an arthrotomy with the patellar tendon. Currently, we prefer an initial arthroscopic step in which the indication is tested, after which the bone tunnel is prepared. Once the graft is positioned, it is fixed to the femur and the bi-UKR technique is then continued. Tibial fixation with screws or staples is done after cementation (Fig. 9.8) [6].

9.5 Graft Selection

We started our experience in 1996, with the patellar tendon. Since 2001, we have implanted UKR and bi-UKR + ACL as first implants in patients with selective indications. We then switched from the patellar tendon to the hamstrings in order to reduce the risk of complications, particularly the risk of joint stiffness and anterior knee pain, as well as the challenges posed by an eventual patellar implant in case of revision with TKR. The first cases, in 2001, involved an arthrotomy with the hamstrings fixed with Rigidfix at the femur and staples at the tibia. Since 2008, we have used cadaver grafts [7], which has reduced the risk of hematoma and medial and posterior thigh pain. The disadvantages are, in addition to the costs, potential problems with osseo-integration and the transmission of an infectious disease from the graft.

9.6 Biomechanics

The preservation of both cruciate ligaments in unicondylar knee arthroplasty is more likely to confer normal knee mechanics and thus enhanced functional improvements, as shown in our recent study carried out at the Istituto Ortopedico Galeazzi in Milano by Romagnoli and Banks [8]. With both cruciate ligaments preserved, total knee arthroplasty should provide better functional benefits than achieved following arthroplasty, which sacrifices one or both cruciates. We compared knee kinematics in patients with well functioning, cruciate-preserving, medial unicondylar and bi-unicondylar arthroplasties in order to determine whether there were differences in knee motion. Eight consenting patients with seven medial unicondylar and five bi-unicondylar arthroplasties were studied using lateral fluoroscopy during treadmill gait, stair climbing, and maximum flexion activities. Custom computed tomography and CAD based models of each knee were used for shape matching to determine the 3D kinematics of the medial unicondylar vs. the bi-unicondylar group (Fig. 9.9).

Maximum flexion in kneeling was 135° ± 14° for unicondylar knees and 123° ± 14° for bi-unicondylar knees ($p = 0.22$). For 0–30° flexion during stair climbing, the medial condyle translated posteriorly 3.5 ± 2.5 mm in unicondylar knees and 4.7 ± 1.9 mm in bi-unicondylar knees ($p > 0.05$). Lateral posterior translation was 5.0 ± 2.3mm in bi-unicondylar knees for 0–30° flexion. For the medial condyle, posterior translation was 1.5 ± 1.6 mm while for bi-unicondylar knees it was 5.1 ± 2.2 mm ($p << 0.05$). Posterior lateral condylar translation in the bi-unicondylar knees was 3.8 ± 3.4 mm (Fig. 9.10).

Retaining both cruciate ligaments in a resurfacing knee arthroplasty appears to maintain the essential features of normal knee motion: femoral rollback and tibial internal rotation with flexion. There were no differences in medial kinematics during stair climbing, indicating similar knee function for the unicondylar and bi-unicondylar groups. The close similarity in the pattern and magnitude of medial and lateral condylar translation in the bi-unicondylar knees was surprising and suggested that a larger lateral translation is typical of the cruciate-intact knee. Both condyles moved 5 mm posteriorly on the tibia at heel-strike, indicating a dynamic posterior slide of the femur with impact and weight-bearing. These observations suggest that dynamic stabilizers do not eliminate the envelope of passive laxityof the intact knee caused by external knee loads.

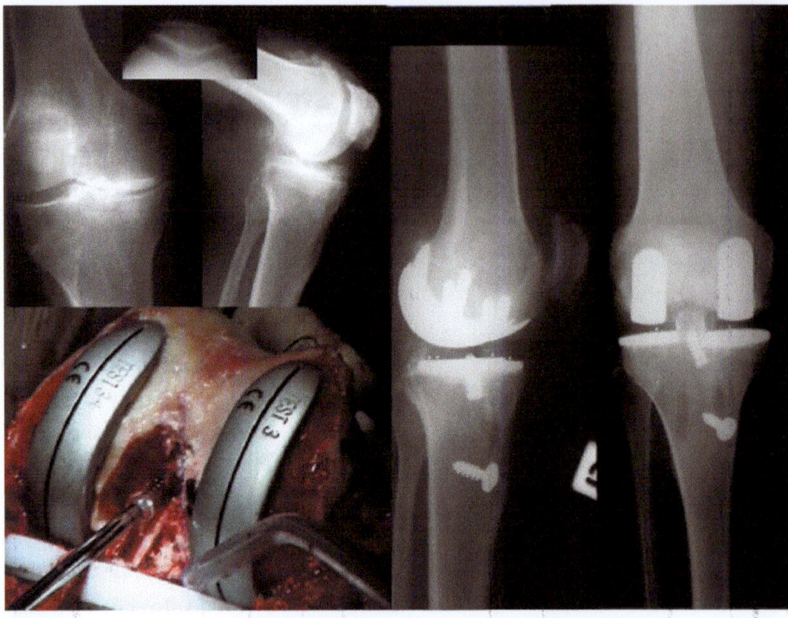

Fig. 9.7 Bi-unicompartmental implant plus ACL reconstruction performed in 1996 with the patellar tendon in a 54-year-old male patient, an ex-professional soccer player

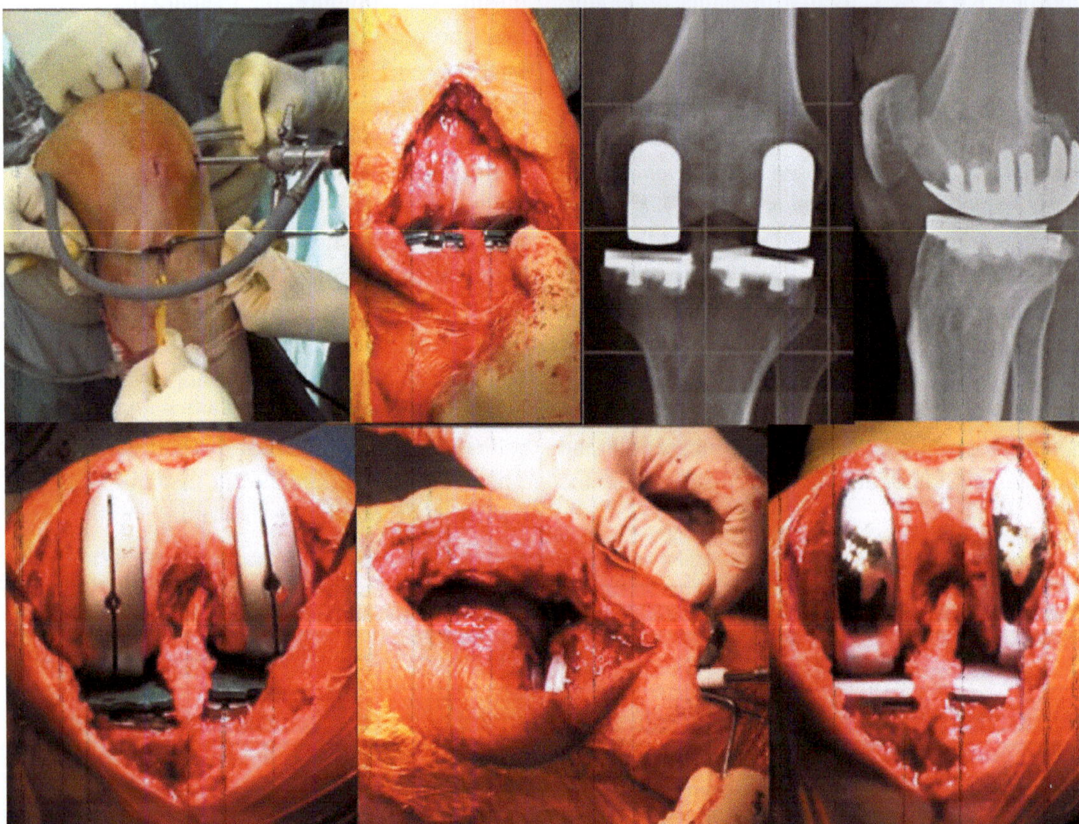

Fig. 9.8 Bi-unicompartmental implant plus contemporary ACL reconstruction: surgical steps

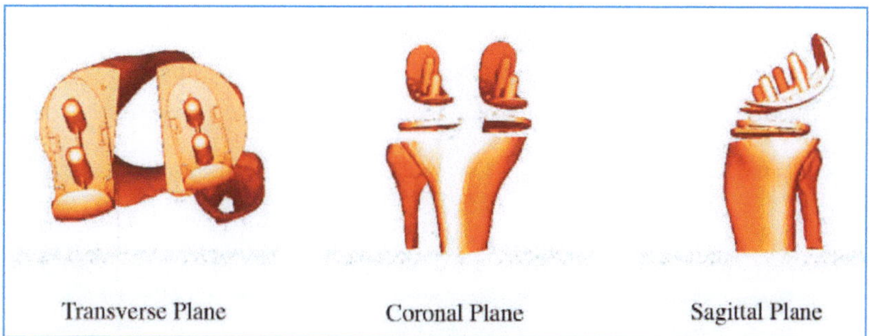

Fig. 9.9 Computed tomography and CAD based models: the knee is in the "neutral" position with respect to the tibial anatomic planes

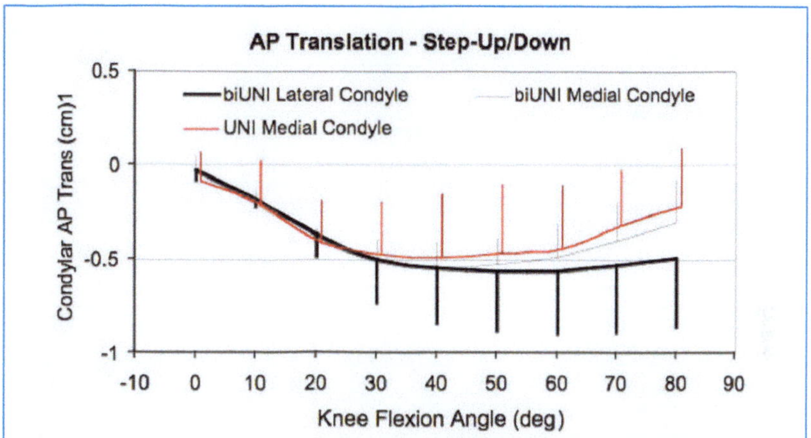

Fig. 9.10 Anteroposterior (AP) condylar translation during step activity in seven unicondylar (UNI) and five bi-unicondylar (biUNI) knees. There were no significant differences in medial translations between UNI and biUNI knees, nor was either medial or lateral translation different in the biUNI knees

9.7 Complications

Causes of failure in this procedure can be intraoperative or postoperative. Intraoperatively, malpositioning of the components, intercondylar eminence fracture, incorrect ligament balance, and cementation mistakes are possible complications during surgery. A tibial eminentia fracture that occurs intraoperatively can be stabilized with two divergent cortical screws, which must be fixed before cementation. Complications following surgery include patellofemoral joint degeneration or secondary ligamentous degeneration-laxity, aseptic component loosening, and polyethylene wear. Septic loosening has the same incidence as in other prosthetic procedures [3-4].

9.8 Patients and Methods

From January 2001 to January 2010, 71 bi-unicompartmental knee arthroplasties were performed by the senior surgeon of our institution in 68 patients, who were followed-up prospectively. The average follow-up was 6 years (maximum 11). The patients were selected based on clinical and radiological symptoms and signs. Clinically, indications for surgery were: knee pain, no femoropatellar joint symptoms, < 10° fixed flexion contracture, and range of motion > 90°. The patients did not have inflammatory arthritis, hemochromatosis, hemophilia, parapatellar tenderness, patellofemoral joint symptoms, or joint instability. The patient population consisted of 41 females and 27 males with an average age at surgery of 67 years (range: 47–81 years). Their average height was 167.3 cm (156–183 cm) and their average weight was 74 kg (53–92 kg) (Fig. 9.11).

One patient was previously treated by high tibial osteotomy (HTO), two had necrosis of both femoral condyles, one had a post-tibial plateau fracture, one had spina bifida, one had poliomyelitis but with good muscle control, and one had an ACL lesion treated with a contemporary reconstruction using a cadaver graft. At surgery, the patients had no more than type I femorotibial involvement and degeneration according to the Ahl-

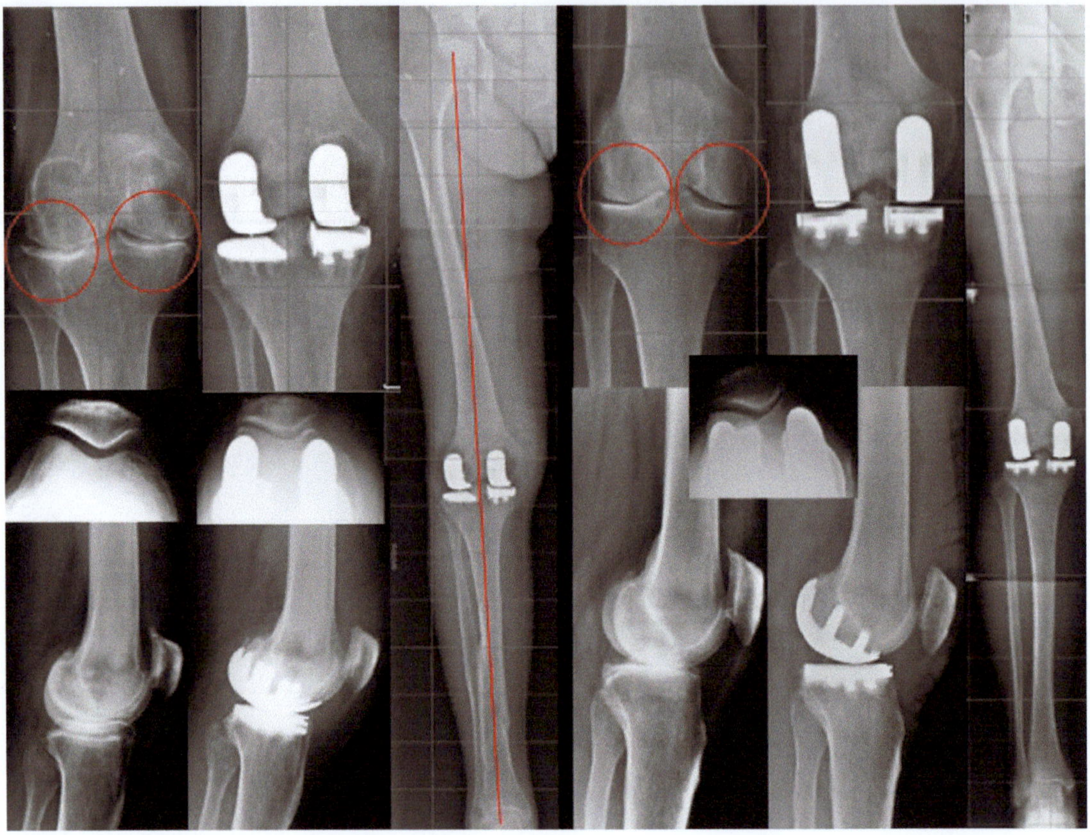

Fig. 9.11 Two cases of bi-unicompartmental implants: *left* a 69-year-old female; *right* a 64-year-old male

back classification. The patients were followed-up yearly for a period of 3 years and then every 2 years. At the most recent follow-up of 71 knees, all 68 patients were evaluated: 65 (68 knees) clinically and radiologically and three only by phone interview as they were not able to visit the clinic. All patients expressed personal satisfaction. Postoperative knee function was evaluated using the Hospital for Special Surgery Knee Score before surgery and at last follow-up. An X-ray was taken for AP weight-bearing, lateral, and patellar skyline views of the knee. Radiographic evaluation included the mechanical and anatomical axes, the cement interface, and the prosthesis-cement interfaces in each of 11 zones, searching for the presence and extent of radiolucencies. These were considered to be progressive if there was either an increase in size or the radiolucency had progressed from one zone to an adjacent zone with time. Radiographically, in addition, the opposite compartment and the patellofemoral joint were evaluated Preoperative X-rays served as the baseline for the evaluation of radiographic progression of the patellofemoral joint, which if present was graded on a four-point scale. Grade 1 radiographic change was defined as no measurable joint-space loss but with radiographic changes such as osteophytes. Grade 2 radiographic changes were defined as up to 25% joint space loss. Grade 3 radiographic changes were defined as up to 50% joint-space loss. Grade 4 radiographic changes were defined as > 50% joint-space loss. Kaplan survival analysis was used to assess the long-term results using revision as the end point.

9.9 Results

Clinically, the average preoperative Hospital for Special Surgery Knee Score was 59 points (range: 42–68 points), which postoperatively improved to 92 points (range 70–100 points). The

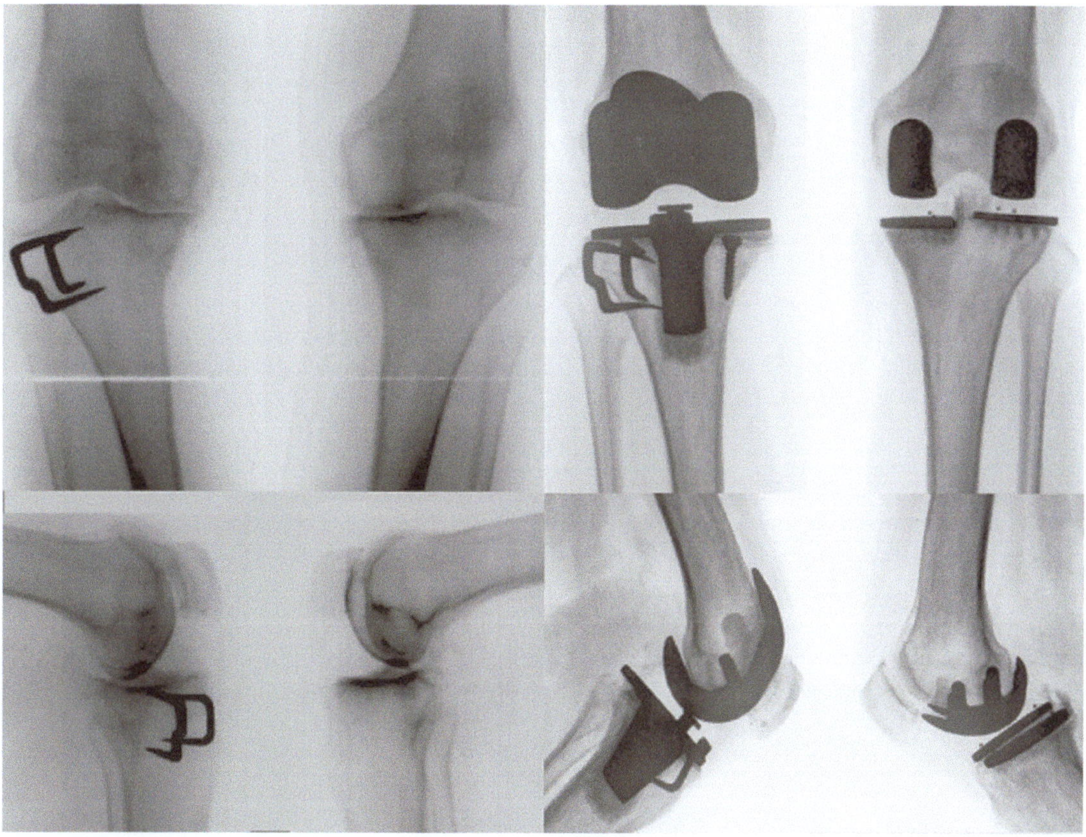

Fig. 9.12 Bilateral implant (Bi-Uni) in a left knee at 16 years of follow-up

average preoperative ROM was 104.7° (range: 80–130°) At the final follow-up, the average ROM was 124.7° (range: 102–136°). In 58 knees, the ROM was > 120°. Sixty-four patients had no pain (94%), while two had slight or occasional pain (3%) (Fig. 9.12).

At the time of the latest follow-up, 64 patients (94%) were enthusiastic regarding the procedure, two patients (3%) were satisfied with the procedure, and in two patients (3%) the procedure failed at 5 and at 5.5 years after surgery.

Radiographically, no component showed evidence of loosening, defined as no change in the position of the components on sequential radiographs. There was no radiographic evidence of osteolysis. The average preoperative deformity ranged from 12° varus to 7° of mechanical axis valgus. The average postoperative alignment was 2,2° of mechanical axis valgus (range: from 3° varus to 2° valgus).

There was no radiographic progression of the patellofemoral joint in 57 knees (80.2%) but 14 knees (19.7%) had grade 2 progression.

There were two revisions (Table 9.1). One, 5 years after surgery, for anterior instability and femoropatellar joint degeneration and the other, 5.5 years after implantation, for continuous anterior knee pain; In the first case, which was probably due to the acquired instability caused by the progressive ACL degeneration, the patient underwent revision because of continuous anterior knee pain. Capsuloligamentous instability was evident as an ACL deficiency; femoropatellar joint degeneration was determined during surgery (Fig. 9.13).

In the second case, rheumatoid arthritis was determined based on a biopsy during revision. In neither case was there component instability or polyethylene wear. No failure was registered among the patients with HTO (n =1), tibial pla-

Table 9.1 Survival of 61 bi-unicompartmental knee replacements

Years since surgery	N. at start	Failure	Width	Lost to FU	N. at risk	Fail %	Succ %	Surv rate	%var	% SE	Cause of failure: rev
0-1	71	0	0	0	71	0.00	100.00	100.00	0.00	0.00	
1-2	71	0	7	0	67.5	0.00	100.00	100.00	0.00	0.00	
2-3	64	0	7	0	60.5	0.00	100.00	100.00	0.00	0.00	
3-4	57	0	10	0	52	0.00	100.00	100.00	0.00	0.00	
4-5	47	1	8	0	43	2.23	97.67	97.67	5.16	2.27	Instability
5-6	38	1	4	0	36	2.78	97.22	94.90	12.77	3.57	Instability
6-7	33	0	7	0	29.5	0.00	100.00	94.90	15.58	3.95	
7-8	26	0	6	0	23	0.00	100.00	94.90	19.98	4.47	
8-9	20	0	9	0	15.5	0.00	100.00	94.90	29.65	5.45	
9-10	11	0	6	0	8	0.00	100.00	94.90	57.45	7.58	
10-11	5	0	5	0	2.5	0.00	100.00	94.90	183.83	13.56	
Total		2	69	0							

FU, follow-up

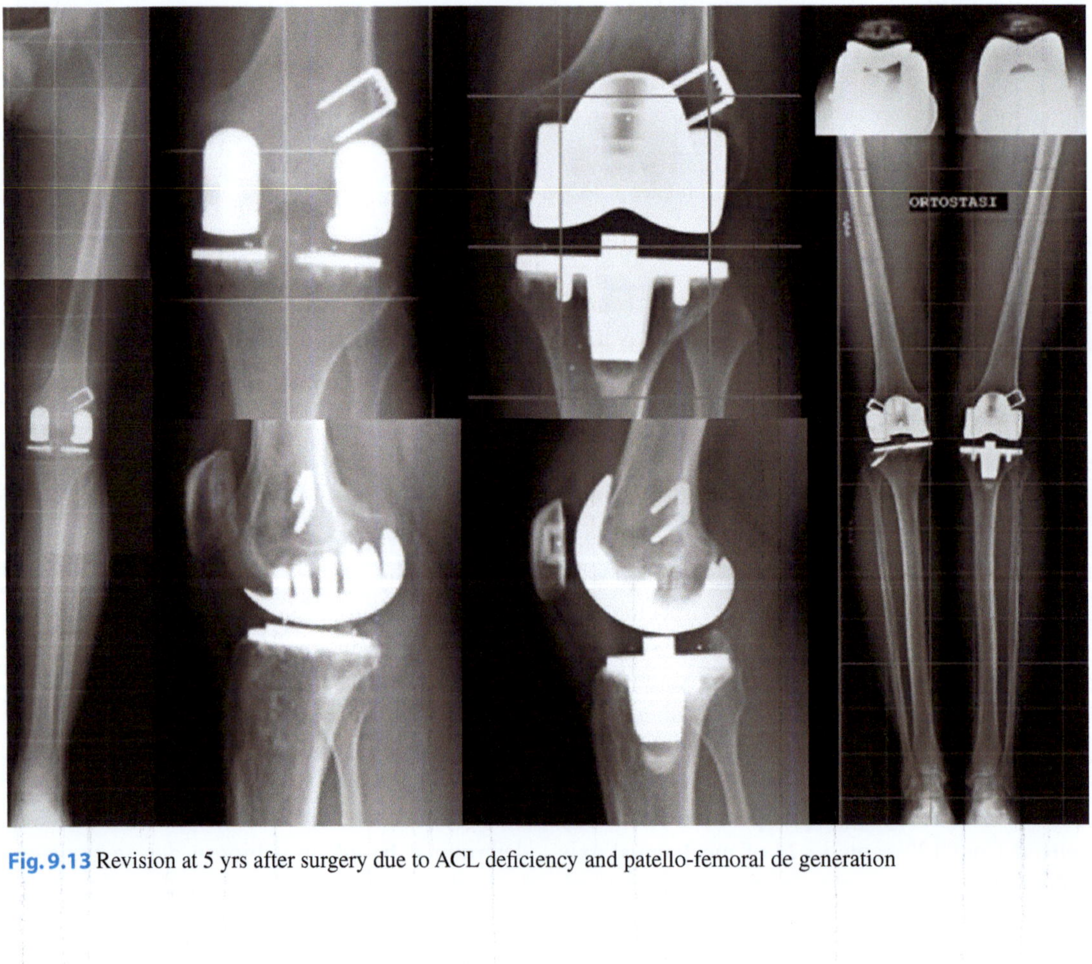

Fig. 9.13 Revision at 5 yrs after surgery due to ACL deficiency and patello-femoral de generation

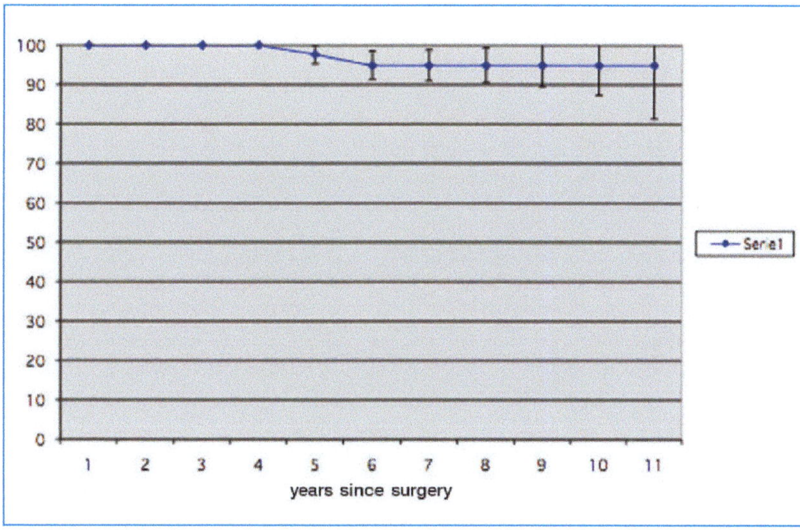

Fig. 9.14 Kaplan-Meier survival curve of bi-unicompartmental knee replacement. See Table 9.1 for details

teau fracture (n =1), femoral condyle necrosis (n = 2), spina bifida (n = 1), poliomyelitis (n = 1), and contemporary ACL reconstruction (n = 1). The cumulative survival rate at 11 years was 94.90% (Table 9.1, Fig. 9.14).

9.10 Conclusions

In attempts to perform truly mini-invasive and tissue-sparing surgery, defined as the preservation or reconstruction of the intact and functional structures of the knee during the implant procedure, Bi-UKR is a possible solution. It is strongly indicated in young, active patients, especially males < 60 years with femorotibial arthritis but an asymptomatic patella and a stable ACL. In these patients, who typically have a high functional demand, this solution allows rapid recovery of daily activity with a very nearly normal gait and a ROM wider than achieved in the best series of TKA. Moreover, the survival curve demonstrates results very similar to those of TKA.

Bicruciate-retaining knee arthroplasty, even if not commonly performed, can provide a high level of function as well as knee kinematics that retain the essential features of the normal knee.

References

1. Romagnoli S, Boniforti F, Cavazzuti G, Castelnuovo N, Verde F (2005) Biomechanik und Arthrose. In: Buckup K (ed) Die unicondylare Schlittenprothese (Unicompartmental Knee Arthroplasty). Steinkopff, Darmstadt
2. Romagnoli S, Verde F, Bibbiani E, Castelnuovo N (2008) La Bimono. G.I.O.T. 34 (suppl. 1)
3. Romagnoli S et al (2007) Bi-uni knee replacement. Basic science, Clinical Repair and reconstruction of articular cartilage defect: current status and prospect. Timeo Editore, Bologna
4. Romagnoli S, Verde F, Bibbiani E et al (2010) Bi-unicompartmental knee prostheses. In: Scuderi GR, Tria AJ (eds) Minimally invasive surgery in orthopaedics. Springer, Heidelberg, pp 327-40
5. Romagnoli S, Camera A, Bertolotti M, Arnaldi E (2000) La protesi Bimonocompartimentale con rispetto ricostruzione del LCA. Il Ginocchio, vol.19
6. Romagnoli S, Verde F, Eberle RW (2006) 10 year minimum follow-up of medial unicompartmental knee arthroplasty with the allegretto prosthesis. JBJS-BR 88-B, Suppl I:100
7. Romagnoli S, Verde F et al (2011) La protesi monocompartimentale con ricostruzione del LCA. In: Confalonieri N (ed) La protesi monocompartimentale del ginocchio. CIC Editore
8. Romagnoli S, Banks SA, Fregly BJ, Boniforti F, Reinschmidt C (2005) Comparing in vivo kinematics of unicondylar and bi-unicondylar knee replacement. Knee Surgery, Sports Traumatology, Arthroscopy. Springer, Berlin

10 Tissue-Sparing Surgery (TSS) and Computer-Assisted Surgery (CAS) in Knee Reconstruction: Bi-Unicompartmental vs Total Knee Arthroplasty

Norberto Confalonieri and Alfonso Manzotti

10.1 Introduction

In the beginning of this century, a new ideal of a renewed, less invasive, reconstructive surgery began to grow in the whole orthopedic world, moving firstly from USA. Likewise, minimally invasive total knee replacement is growing in popularity because of faster recoveries, theoretical reduced blood losses, and reduced economical costs [1–3]. Nevertheless, economical pressures by companies interested in an increasing market have played an important role in developing these new trends. However, less-invasive surgery has been often identified both by surgeons and manufacturers as requiring shorter surgical approaches to implant the same prostheses used with traditional approaches, performing the so called "key-hole surgery" even with new potential risks (malalignment, avulsions, and local wound problems). More recently, different authors recommend caution toward these mini-incision techniques in total joint replacement [4, 5].

In Europe, even before mini-invasive surgery, it was hypothesized that real mini-invasive surgery should not be identified with shorter skin incision but both with a new respect for all the tissues, including the cruciate ligaments, and with a preserved joint kinematics using new tools and smaller implants. This was recently redefined as tissue-sparing surgery [6].

A brave comparison could be done with the philosophical thinking called Humanism, born in Italy in 1400 with thinkers like Cusano, Savonarola, Lorenzo de Medici under the influences of Pitagora, Zenone, Socrates-all ancient Mediterranean philosophers-considering for the first time the human being as the center of all the universe. Similarly, from USA in the beginning of 1900. a "new" ideology named New Humanism invaded Europe to influence the entire century by bringing the same philosophy developed 500 years before.

Even before the mini-invasive age in Europe, unicompartmental knee replacement (UKR) and patellofemoral replacement (PFR) were well-accepted surgical procedures for the treatment of knee arthritis aiming to replace only the damaged compartment and preserving ligaments and maintaining physiological kinematics [7–10]. Recently, even in literature, good results supports this increased popularity among orthopedic surgeons to offer a relatively less-invasive as well as a more physiological approach to the arthritic knee [11–13].

Likewise in Europe, a few surgeons have been experiencing association of different small implants to achieve a genuine patient-customized procedure over several years but with not many reports in the literature regarding long-term results [14–17]. In 2010, Heyse et al. reported 12-year follow-up results of the association of UKR

N. Confalonieri (✉)
Orthopedic, Traumatology and Hand Surgery Department
CTO Hospital
Milan, Italy
E-mail: norberto.confalonieri@icp.mi.it

N. Confalonieri, S. Romagnoli (eds.), *Small Implants in Knee Reconstruction*,
DOI 10.1007/978-88-470-2655-1_10, © Springer-Verlag Italia 2013

+ PFR, reporting both excellent clinical results and patients satisfaction but defining this as a high-demanding procedure [18]. In 2010, Parratte et al. published 17-year follow-up results of both bi-UKRs and UKR + PFR with, respectively, 78% and 54% survivorships [19]. Likewise, all the authors underline how this high-demanding procedure based on a customized approach to knee arthritis should be reserved to selected patients and performed in specifically trained centers [17, 20, 21].

Nevertheless, the entire orthopedic community is looking at these combined implants with an increasing interest. In 2010, Köck et al. published the results of an anonymous survey in 220 departments of orthopedics and 230 departments of trauma surgery, reporting that 43.4% of the surgeons involved believe that bicompartmental arthroplasty in case of additional involvement of the femoropatellar joint could be an attractive option [22].

Computer-assisted surgery has been developed to help surgeon in reconstructive procedures improve implant alignment and performance. In the literature, different authors have already demonstrated its efficacy in traditional knee replacement surgery despite different systems available, achieving better aligned implants despite longer surgical time [23–26].

Nevertheless, very few studies have analyzed the application of navigation in small implants, mainly in UKR, demonstrating results similar to TKR only with a superior final implant alignment even in these implants [27–30].

Computer/robotic-assisted surgery could offer further advantages in highly demanding surgeries: it could help surgeons in achieving a restored joint line and slope, and the surgeons is always aware about the amount of bone cuts, even according to the limb alignment and soft tissue balancing, and this could be more evident in performing small implants [30, 31].

On the basis of their positive experience in computer-assisted (CAS) TKR with more than 1,000 implants with the adoption of new improved dedicated software, the authors explored even these bicompartmental implants (bi-UKR and UKR + PFR) to reproduce more easily this highly demanding surgery [30]. Since 1988, they implanted >900 UKRs using almost all the designs available: bi-UKR since 1998, UKR + PFR since 2005, and since 2007 UKR + PFR using a monobloc femoral shield, with an experience of >200 combined implants. Furthermore, in 2003, they adopted navigation to improve the accuracy and to make reproducible the surgical technique and, more recently, even patient-specific instrumentation even more useful than in TKR.

In this chapter, the authors present their experiences together their own interpretation of less invasive surgery in knee reconstruction using an analysis of these "customized implants," their performance, and the potential advantages of their association to CAS.

10.2 Bi-Unicompartmental Knee Replacement

Bicruciate ligament retention in TKR has been evaluated since the earliest nonhinged implants in the late 1960s. In gait studies by Andriacchi et al. the knees in which both cruciate ligaments were retained were the only arthroplasty that had normal flexion [9]. As well, Stiehl et al. demonstrated that bicruciate-retaining TKR typically experienced a physiological posterior femoral rollback during a deep knee bend with a limited anterior–posterior translation and remained posterior to the mid-sagittal line in all positions [32].

Despite all these biomechanical studies, the first results reported in the literature were quite poor with the first designs, with higher rates of failure with respect to the traditional implants. Lewallen et al. reported in a 10-year follow-up study of polycentric TKR only 66% survivorship [16]. Likewise, Morrison et al. recently reported early adverse results in a 2-year compared to TKR prospective study but showing better early stiffness [21]. However more recently, new designs with modified surgical techniques have been introduced. Cloutier et al. in 1991 reported a 96% success rate in a 9- to 11-year follow-up study with bicruciate-retaining implants [33].

A few surgeons around the world have been using an even less invasive implant than the above-mentioned bicruciate-retaining TKR for several years using two UKRs to address the two tibiofemoral compartments simultaneously. The benefits of this approach when compared to TKR include greater tissue sparing, reduced surgical morbidity, and easier revision surgery. In addition, a recent study has demonstrated that bi-UKR more closely resembles the biomechanics of an intact knee than does a TKR [7–9]. Fuchs et al. reported that implants preserving both cruciate ligaments can achieve functional results at least similar to TKR without any arthritis progression [8]. Current patient's expectations following knee replacement surgery include a knee that resembles normal and allows an unrestricted active life, and the superior biomechanical resemblance of the bi-UKR to a normal knee might better match these expectations.

10.2.1 Surgical Technique for Computer-Assisted Bi-UKR

Since 2001, in our department, different systems based on computer-assisted navigation systems without use of computed tomography (CT) have been used in >1,000 joint replacements (knee and hip), and according to these navigation systems, all data have been acquired in the operating theater during the procedures. We consider the procedure as two different unicompartmental replacements. We repair first the most damaged compartment, usually medial in varus and lateral in valgus.

Step 1: Prepare the surgical field according to your preferences. However, the patient should be in supine position just with the feet outside allowing the knee to be easily flexed at 90°. Place a support by the side of the thigh to maintain lower limb position even with the knee flexed. The surgeon is supposed to be in front of the patient and able to check the mechanical axis constantly.

Step 2: We always position a metal locator in the center of the hip as further limb alignment reference during the surgery in order to keep a constant check on axial adjustment and on the correct positioning of the prosthetic femoral component (an X-ray of the hip should give you the position of the metal locator).

Step 3: With the patient under anesthesia, the surgeon should evaluate clinically the limb deformity and how much can be reduced manually acting on the knee.

Step 4: The skin incision with the limb flexed at 90° should not exceed 12–14 cm in a median or paramedian medial direction. The patella should be only retracted and not dislocated.

Step 5: First approach the most damaged compartment, remove the meniscus but leaving its posterior wall intact. We consider two different implants (medial first in varus and lateral first in valgus) with two different slopes, tibial cuts, and joint spaces (Fig. 10.1).

Step 6: Insert the screws for the infrared-reflecting diodes (LED) of the computer scanner with tiny skin incision of <1 cm. One diode should be located on the femur and one on the tibia both 10 cm away from the joint line. A third diode will be applied to the foot, clipping it to an external metal support fixed by an elastic band. Proceed with the lower limb data acquisition using the computer. Just moving the limb and using mathematical models, the navigator determines the axis, which goes through the rotation center of the femoral head, the center of the knee and ankle. Acquire the deepest point in the more damaged tibial plateau with a mobile pointer, then the deepest point of other tibial compartments, the centre of the tibial plateau, both posterior femoral condyles, the superior femoral cortex, and medial and lateral epicondyles, always according to the indications on the screen step by step (Fig. 10.2).

Step 7: With the data reported on the screen, the surgeon can recalculate with numbers the deformity and how much can be corrected. Data processing empowers the system to produce on-screen information related to the mechanical function in frontal and lateral projection within the entire given range of movement. It suggests

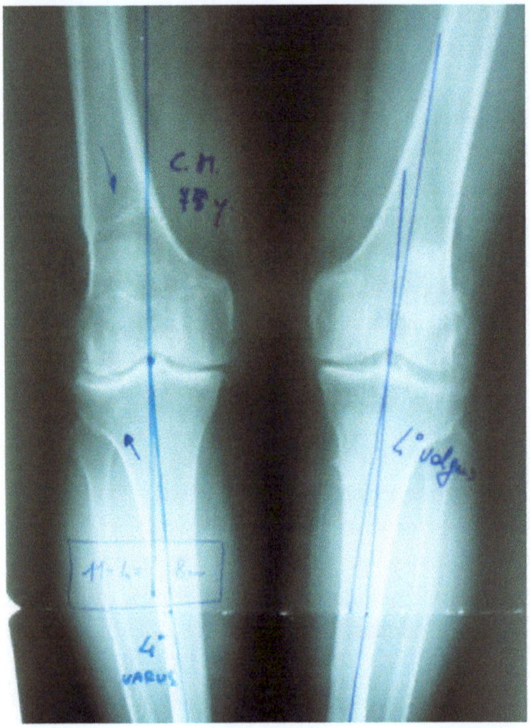

Fig. 10.1 Active woman golfer with posttraumatic right knee arthritis

implant size, amount of bone according to the deformity, and tridimensional implant alignment.

Step 8: The deformity should always be reducible manually; otherwise, the surgeon should proceed with a slight release of the ligaments under the direct control of the system.

Step 9: Position the tibial cut guide and connect with a mobile diode to the computer. The height of the resection is based on preoperation planning calculations, its orientation (varus–valgus), guided and checked on the display. The slope will be almost normal, about 5°, even according to the implant slope. Considering that in knees with an intact anterior cruciate ligament (ACL) the articular space is reduced in flexion, the surgeon should always consider that both slope and posterior resection could act on this value. After fixing the guide, use an oscillating horizontal blade for the vertical cut, near the ACL insertion point, moving in an anterior–posterior direction. Then change to a "lamellate" blade for the horizontal bone cut.

Step 10: After the removal of the bone block, insert the tibial trial component. The size of the component should be equal to the amount of resected bone, and the height depends on the deviation axis correction either in flexion or in extension. The computer permits checking for correct alignment during the entire range of motion. With the knee in full extension, mark the front edge of the tibial trial component on the femoral condyle to check the size of the femoral component.

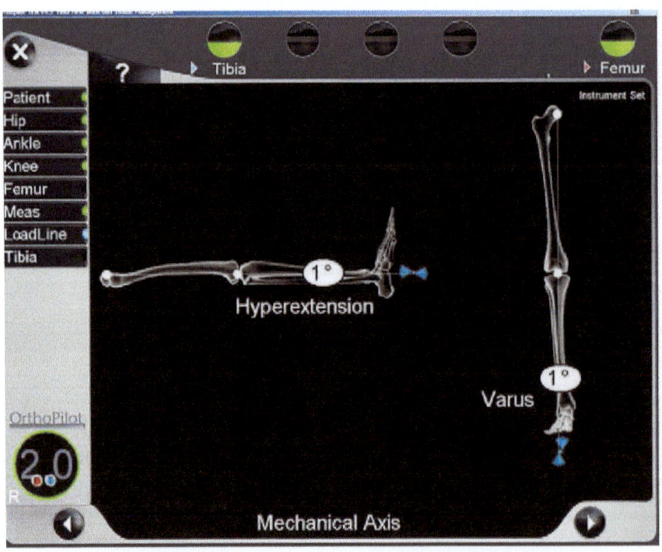

Fig. 10.2 Computer feedback of mechanical axis and arthritis deformity

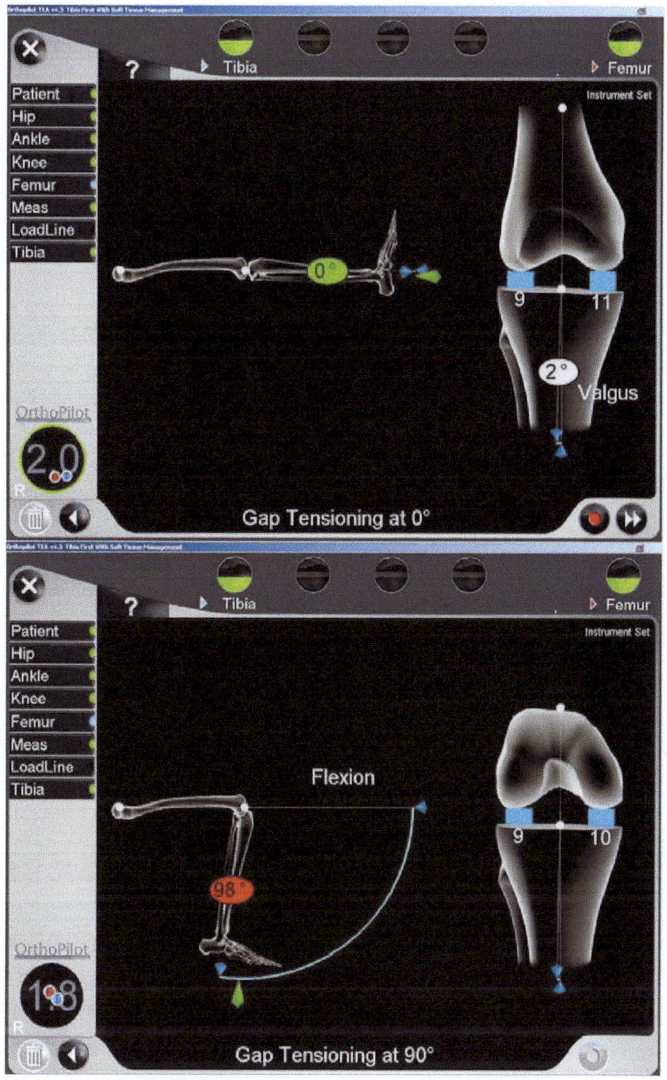

Fig. 10.3 Joint spaces in flexion and extension in medial and lateral compartments

Step 11: A dedicated cutting guide is used for the femoral side. It must be positioned parallel to the tibial component and perpendicular to the mechanical femoral axis just to achieve the largest contact surface between the components for the whole knee range of motion. Remove the femoral–condylar cartilage, and prepare the holes for the pegs of the femoral implant.

Step 12: Position the trial components, check the mechanical axis and the ligament balance, always reading the values and the morphology of the inferior limb in motion on the computer screen.

Step 13: Restore a correct limb alignment without ligament tension. The opposite femorotibial compartment should be approached under the control of the navigation system. Choose the height of the cut on the basis of space (in terms of flexion and extension). In any case, it must be <11 mm (prosthesis thickness – deviation angle – articular space = minimum cut). The latest version of our navigation system provides distractors which tense the ligaments and open the articular space according to values expressed in millimeters. This is particularly helpful in flexion where the joint space is reduced, and we have to act both upon the posterior slope and the osseous resection of the posterior femoral condyle (Fig. 10.3).

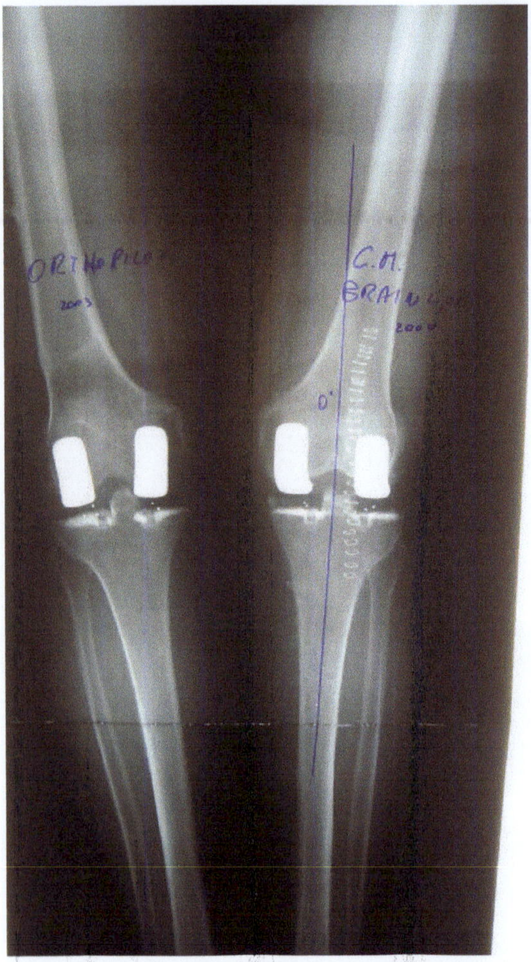

Fig. 10.4 Same patient as in Fig. 10.1: 2 years later, she chose the same implant for the left knee

Step 14: Position the femoral trial components and decide on the definitive tibial thickness and base you decision on the optimal ligament balance in terms of extension and flexion and the mechanical axis close to 180°, without procurvation or recurvation. Everything is shown on the computer in numeric values and visualized by a scheme of the inferior limb.

Step 15: We first implant the two tibial components and then the femoral ones; the limb should be extended and compressed securely against the chest of the operator to complete the operation. Final recording of data is performed for the personal computerized patient file charts (Fig. 10.4).

10.2.2 Our Experience with Bi-UKRs

We have been performing bi-UKRs since 1999 in highly selected cases (<5% of our volume of knee replacement per year). Our approach involved an approximately 12- to 13-cm midpatellar skin incision with a single anteromedial arthrotomy and lateral patella retraction. In all cases, the medial UKR was performed first. This allowed for correct realignment of the limb by replacing the most severely diseased compartment. The amount of bone to be resected from the medial compartment of the tibia necessary to correct the limb alignment was determined preoperatively. This calculation was based on the amount of axial deformity and the thickness of the implanted components. The minimum tibial bone cut was given by the difference between the prosthesis thickness and the axial deviation angle [6]. For example, if a patient had a varus deformity of 8° and the prosthesis being used had a thickness of 11 mm, the planned minimum medial tibial bone to be resected would be approximately 3 mm. Using this technique, the amount of bone to be resected from the lateral compartment corresponds to the thickness of the implant. In 2006, we reviewed, at a minimum follow-up of 3 years (mean: 57.8 months), our experience with these implants in 23 patients enrolled prospectively for a bi-UKR [17]. Preoperatively, patients were evaluated with both the Western Ontario and McMaster Osteoarthritis Index (WOMAC) and the Knee Society score. At latest follow-up, the mean WOMAC score was 1.9 for pain, 0.6 for stiffness, and 4.8 for function. The mean Knee Society score was 84.6, a mean functional score of 86.3 was recorded, and a mean UKR dedicated outcome score [Italian Orthopedic UKR Users Group (GIUM)] was 78.1 with no abnormal results. All the patients were satisfied with the outcome and would undergo the same procedure again. No implant has required revision. The most common complication occurred intraoperatively. In three cases (12.5%) an intraoperative fracture of the tibial spines occurred during implantation of the prosthesis, possibly related to excessive tension on the ACL. All fractures were managed successfully with intraoperative internal fixation. This fracture did not adversely affect the final result. In an attempt to overcome this complication, a more precise computer-assisted technique for bi-UKR has been introduced since 2003 [30] to achieve a well-balanced implant both in extension and flexion and with no tension on the ACL tibial insertion.

10.3 Patellofemoral and Unicompartmental Replacement

The association of a unicompartmental with a patellofemoral implant is one of the hottest topics today [18–20]. Likewise for bi-UKRs leaving intact the ACL and treating simultaneously the worn patellofemoral and one of the tibiofemoral compartments may be an attractive option for the modern knee surgeon. A minimally invasive surgical technique is well suited for this procedure and allows for a quicker recovery when compared with TKR [20]. Treatment specifically targeted at the pathologic compartments without loss of normal bone and ligaments results in a rapid return to normal activity, increased stability, and decreased pain. Even for this association, the objective is to extend indications for unicompartmental techniques in knees with an intact ACL to preserve the normal knee biomechanics.

10.3.1 Surgical Technique for Computer-Assisted UKR + PFR

The surgical approach starts with an anteromedial or anterolateral parapatellar approach according to the tibiofemoral compartment to be addressed. The damaged tibiofemoral compartment is the first to be replaced, correcting the axis deformity using both the bone cut and a tibial component height to restore a mechanical axis close to 180° (e.g., 11° of varus deformity can be corrected with 3 mm of bone cut associated with 8 mm tibial component height) . Likewise, a correct limb alignment permits a better patellofemoral kinematic with reduce patellar tilt. Attention should be paid to the selection of the femoral condyle component size to avoid a potential conflict between this component and the femoral component in the trochlea groove. Leaving the trial component in situ in the tibiofemoral compartment, subsequently the surgeon addresses the patellofemoral joint dislocating the patella. The femoral trochlea is resurfaced, looking carefully at the size and rotation following an accurate osteophytes removal.

Patellar resurfacing is always performed using an alloy component of the correct size and always reducing patellar width and in some cases in association to release of the retinaculum to improve patellar tracking. In the latter case, the authors did not perform any patellar replacement but limited the procedure to a complete and accurate osteophyte removal associated with a circumferential cauterization. Both components were implanted with cement. Dedicated software for UKR and PFR implantation in association can improve the surgical technique. Likewise, it is possible as in TKR to know limb alignment, bone cuts, patella tracking, and tilting during the entire surgery, greatly helping the surgeon to reconstruct a more "physiological" joint.

10.3.2 Our Experience with PFR and UKR

Our experience is limited to 54 cases. We reviewed 21 cases (Acuris + Journey, Smith & Nephew, Memphis, TN, USA), all performed in the last 2 years using a computer-assisted technique to assess the patella tracking, supposing that this bicompartmental implant could achieve comparable results. Fourteen anteromedial and seven anterolateral implants in 21 patients were prospectively involved in the study. All knees were stable and underwent selective reconstruction simultaneously using UKR and PFR.

All bicompartmental implants were performed by the same surgeon. Surgical time, hospital stay, and all intra- and post-operative complications were registered. At a minimum follow-up of 20 months, every single case was matched to a similar case where a cruciate-retaining TKR had been implanted. In both surgical procedures, computer assistance was used (Vector Vision, BrianLAB, Munich, Germany). Criteria of matching were: sex, age, preoperative range of motion, and arthritis grade. In both the groups all the cases were assessed clinically using WOMAC, Korean Knee Score (KKS), and GIUM. All the knees were radiologically investigated using the same radiological protocol. Patella were resurfaced in the first ten and just decauterizied in the last cases. Intraoperatively, the authors did not registered any complication. There was no revision in either group. The mean surgical time was 86 min (range: 78–121) in UKR + PFR group and 81 min (range: 71–112) in TKR-CAS group. There were no statistical significant differences in the hospital stay. No statistically significant differences were seen for the Knee Society, Functional, and GIUM scores between the two groups. Statistically significantly better WOMAC Function/Stiffness indexes were registered for the UKR + PFR group. TKR implants achieved statistically better aligned mechanical axes.

10.4 UKR + PFR Using a Monobloc Femoral Shield

In 2007, a revolutionary bicompartmental design was proposed specifically to address the joint involvement of these patients with a monolithic device that resurfaces both the medial and the patellofemoral compartments aiming to reduce the femoral components to a whole element while preserving both the lateral bone/cartilage areas and cruciate ligaments. Up to now, there are only two short-term follow-up studies reported in the literature (respectively, 95 and 36 cases) with this unique new implant [34, 35]. Engh et al. reported no revision, with a high level of satisfaction following this implant [34]. Palumbo et al. reported a unacceptable short-term survivorship and discouraged its adoption [36]. Obviously, longer follow-up and major prospective studies are needed to assess its efficacy in selective treatment of knee arthritis

10.4.1 Our Experience with UKR + PFR Using a Monobloc Femoral Shield

Our experience of this implant (Deuce, Smith and Nephew, Memphis, TN, USA) is limited to 21 cases in 20 patients all performed by two surgeons of our department in the last 4 years. Up to now, no navigation system is available on the market to help the surgeon during the surgery, and all our cases were implanted using a short intramedullary guide for the femoral component and an extramedullary guide for the tibia.

At a minimum follow-up of 18 months, even for this specific dedicated anteromedial ACL-sparing implant, the authors performed a short-term prospective study matching every single case to a similar TKR group implanted for isolated anteromedial bicompartmental knee arthritis. In the first nine cases, the patellar was resurfaced and was decauterized in all the other cases. Criteria of matching (sex, age, preoperative range of motion and arthritis grade) and parameters assessed (surgical time, hospital stay and all intra- and postoperative complications) were the same used for the UKR + PFR study. Likewise, all the cases were assessed clinically using WOMAC, KKS, and GIUM and radiologically investigated using the same radiological protocol. Even for this new implant, we did not register any complication. One Deuce case at 7 weeks postoperatively underwent a closed manipulation under anesthesia because of insufficient flexion (95°). One implant was revised in another hospital because of unclear pain without signs of loosing or sepsis and without any significant improvement after the revision.

The mean surgical time was 64 min (range: 48–104) in Deuce group and 74 min (range: 59–110) in TKR. There were no statistically significant differences in the hospital stay. No statistically significant difference was seen for the Knee Society and GIUM scores between the two groups. Statistically significantly better Functional score and WOMAC Function/Stiffness indexes were registered for the Deuce group. Even in this study, computer assistance permitted a statistically better aligned mechanical axis in the TKR group.

However, the results of these two short-term prospective studies suggest that both the association of UKR + PFR and a dedicated anteromedial implant are viable options for arthritis involving simultaneously a tibiofemoral and patellar femoral joint at least as well as TKR but maintaining an higher level of function.

10.5 Conclusions

The shifting demographics of patients with localized knee arthritis, including younger, more active patients, is a major impetus for growing interest in conservative surgical alternatives such as UKR, PFR and their association [20, 21]. Even our arthritis localizations is moving toward more localized scenarios often following surgical procedures like meniscectomized ligament reconstructions in highly motivated patients.

The role of minimally invasive techniques for the treatment of knee arthritis continues to evolve toward a concept of tissue-sparing surgery [6]. The first enthusiasm toward shorter surgical approaches has been mitigated by nonpermanent advantages together with new complications, and the surgeon cannot announce a new mini-invasive approach just because a of a shorter incision to implant the same prostheses and sacrificing ligaments.

Small implants and preserved joint biomechanics could represent a new development in reconstructive surgery, and the approach described in this chapter could be a very attractive approach [6–8]. Using computer assistance may help the surgeon in reproducing this highly demanding surgery in a standardized technique. The authors strongly believe that this "personalized at the time treatment" for each patient according to severity of the disease using different implant option in association with computer assistance could be one of the newest and most interesting improvements in the following years.

References

1. Haas SB, Cook S, Beksac B (2004) Minimally invasive total knee replacement through a mini midvastus approach: a comparative study. Clin Orthop Relat Res 428:8-73
2. Laskin RS (2005) Minimally invasive total knee arthroplasty: the results justify its use. Clin Orthop Relat Res 440:54-9
3. Lonner JH (2006) Minimally invasive approaches to total knee arthroplasty: results. Am J Orthop 35 (7 Suppl):27-33
4. Berend KR, Lombardi AV Jr (2005) Avoiding the potential pitfalls of minimally invasive total knee surgery. Orthopedics 28(11):1326-30
5. Dalury DF, Dennis DA (2005) Mini-incision total knee arthroplasty can increase risk of component malalignment. Clin Orthop Rel Res 440:77-81
6. Confalonieri N, Manzotti A (2006) Tissue-sparing surgery with the bi-unicompartmental knee prosthesis: retrospective study with minimum follow-up of 36 months J Orthopaed Traumatol 7:108–112
7. Banks SA, Frely BJ, Boniforti F, Reischmidt C, Romagnoli S (2005) Comparing in vivo kinematics of unicondylar and bi-unicondylar knee replacement. Knee Surg Sports Traumatol Arthrosc 13:551-6
8. Fuchs S, Tibesku CO, Frisse D, Genkinger m, Laaß H, Rosenbaum D (2005) Clinical and functional of uni-and bicondylar sledge prostheses. Knee Surg Sports Traumatol Arthrosc 13:197-202
9. Andriacchi TP, Andersson GB, Fermier RW, Stern D, Galante JO (1980) A study of lower-limb mechanics during stair-climbing. J Bone Joint Surg Am 62(5):749-57
10. Weale AE, Halabi OA, Jones PW, White SH (2001) Perceptions of out-comes after unicompartmental and total knee replacements. Clin Orthop 382:143-153
11. Eickmann TH, Collier MB, Sukezaki F, McAuley JP, Engh GA (2006) Survival of medial unicondylar arthroplasties placed by one surgeon 1984-1998. Clin Orthop Relat Res 17:167-175
12. O'Rourke MR, Gardner JJ, Callaghan JJ, Liu SS, Goetz DD, Vittetoe DA, Sullivan PM, Johnston RC (2005) The John Insall Award: unicompartmental knee replacement: a minimum twenty-one-year followup, end-result study. Clin Orthop Relat Res 440:27-37
13. Swienckowski JJ, Pennington DW (2004) Unicompartmental knee arthroplasty in patients sixty years of age or younger. J Bone Joint Surg 86-A Suppl 1(Pt 2):131-42
14. Swanson AB, Swanson GD, Powers T, Khalil MA, Maupin BK, Mayhew DE, Moss SH (1985) Unicompartmental and bicompartmental arthroplasty of the knee with a finned metal tibial-plateau implant. J Bone Joint Surg Am 67(8):1175-82
15. Goodfellow JW, O'Connor J (1986) Clinical results

of the Oxford knee. Surface arthroplasty of the tibiofemoral joint with a meniscal bearing prosthesis. Clin Orthop Relat Res 205:21-42
16. Lewallen DG, Bryan RS, Peterson LF (1984) Polycentric total knee arthroplasty. A ten-year follow-up study. J Bone Joint Surg Am 66(8):1211-8
17. Confalonieri N, Manzotti A, Cerveri P, De Momi E (2009) Bi-unicompartmental versus total knee arthroplasty: a matched paired study with early clinical results. Arch Orthop Trauma Surg 129(9):1157-63
18. Heyse TJ, Khefacha A, Cartier P (2010) UKA in combination with PFR at average 12-year follow-up. Arch Orthop Trauma Surg 130(10):1227-30
19. Parratte S, Pauly V, Aubaniac JM, Argenson JN (2010) Survival of bicompartmental knee arthroplasty at 5 to 23 years. Clin Orthop Relat Res 468(1):64-72
20. Tria AJ Jr (2010) Bicompartmental arthroplasty of the knee.Instr Course Lect 59:61-73
21. Morrison TA, Nyce JD, Macaulay WB, Geller JA (2011) Early adverse results with bicompartmental knee arthroplasty a prospective cohort comparison to total knee arthroplasty. J Arthroplasty 26(6 Suppl):35-9
22. Köck FX, Weingärtner D, Beckmann J, Anders S, Schaumburger J, Grifka J, Lüring C (2011) Operative treatment of the unicompartmental knee arthritis - results of a nationwide survey in 2008. Z Orthop Unfall 149(2):153-9
23. Huang TW, Hsu WH, Peng KT, Wen-Wei Hsu R, Weng YJ, Shen WJ (2011) Total knee arthroplasty with use of computer-assisted navigation compared with conventional guiding systems in the same patient: radiographic results in asian patients. J Bone Joint Surg Am 93(13):1197-202
24. Zhang GQ, Chen JY, Chai W, Liu M, Wang Y (2011) Comparison between computer-assisted-navigation and conventional total knee arthroplasties in patients undergoing simultaneous bilateral procedures: a randomized clinical trial. J Bone Joint Surg Am 93(13):1190-6
25. Khan MM, Khan MW, Al-Harbi HH, Weening BS, Zalzal PK (2011) Assessing short-term functional outcomes and knee alignment of computer-assisted navigated total knee arthroplasty. J Arthroplasty [Epub ahead of print]
26. Pang HN, Yeo SJ, Chong HC, Chin PL, Ong J, Lo NN (2011) Computer-assisted gap balancing technique improves outcome in total knee arthroplasty, compared with conventional measured resection technique. Knee Surg Sports Traumatol Arthrosc 19(9):1496-503
27. Konyves A, Willis-Owen CA, Spriggins AJ (2010) The long-term benefit of computer-assisted surgical navigation in unicompartmental knee arthroplasty. J Orthop Surg Res 31:94
28. Jung KA, Kim SJ, Lee SC, Hwang SH, Ahn NK (2010) Accuracy of implantation during computer-assisted minimally invasive Oxford unicompartmental knee arthroplasty: a comparison with a conventional instrumented technique. Knee 17(6):387-91
29. Jenny JY (2005) Navigated unicompartmental knee replacement. Orthopedics 28 (10 Suppl): s1263-7
30. Confalonieri N, Manzotti A (2005) Computer Assisted bi-unicompartimental knee replacement. Int J Medical Robotics and Computer Assisted Surgery 1(4):1-6
31. Lonner JH (2009) Modular bicompartmental knee arthroplasty with robotic arm assistance. Am J Orthop (Belle Mead NJ) 38(2 Suppl):28-3
32. Stiehl JB, Komistek RD, Cloutier JM, Dennis DA (2000) The cruciate ligaments in total knee arthroplasty: a kinematic analysis of 2 total knee arthroplasties. J Arthroplasty 15(5):545-50
33. Cloutier JM, Sabouret P, Deghrar A (1999) Total knee arthroplasty with retention of both cruciate ligaments. A nine to eleven-year follow-up study. J Bone Joint Surg Am 81(5):697-702
34. Engh GA (2007) A bicompartimental solution: what the Deuce? Orthopedics 30:770
35. Rolston L, Bresh J, Engh GA, Alois F, Kreuzer S, Nadaudad M, Puri L, Wood D (2007) Bicompartimental knee arthroplasty: a bone-sparing, ligament sparing, and minimally invasive alternative for active patients. Orthopedics 30(8 Suppl):70-3
36. Palumbo BT, Henderson ER, Edwards PK, Burris RB, Gutiérrez S, Raterman SJ (2011) Initial experience of the journey-deuce bicompartmental knee prosthesis a review of 36 cases. J Arthroplasty 26(6 Suppl):40-5

Bicompartmental Prosthesis

11

Sergio Romagnoli, Francesco Verde, Michele Corbella, and Sara Zacchetti

11.1 Introduction

In the last few years, on the basis of the excellent long-term results achieved with unicompartmental knee replacement (UKR), there is growing interest in single or combined compartmental substitutions of the knee while preserving the anterior cruciate ligament (ACL) [1] (Fig. 11.1). This kind of prosthesis is consistent with tissue-sparing surgery (TSS), the aim of which is to reduce local and general surgical aggression and thereby to optimize the patient's postoperative course and functional recovery.

Today, the term "bicompartmental" refers to a surgical procedure that replaces one of the tibiofemoral compartments in association with the patellofemoral compartment while respecting

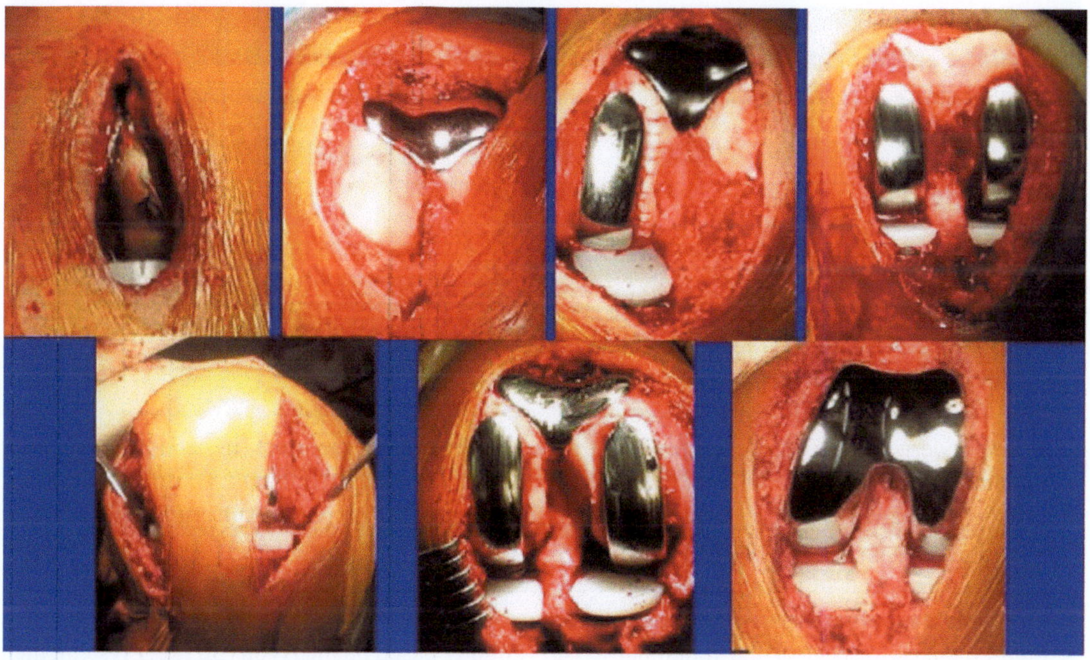

Fig. 11.1 Pre total knee replacement implants: 27 years of experience (1985–2012)

S. Romagnoli (✉)
Galeazzi Orthopedic Institute
Milan, Italy
E-mail: sergio.romagnoli@libero.it

N. Confalonieri, S. Romagnoli (eds.), *Small Implants in Knee Reconstruction*,
DOI 10.1007/978-88-470-2655-1_11, © Springer-Verlag Italia 2013

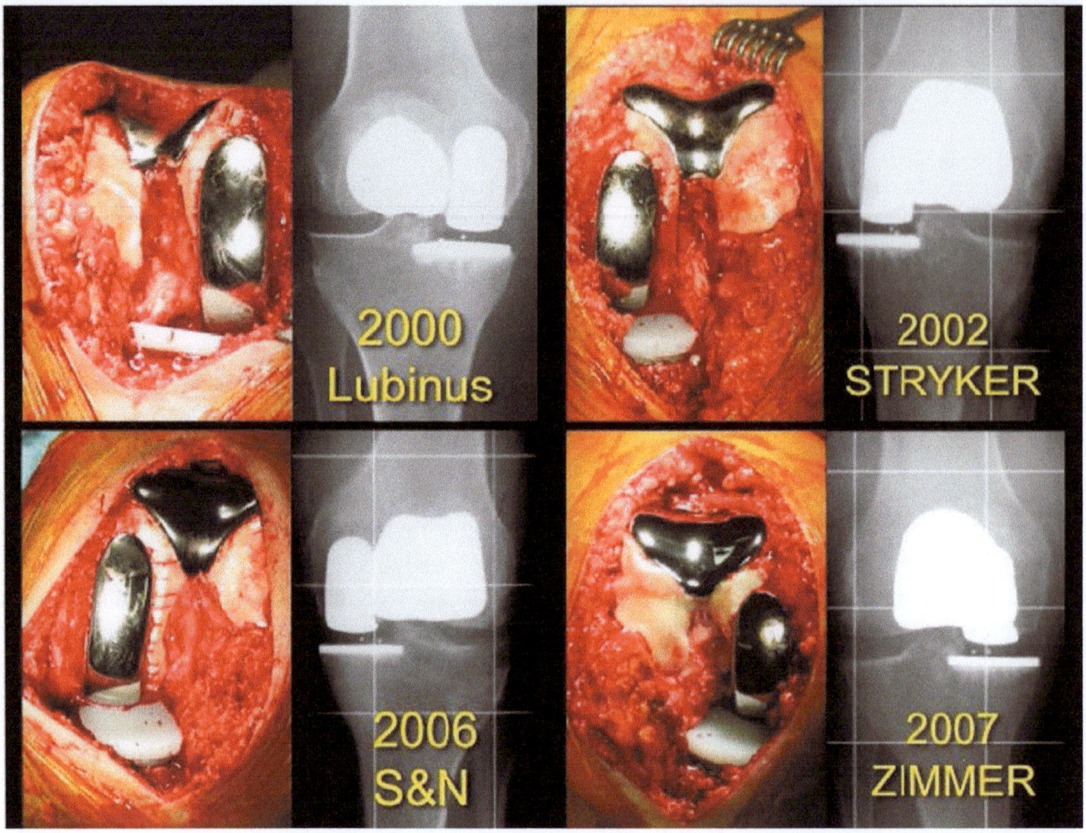

Fig. 11.2 Several patellofemoral implants associated with the Allegretto (Zimmer) unicompartmental knee

the ACL. Improvements in screening for the correct indications and in the quality of treatment of knee arthritis in terms of prosthetic designs and surgical technique are such that even young patients are undergoing prosthetic surgery. In this population, in which expectations are high, mini-invasive conservative solutions that can guarantee maximum results are needed. The advantages of a bicompartmental implant combining UKR and a patellofemoral prosthesis are: preservation of both cruciates, respect of the rotational axis, preservation of bone stock, patellar height and tracking, reproduction of the normal joint kinematics, and morphotype respect. The problems in this surgical procedure are still linked to the poor results obtained with the first series of patellofemoral prosthetic implants.

11.2 Patellofemoral Prosthetic Design

In the 1980s, incorrect indications and poor prosthesis design (Lubinus, Grammont, Cartier, Bousquet) led to poor results and a high failure rate. However, in the last 15 years new designs have yielded more favorable results.

Our experience with these new designs was initially based on the Avon (Stryker) system, then on the Journey system (Smith and Nephew), and more recently on the NexGen system (Zimmer) (Fig. 11.2) [2, 3]. The NexGen relies on left and right anatomical implants and takes into account gender differences by offering a smaller size design specific for females. In fact, among the five

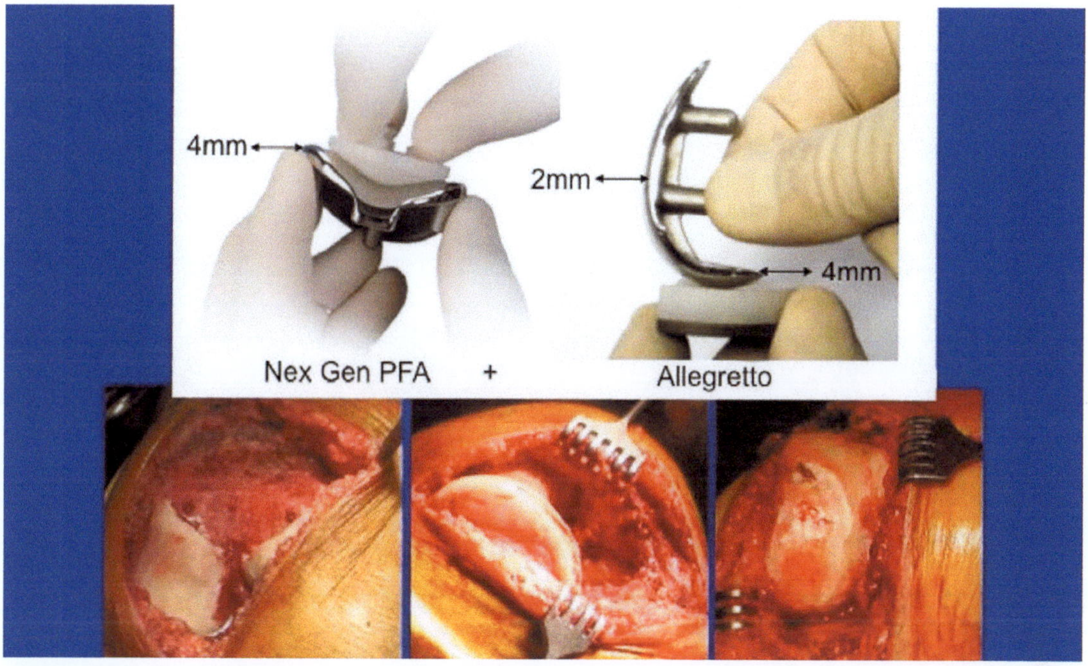

Fig. 11.3 Bicompartmental implant with two resurfacing implants

sizes of NexGen prostheses, the first four have a gender-specific design (Fig. 11.3).

As shown in the literature, in the last years the principal anatomical difference in the knees of males and females is the patellofemoral joint. This could explain the significant patellofemoral arthritis and the chronic anterior knee pain in women who receive a total knee replacement (TKR). In the NexGen patellofemoral system, the gender-specific adjustments are [4-7]: lateralization of the trochlear sulcus by 1.5–2 mm and an obliquity of 3° [8-11] in addition to a reduced anterior flange thickness.

11.3 Indications

Knee arthritis often involves only one of the femorotibial compartments together with the symptomatic patellofemoral joint degeneration. Among our patients, this pattern comprises only 15% of our knee arthritis cases while in 4% there is isolated femoropatellar involvement. In the former, bicompartmental arthritis treatment is based on a lateral or medial UKR and the use of a patellofemoral prosthesis. This combined prosthetic procedure widens the indications and reduces the limits to UKR and an isolated patellofemoral prosthesis. Moreover, the procedure is suitable for patients with a borderline UKR indication, in which there is femorotibial compartmental arthritis and a symptomatic patellofemoral joint, and in patients with borderline indications for a patellofemoral prosthesis due to isolated patellofemoral arthritis, mechanical axis deviation, and initial femorotibial unicompartmental involvement (varus > 3° or valgus > 5°) (Figs. 11.4–11.6) [12].

Radiographic evaluation is based on standard anteroposterior, lateral, and sky-view projections that demonstrate femorotibial degeneration higher than grade I and a femoropatellar involvement according to the Ahlback scale. Also, on a weight-bearing long anteroposterior X-ray view, the mechanical axis can be calculated in order to correctly determine the range of the deformity. Magnetic resonance imaging in some cases shows instability features, such as ACL deficiency, and the patellofemoral status. Femorotibial and/or patellofemoral signs of disease are generally present, including pain while walking and doing stairs or effusion. Age and weight are not a limit.

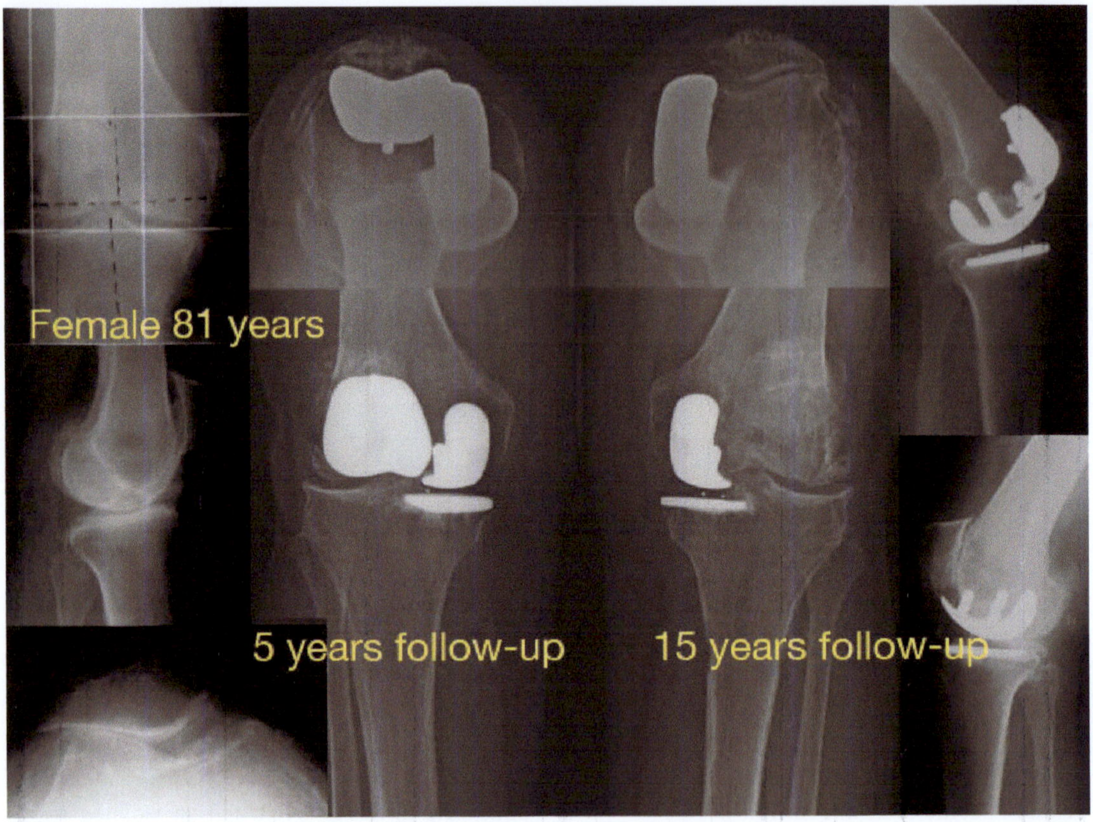

Fig. 11.4 Borderline indication: primary varus or valgus femorotibial arthritis secondarily involving the patellofemoral joint

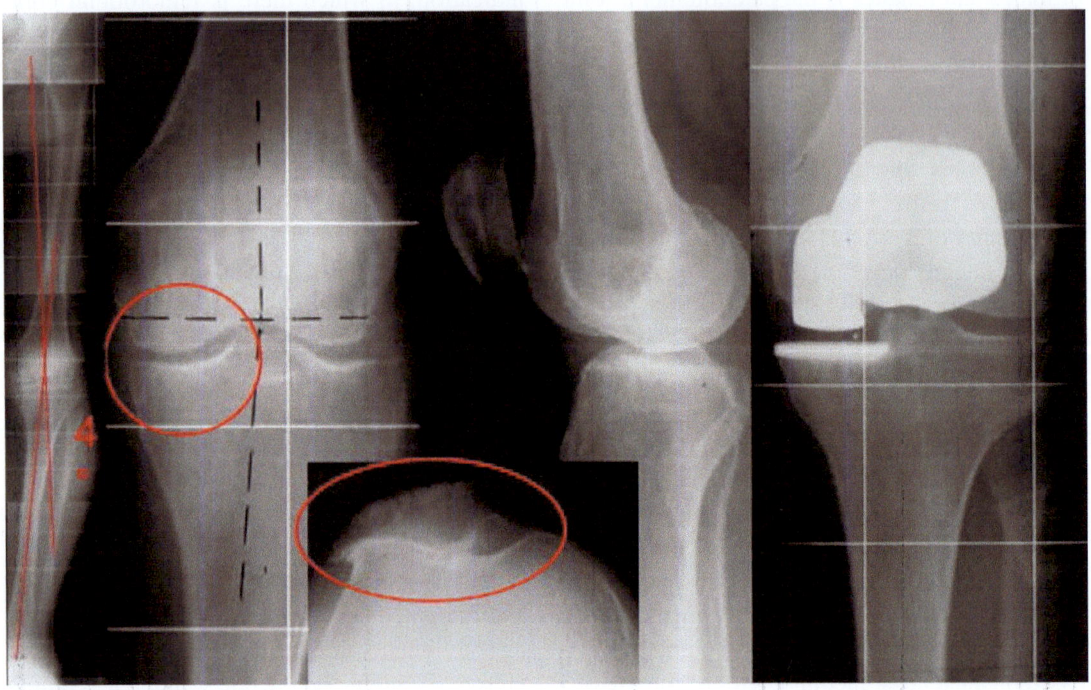

Fig. 11.5 Borderline indication: patellofemoral primary knee arthritis with a moderate mechanical axis deviation in varus > 3° or in valgus > 5°

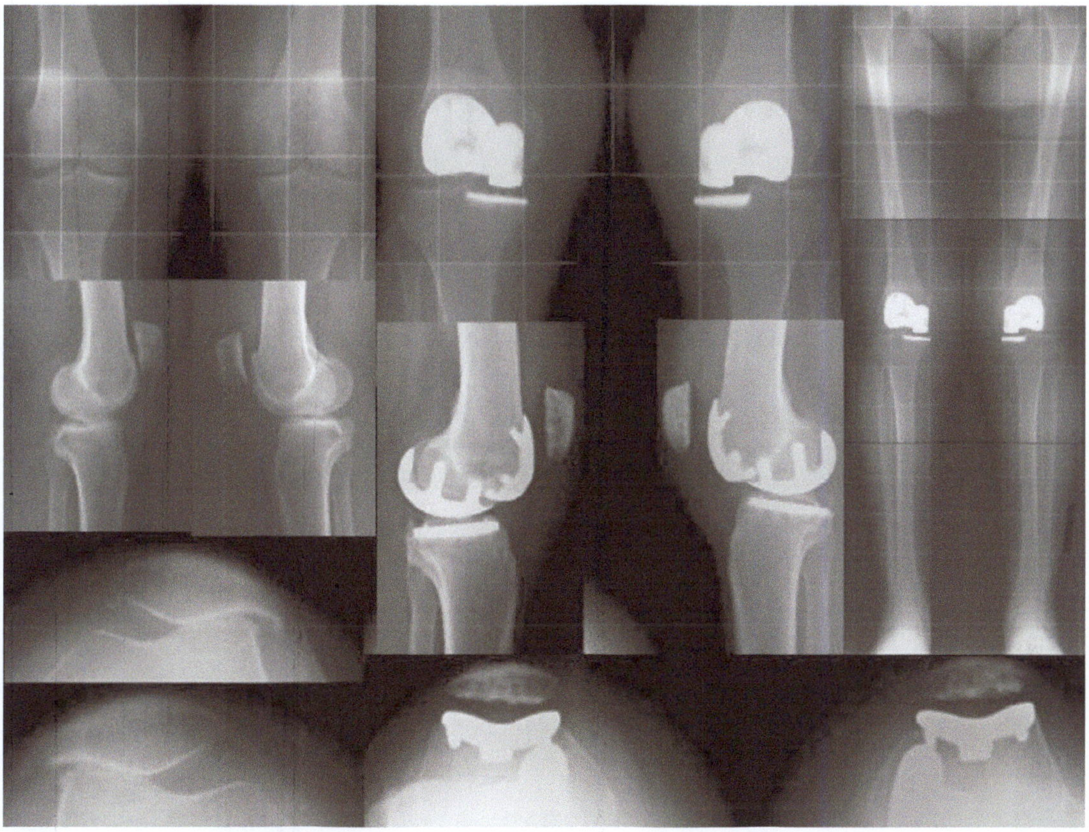

Fig. 11.6 Simultaneous bilateral UKR + patellofemoral implant

11.4 Surgical Technique

The surgical approach is the same as in a UKR, medial in varus or lateral in valgus but 1–2 cm longer [13-16]. In the varus knee we use a mini-mid-vastus approach (Fig. 11.7) whereas in valgus the approach relies on the lateral intermuscular septum, which minimizes damage to the quadriceps and enhances the functional recovery.

Usually the procedure starts with the UKR, following the tibia-first technique and then a distal femoral cut in extension. Once stability has been tested with trials, the implant surface can be prepared for the patellofemoral prosthesis, beginning with the femoral trochlea and then proceeding to the patella. An anterior femoral cut, according to the deformity and possible dysplasia, is made perpendicular to the axis of the joint. The amount of bone-cartilage removed in consideration of tissue damage and wear should be of the same thickness as the prosthesis in patients with arthritis. In those with dysplasia or trochlea aplasia, the existing defect must be considered. The anatomy of both the femoral trochlea and the femoral condyle is related to morphotype, gender, and race. Thus, there is extreme variability in terms of dimension, distance, and the angle between the axis of the medial condyle and that of the femoral trochlea. Furthermore, the sizes of the two joints are not necessarily proportional (Fig. 11.8). Consequently, substitution of the two femoral compartments with a single bicompartmental prosthesis that is not custom-made is unlikely to recreate the correct anatomy and kinematics.

The second step consists of the preparation of the distal condylar trochlea, which is the critical zone of "transition" between the cartilage and the prosthesis. In the NexGen patellofemoral joint

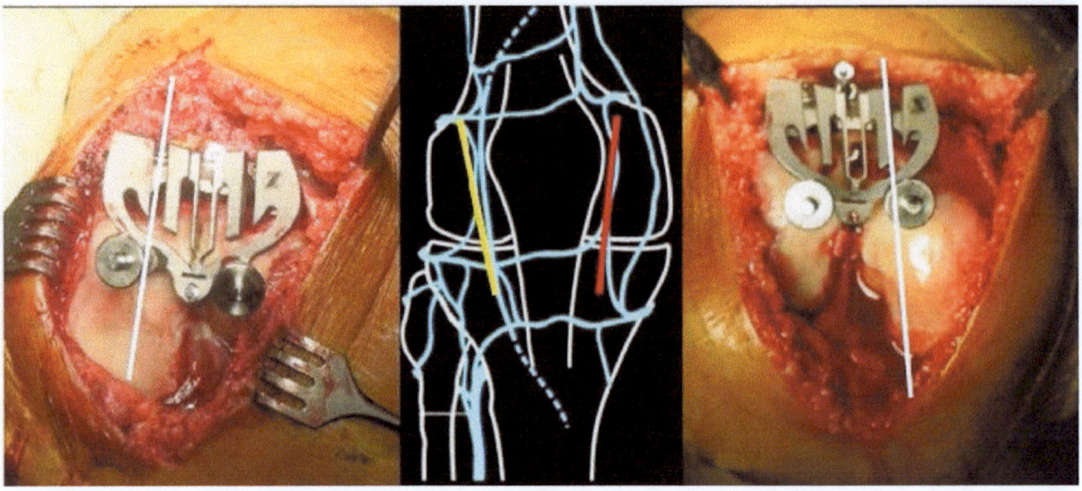

Fig. 11.7 Parapatellar lateral and parapatellar medial mini-invasive approach

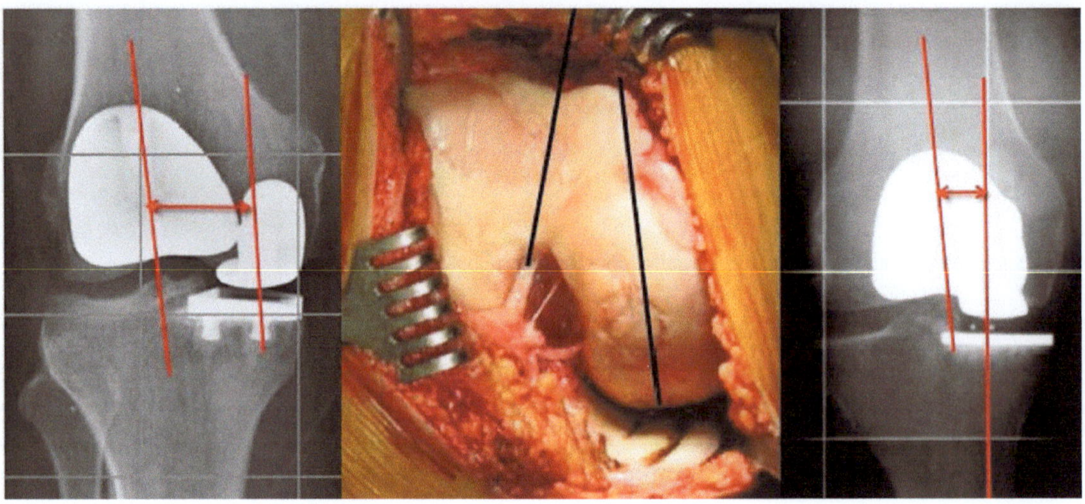

Fig. 11.8 Variability in the angle between the axis of the medial condyle and that of the femoral trochlea

system, this step involves "milling," which relies on a guide for each size and on a high-velocity cutter (Fig. 11.9).

Once the guide is positioned on the femoral resected area, in contact with the distal condylar cartilage, it is centered with respect to the mediolateral trochlear anatomy and then fixed with screws. The high-velocity cutter will remove a minimal amount of cartilage-bone, corresponding to the thickness of the prosthesis. Accurate preparation of the width and depth of this area will avoid the presence of a step at the cartilage-metal transition or exposure of the cement to patellar tracking, which could create impingement and polyethylene wear. The final step is realized with an appropriate guide hole for the implant stems.

The patellar step is done with the patient's knee in extension in order to reduce patellar eversion and consequent stress on the extensor apparatus. We use a standard technique and prefer an all-poly component with an onlay design, sym-

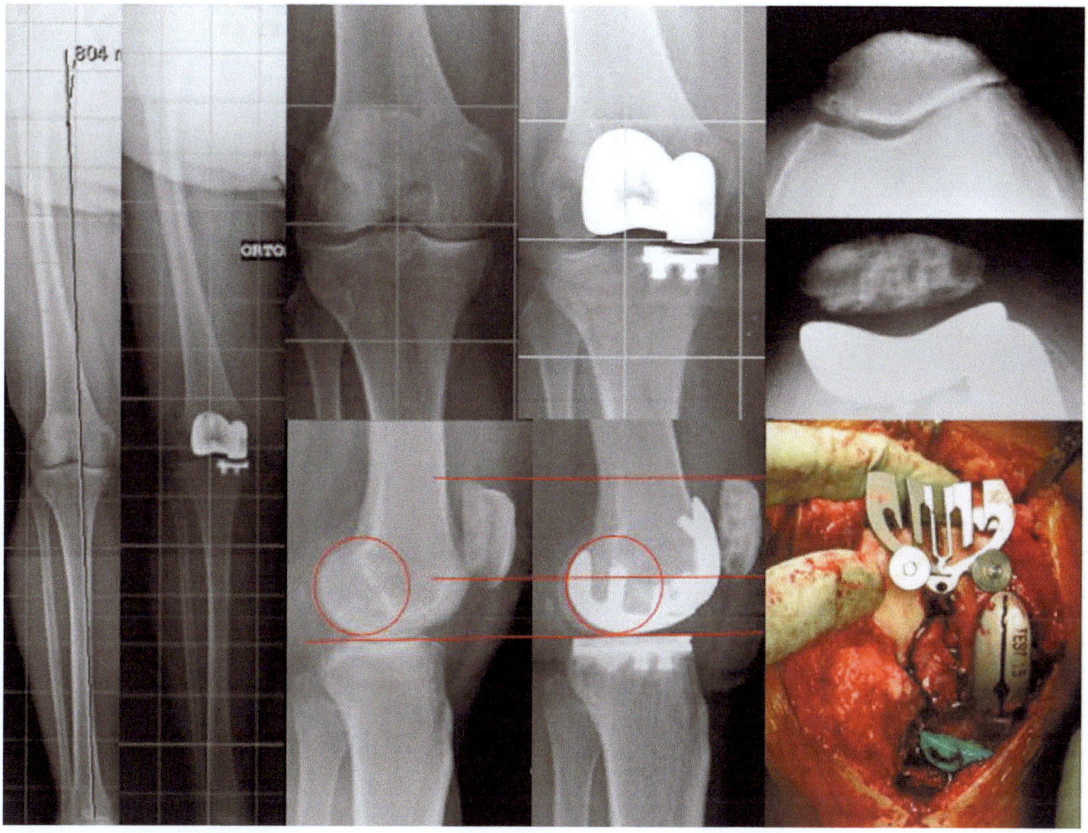

Fig. 11.9 Bicompartmental implant: the guide for milling is positioned on the trochlea

metric or asymmetric. A lateral release is frequently performed. Tibial tuberosity osteotomy is rarely indicated in cases of severe malalignment with trochlear dysplasia and frequent patellar dislocations, or in post-traumatic sequelae with problematic patellar eversion.

In other cases we utilize a patellofemoral inlay solution. This kind of implant follows the existing anatomy and is implanted after a Kirschner wire has been implanted in the center of the joint and the patellar surface (Fig. 11.10). In patients with trochlear dysplasia, the implant does not correct the deformity, avoiding problems in patellar tracking and the consequent necessity of an excessive lateral release.

It is very important to keep the distance at a minimum of 2 mm between the two prosthetic components. Our objective is to respect the femoral surfaces, the rotational axis, and the trochlear depth, avoiding excessive tension on the patella. The implanted trials must achieve a perfect patellofemoral tracking without patellar clunk or tilting in the area of the component transition. We currently use only resurfacing prosthetic designs (Allegretto, ZUK, NexGen, Hemicap).

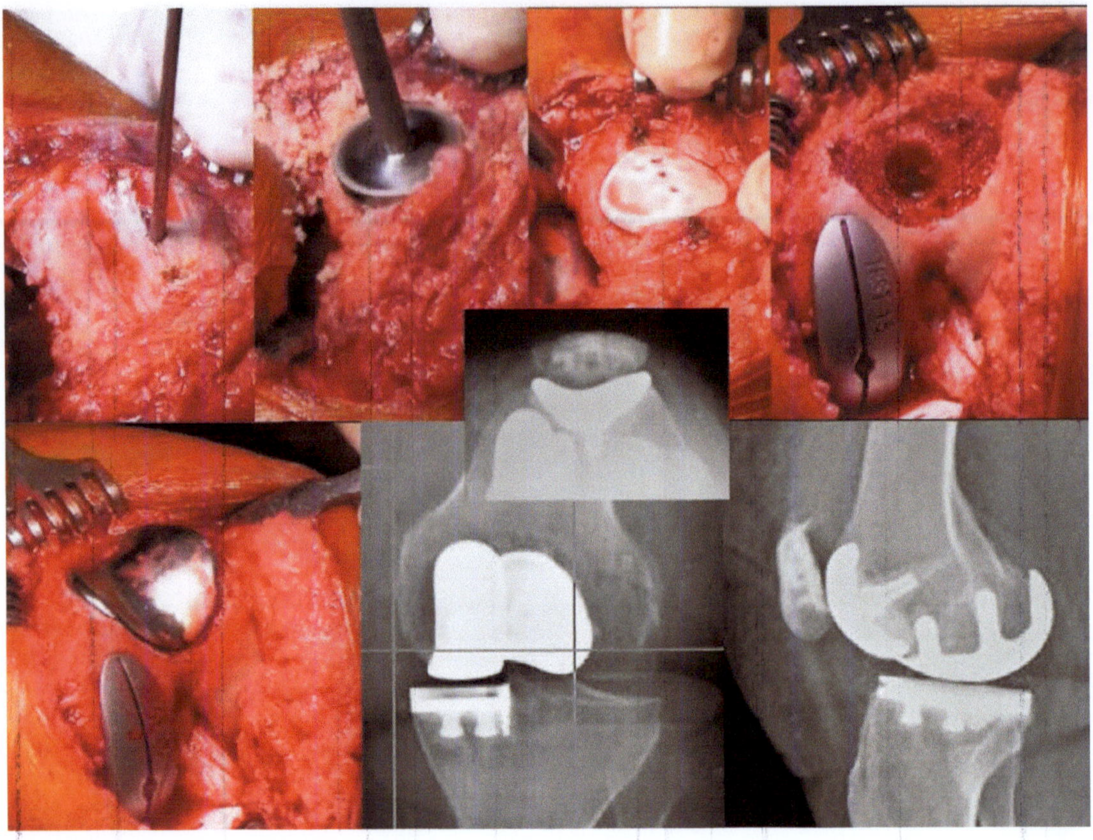

Fig. 11.10 Bicompartmental implant with an inlay patellofemoral solution

11.5 Patients and Methods

From December 2004 to January 2010, 106 bicompartmental knee arthroplasties were performed in 95 patients by the senior surgeon of our institution: 11 cases of lateral and 95 cases of medial femorotibial and patellofemoral resurfacing, followed prospectively for an average of 5 years (maximum 8 years). Patients were selected based on clinical and radiological symptoms and signs. Clinically, the indications for surgery were: knee pain, femoropatellar joint symptoms, fix flexion contracture < 10°, range of motion (ROM) > 80°. The patients did not have inflammatory arthritis, hemochromatosis, hemophilia, or joint instability. The patient population consisted of 69 women and 26 men with an average age at surgery of 69 years (range: 44–86 years). Their average height was 166.9 cm (range: 154–180 cm), their average weight was 73 kg (range: 50–89 kg). One patient was previously treated by high tibial osteotomy (HTO), seven had a postpatellar fracture, and two had trochlear fracture sequelae. The patients were followed yearly for the first 3 years and then every 2 years. One patient died due to unrelated causes.

As of the most recent follow-up, 105 knees in 94 patients (25 men and 69 women) have been evaluated. Of these, 84 patients (95 knees) were evaluated clinically and radiologically while ten patients could only be interviewed by phone because they were not able to attend the clinic. All were interviewed regarding the level of personal satisfaction. Postoperative knee function was evaluated using the Hospital for Special Surgery Knee Score before surgery and at the last follow-up. X-ray images were acquired for anteroposterior weight-bearing as well as lateral and patellar skyline views of the knee. Radiographic measure-

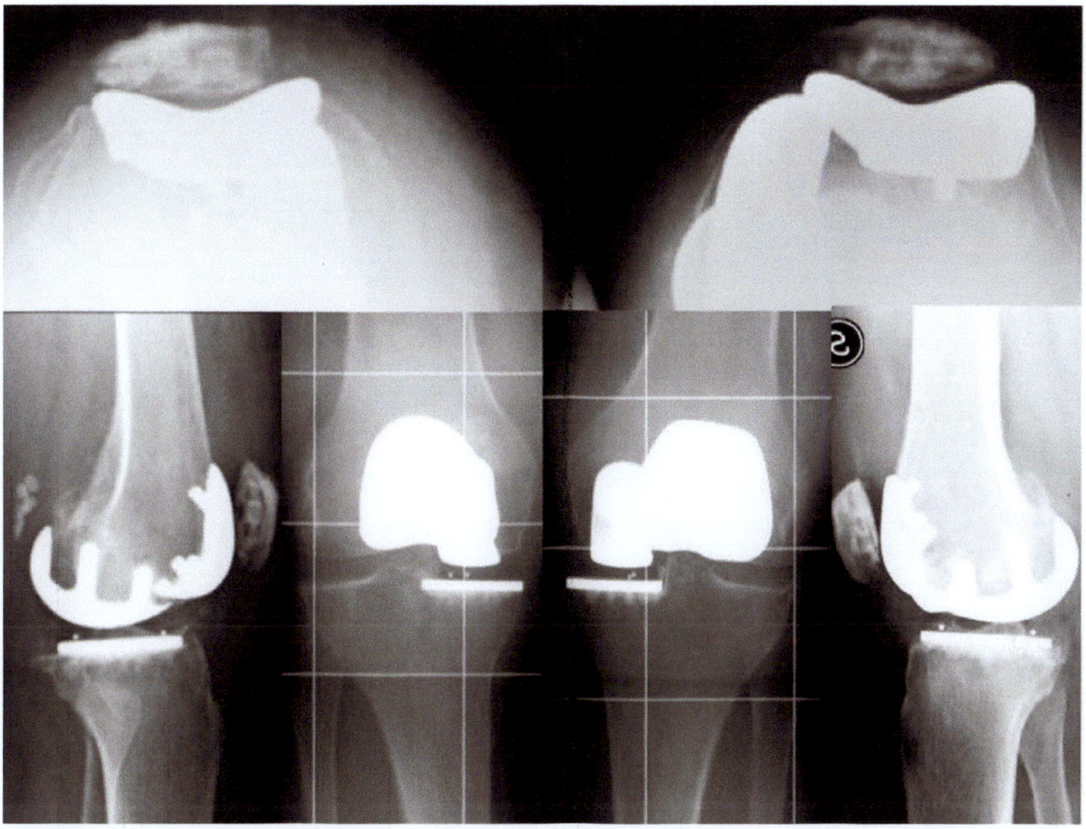

Fig. 11.11 *Left* 5-year follow-up and *right* 8-year follow-up of bicompartmental implants

ments included the mechanical and anatomical axes. In addition, the opposite compartment joint was radiographically evaluated With the preoperative radiographs as the baseline, progression was evaluated. These changes, when present, were graded on a four-point scale. Grade 1 radiographic change was defined as no measurable joint-space loss but with radiographic changes such as osteophytes. Grade 2 radiographic changes were defined as joint-space loss ≤ 25%. Grade 3 radiographic changes were defined as ≤ 50% joint-space loss, and grade 4 as > 50% joint-space loss.

A Kaplan-Meier survival analysis was used to evaluate the long-term results, with revision as the end point (Fig. 11.11).

11.6 Results

Clinically, the average preoperative Hospital for Special Surgery Knee Score was 61 points (range: 52–70 points), which improved to 93 points (range: 72–100 points). The average preoperative ROM was 102.5° (range: 88–135°). At the final follow-up, the average ROM was 125.2° (range: 104–135°). For 89 patients, the ROM was > 120°. Among the 94 patients, 87 (92.5%) had no pain while seven (7.5%) had slight or occasional pain.

At the time of the latest follow-up, 84 patients (89,3%) were enthusiastic regarding the procedure and ten (10.6%) were satisfied. None reported any change or dissatisfaction.

Radiographically, no component showed evidence of loosening, defined as no change in the position of the components on sequential X-rays. There was no radiographic evidence of osteolysis. The average preoperative deformity ranged from 11° varus to 10° of mechanical axis valgus. The average postoperative alignment was 2.5° (range: 3° varus to 2° valgus) of mechanical axis varus.

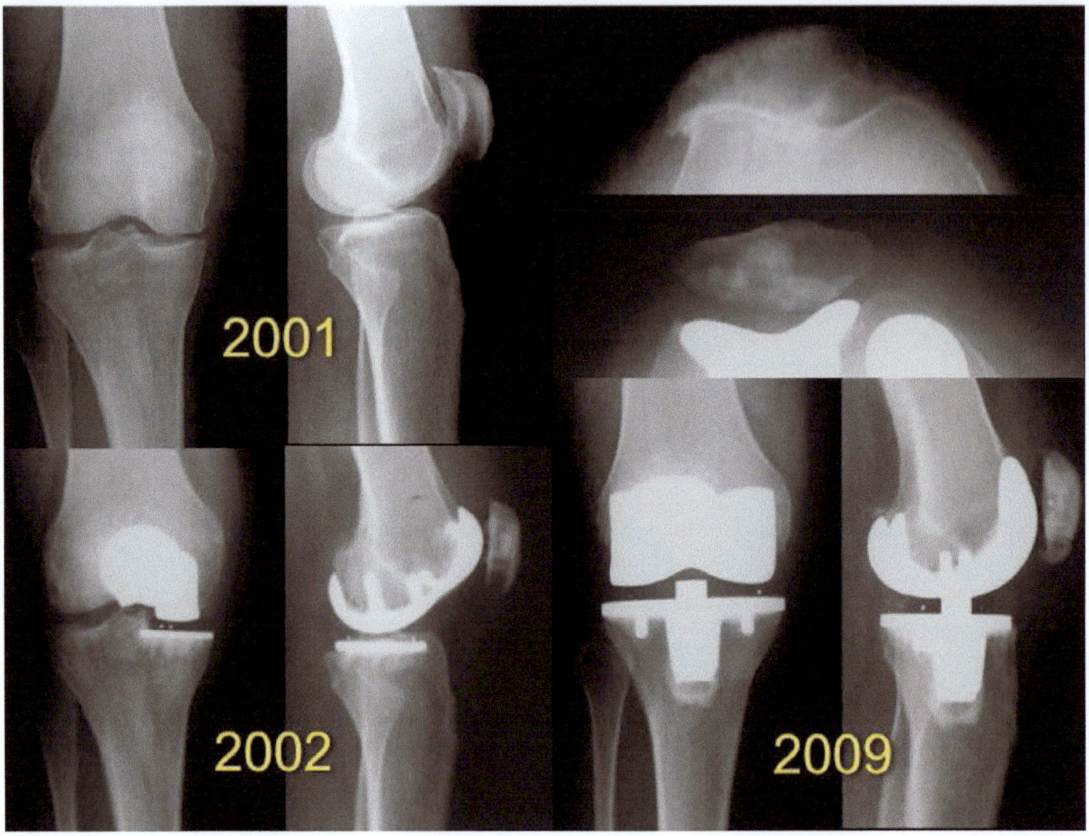

Fig. 11.12 A bicompartmental knee implant failed due to patellar subluxation. Revision with primary TKR

There was no radiographic progression of the other femorotibial compartment joint in 83 knees (87.3%) , but 11 knees (11.6%) had grade 2 progression. Polyethylene wear was evaluated radiographically using the same four-point scale to classify progressive penetration of the femoral component on the tibial aspect of the material. None of the knees showed signs of penetration (100%).

There were four revisions. Two patients (Allegretto+ NexGen patellofemoral joint) underwent revision in the form of a patellar implant, 1 year and 4 years after surgery, but these cases were not considered as failure; the third patient (Allegretto + Lubinus) underwent revision 1 year after implantation for patellar subluxation and clunk, while in the fourth the revision was performed 8 years after implantation for necrosis of the medial femoral condyle. In the first two cases, the revision was performed due to continuous anterior knee pain. Patellar degeneration was clinically evident. In the third case the trochlear inlay design did not correct the patellar subluxation due to dysplasia of the anterior femoral condyles; the revision was a primary TKR (Fig. 11.12).

In the fourth patient, degeneration of the medial femoral condyle necessitated a revision consisting of a medial UKR, such that the final knee prosthesis was tricompartmental (Fig. 11.13).

There was no case of component instability or polyethylene wear.

The cumulative survival rate at 9 years is 96.26% (Table 11.1, Fig. 11.14).

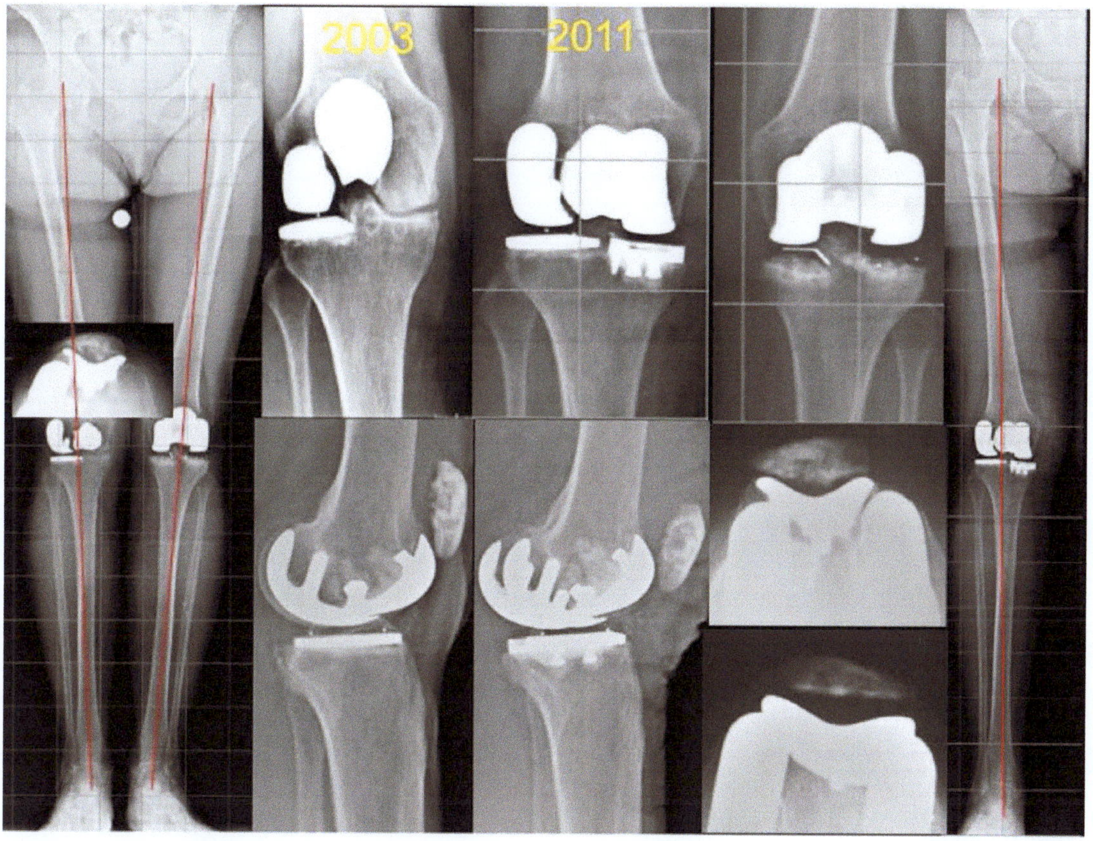

Fig. 11.13 Medial femoral condyle degeneration involving a bicompartmental implant in the left knee. Revision at 8 years with a medial UKR

Table 11.1 Survival of 106 bicompartmental knee replacements

Years since surgery	N. at start	Failure	Width	Lost to FU	N. at risk	Fail %	Succ %	Surv rate	%var	% SE
0-1	106	0	0	0	106	0.00	100.00	100.00	0.00	0.00
1-2	106	0	0	0	106	0.00	100.00	100.00	0.00	0.00
2-3	106	0	15	0	98.5	0.00	100.00	100.00	0.00	0.00
3-4	91	0	14	0	84	0.00	100.00	100.00	0.00	0.00
4-5	77	0	17	0	68.5	0.00	100.00	100.00	0.00	0.00
5-6	60	2	13	0	53.5	3.74	96.26	96.26	6.47	2.54
6-7	45	0	15	0	37.5	0.00	100.00	96.26	9.24	3.04
7-8	30	0	13	0	23.5	0.00	100.00	96.26	14.74	3.84
8-9	17	0	17	0	8.5	0.00	100.00	96.26	40.75	6.38
Total		2	104	0						

11.7 Conclusions

Cruciate-retaining bicompartmental knee arthroplasties currently offer a high level of functionality and the joint kinematics include essential features similar to those of a normal knee and a survivorship comparable to that achieved with TKR. The association of a UKR with a femoropatellar prosthesis reduces the risk of failure due to anterior knee pain and enlarges the indication

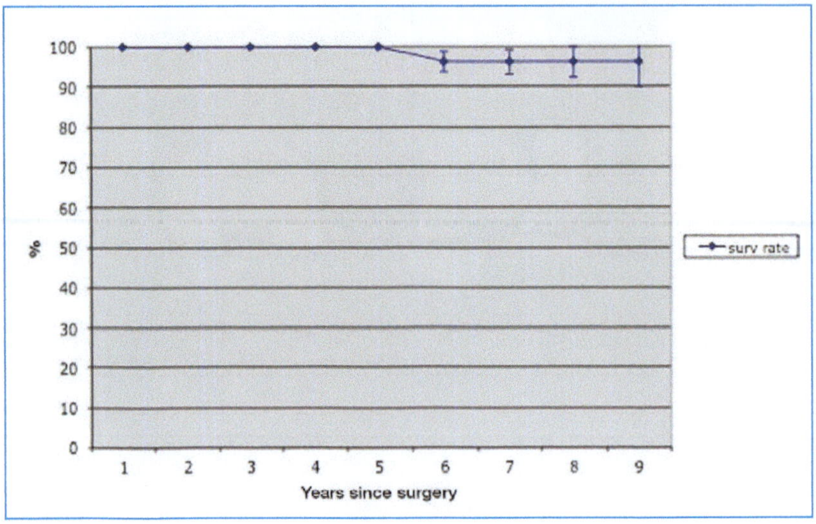

Fig. 11.14 Kaplan-Meier survival curve of bi-unicompartmental knee replacement. See Table 11.1 for details

to treat bicompartmental knee arthritis in young active patients while offering the possibility of the best outcome in terms of functional recovery and return to sports activities. Bicompartmental prostheses (UKR+patellofemoral), in particular the new implant designs, allow further expansion to include an increasing number of patients with good future perspectives.

References

1. Romagnoli S, Banks SA, Fregly BJ, Boniforti F, Reinschmidt C (2005) Comparing in vivo kinematics of unicondylar and bi-unicondylar knee replacement. Knee Surg Sports Traumatol Arthrosc 13(7):551-6
2. Ackroyd CE, Chir B (2005) Development and early results of a new patellofemoral arthroplasty. Clin Orthop 436:7-13
3. Ackroyd CE, Newman JH, Evans R, Eldridge JD, Joslin CC (2007) The Avon patellofemoral arthroplasty: five-year survivorship and functional results. J Bone Joint Surg Br 89(3):310-5
4. Tosi LL, Boyan BD, Boskey A (2005) Does sex matter in muscoloskeletal health? The influence of sex and Gender on muscoloskeletal health. J Bone Joint Surg Am 87:1631-1647
5. Kuhn M, Mahfouz M, ElHak E, Merkl B (2005) Reconstruction of 3D patient-specific bone models from biplanar x-ray images. Int Conf Biomed Engr
6. Csintalan RP, Schulz MM, Woo J, McMahon PJ, Lee TQ (2002) Gender differences in patellofemoral joint biomechanics. Clin Orthop 402:260-269
7. Woodland LH, Francis RS (1992) Parameters and comparisons of the quadriceps angle of college-aged men and women in the supine and standingpositions. Am J Sport Med 20:208–211
8. Tillman MD, Smith KR, Bauer JA, Cauraugh JH, Falsetti AB, Pattishall JL (2002) Differences in three intercondylar notch geometry indices between males and females: a cadaveric study. The Knee 9:41-46
9. Aglietti P, Insall JN, Cerulli G (1983) Patellar pain and incongruence. Clin Orthop 176:217-224
10. Bengs BC, Scott RD (2006) The effect of patellar thickness on intraoperative knee flexion and patellar tracking in total knee arthroplasty. J Arthroplasty 21:650-5
11. Chin KR, Dalury DF, Scott RD (2002) Comparative measurement of male and female distal femurs during primary total knee arthroplasty. J Knee Surg 15:213-217
12. Romagnoli S, Verde F et al (2007) BiUni knee replacement. Basic science, clinical repair and reconstruction of articular cartilage defect: Current status and prospect. Timeo Editore, Bologna
13. Romagnoli S, Verde F, d'Amario F, Castelnuovo N (2006) La protesi femoro-rotulea. Archivio di Ortopedia e Traumatologia 116:12–14
14. Romagnoli S, Verde F, Bibbiani E, Castelnuovo N (2008) Protesi Femoro-Rotulea isolate e mono + FR. Minerva Ortopedica e traumatologica 59(Suppl. 1), n. 5
15. Romagnoli S, Verde F, Bibbiani E, Castelnuovo N, Gioni N (2008) La protesi Femoro-rotulea: a che punto siamo? Archivio di Ortopedia e Reumatologia, 119:29-30
16. Romagnoli S, Verde F et al (2010) Biunicompartmental knee prostheses. In: Scuderi GR, Tria AJ (eds) Minimally Invasive Surgery in Orthopaedics. Springer, Berlin Heidelberg New York

12 Surgical Technique and Long-Term Results of Bicompartmental Reconstruction with Small Implants

Sebastien Parratte, Matthieu Ollivier, Jean-Manuel Aubaniac, and Jean-Noel Argenson

12.1 Introduction

Treatment of limited osteoarthritis of the knee remains a challenging problem [1-4]. While the therapeutic goals are to alleviate pain and restore knee function [1-4], non-operative modalities, including physiotherapy, activity modification (avoiding impact activities), anti-inflammatory medications, and bracing, often provide limited pain relief and functional improvement [1-4]. Surgical management of limited arthritis of the knee can include non-prosthetic treatments such as arthroscopic debridement, meniscus transplantation, cartilage repair, high tibial osteotomy (HTO), and tibial tubercle transposition [1-6]. Arthroplasty solutions consist of unicompartmental knee arthroplasty (UKA) and conventional total knee arthroplasty (TKA) [1-6], both of which are expected to be efficient, durable and safe but should preserve the bone stock when possible [3]. TKA may offer durable and satisfying clinical and radiological results when arthritis involves the three compartments of the knee; however, it does not preserve either the bone stock or the ligaments [7, 8]. UKA is a bone- and ligament-sparing technique that can reliably restore knee kinematics and function in patients with arthritis limited to one compartment of the knee [9-12]. The outcomes of UKA have improved since its introduction more than 30 years ago due to improvements in design, indications, materials, and surgical techniques [13, 14]. The results of UKA are reportedly better when the anterior cruciate ligament (ACL) is intact [15, 16]. Similarly, outcome and kinematic studies suggest that maintaining the ACL in bi- and tri-compartmental knee arthroplasty may be advantageous in terms of survivorship [17, 18], stair climbing ability[19], patient satisfaction, and joint kinematics [9, 17, 19-22].

Bicompartmental arthritis of the knee is not rare and bicompartmental knee arthroplasties have been proposed to bridge the gap between UKA and TKA [10, 21]. Indeed, there is a high level of interest in bicompartmental knee arthroplasties that combine medial and lateral UKAs [9, 10, 21]. The advantages of this approach over total knee replacement (TKR) include a smaller implant size, reduced operative trauma, preservation of both cruciate ligaments and bone stock, and a more physiological knee joint [8, 17, 21, 23]. In response to the growing relevance of combined compartmental implants, including medial UKA and lateral arthroplasties, this chapter provides a description of the surgical technique used in bicompartmental knee arthroplasty, including tips and tricks, and reports the long-term results of a consecutive series of these patients.

J. N. Argenson (✉)
Service de Chirurgie Orthopédique
Hôpital Sainte-Marguerite
Marseille, France
E-mail: jean-noel.argenson@ap-hm.fr

12.2 Surgical Technique

The indications for the procedure were: a confirmed diagnosis of bicompartmental osteoarthritis [24]. (Ahlback1 ≥ grade 2) and a preserved

N. Confalonieri, S. Romagnoli (eds.), *Small Implants in Knee Reconstruction*,
DOI 10.1007/978-88-470-2655-1_12, © Springer-Verlag Italia 2013

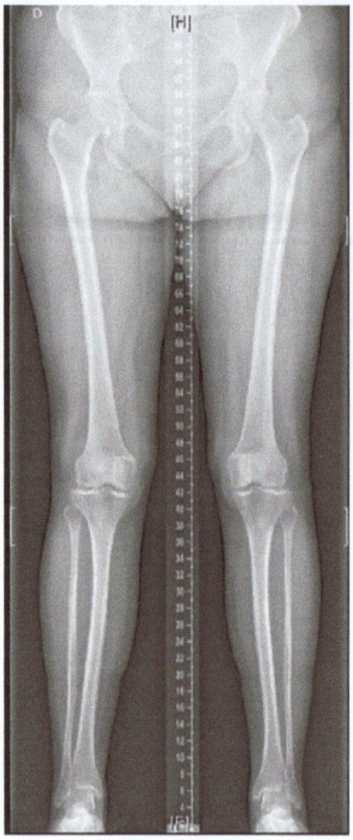

Fig. 12.1 The preoperative radiograph of this 60-year-old woman shows bicompartmental arthritis of the right knee without any major deformation

status of the patellofemoral joint, based on clinical evaluation and sky-view radiographs.(Fig. 12.1) Both a preoperative range of knee flexion > 100º associated with a full range of knee extension and a knee clinically stable in the frontal and sagittal planes were considered as crucial indications. A valgus or varus deformity > 10°, as measured on long-leg X-rays, or a metaphyseal tibial varus > 7° is also considered as a contraindication. We systematically obtained varus and valgus stress radiographs (Fig. 12.2) to evaluate deformity correction [25]. A fixed deformity observed on the stress radiograph was considered as a contraindication.

12.3 Approach

It is important to maintain proper visualization throughout the procedure in order to optimize implant positioning, even when a minimally invasive technique is used. Therefore, the length of the skin incision varies from 10 to 14 cm depending on patient morphotype and skin elasticity. The upper limit of the incision is 1–2 cm over the proximal pole of the patella, extending distally toward the medial side of the tibial tuberosity and ending 2 cm under the joint line, previously located. We first realize the medial UKA by a medial subvastus approach. Once the synovial cavity is opened, proper visualization of the condyle, the ACL, and the corresponding tibial side of the tibial plateau is achieved by excising the obscuring portion of the fat pad.

Before proceeding to the bone cuts, we evaluate the ACL, with the patient's knee in 60° of flexion in order to examine the joint by checking the resistance of the ligament with an appropriate hook. We then evaluate the state of the patellofemoral joint. Osteophytes are removed on the medial femoral condyle, which results in a relative lengthening of the medial collateral ligament and capsule and thus allows passive correction of the deformity. Next, osteophytes located in the intercondylar notch are also carefully removed to avoid late impingement with the ACL on the notch (Fig. 12.3).

The frontal tibial and the distal femoral cuts are linked together and made using an extramedullary alignment. We try to reproduce the natural slope of the medial tibial plateau, usually between 5° and 7° of posterior slope. The sagittal tibial cut is then performed manually, using a reciprocating bone saw and following the line crossing the point at the foot of the ACL and the anterior tibial point. The size of the femoral implant is determined using the cutting block, positioning the femoral finishing guide on the distal femoral cut and searching for the best compromise between an anatomically centered position on the femoral condyle and a long axis perpendicular to the resected tibial plateau. The top of this finishing guide should be placed at least 1–2 mm above the deepest layer of the cartilage to avoid a potential notch between the femoral implant and the patella. To control the mediolateral position of the femoral cutting guide, which determines the position of the final implant, tibial referencing based on the previously made tibial cut is a very helpful landmark. Since the divergence of the medial condyle is different from one knee to another, checking the mediolateral posi-

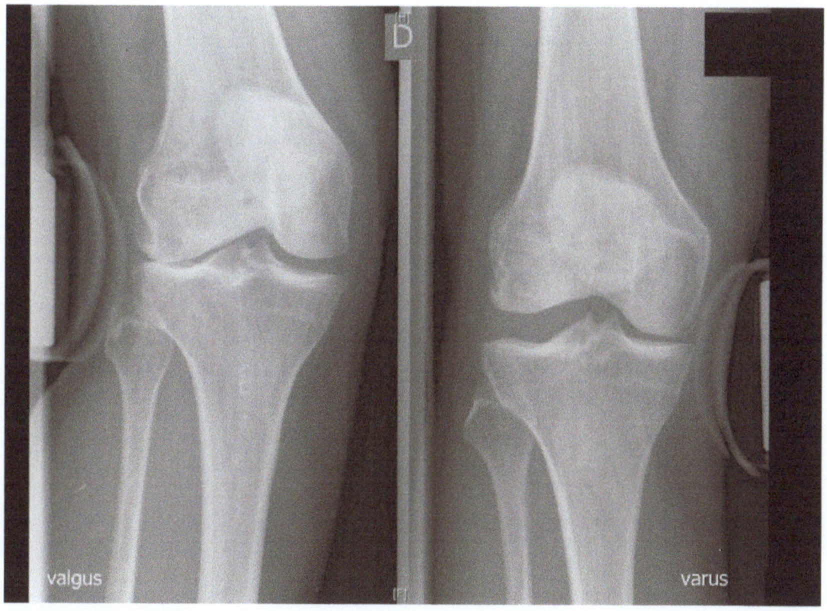

Fig. 12.2 Stress X-rays on the same patient as in Fig. 12.1 confirm the bone on bone contact, reduction of the deformation in each compartment, and correct ligament balance

tion of the guide on the femoral condyle is also recommended. The size of the tibial tray should then be determined, achieving the best compromise between maximal tibial coverage and overhang, which might induce pain. The knee is then brought into maximal flexion and externally rotated. The final preparation of the tibia is completed with the appropriate guide, with the underlying keel impacted in the subchondral bone. Flexion-extension gaps should be tested with the trial components in place. A 9-mm polyethylene trial is used, aiming for a 2-mm laxity at 10° of flexion. At the same time, it should be confirmed that the middle of the femoral component is placed in the middle of the tibial component in flexion and in extension.

The lateral UKA is then realized through a lateral subvastus arthrotomy. In a lateral UKA, osteophytes on the lateral condyle should not be removed; leaving them in place will optimize positioning of the femoral implant, considering the femoral divergence of the condyle. The tibial resection is performed using the same extramedullary ancillaries, making the frontal tibial and distal femoral cuts at the same time. On the lateral side, a tibial slope is not included in the cut, which should stay minimal since the disease is more often on the femoral side. To respect

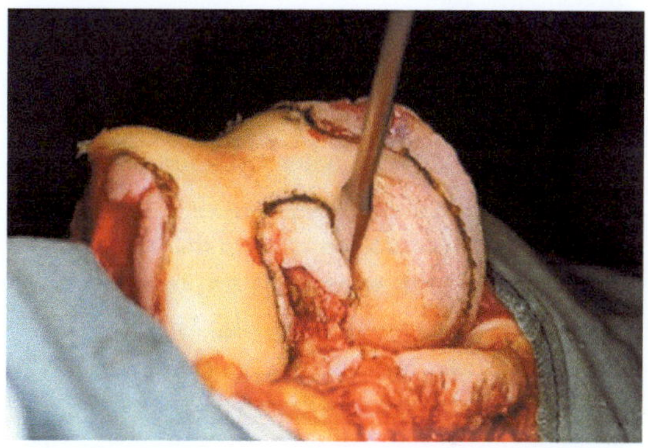

Fig. 12.3 Osteophytes should be carefully removed to avoid late impingement with the ACL, as shown on this intraoperative view of the intercondylar notch observed through an old-fashion approach

the anatomy of the lateral tibial plateau, the cut should be made without any posterior slope. In case of femoral dysplasia, it is often necessary to use a "more proximal" distal femoral cut and a dedicated femoral cutting guide to increase its thickness. The alignment of the femoral cutting guide on the tibial cut is crucial due to the natural shape of the lateral femoral condyle. It is frequently necessary to mark the correct alignment in extension rather than in flexion in order to avoid medial edge loading and impingement between the femoral implant and the tibial spines due to the screw-home mechanism. The polyeth-

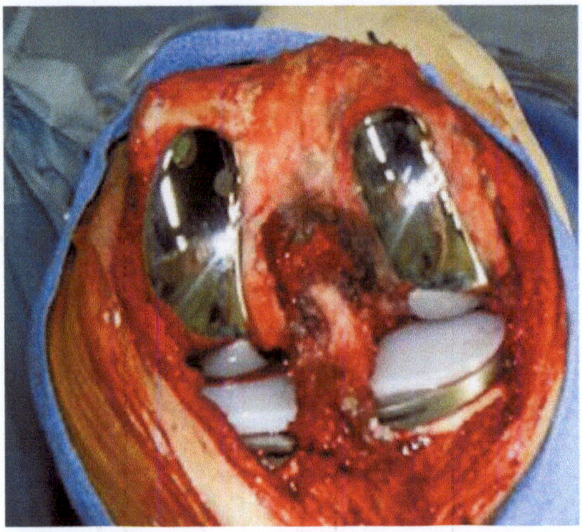

Fig. 12.4 Preservation of the ACL, restoration of the joint line, and correct alignment of the components in each compartment are the most important points to follow in obtaining a well functioning bicompartmental knee arthroplasty

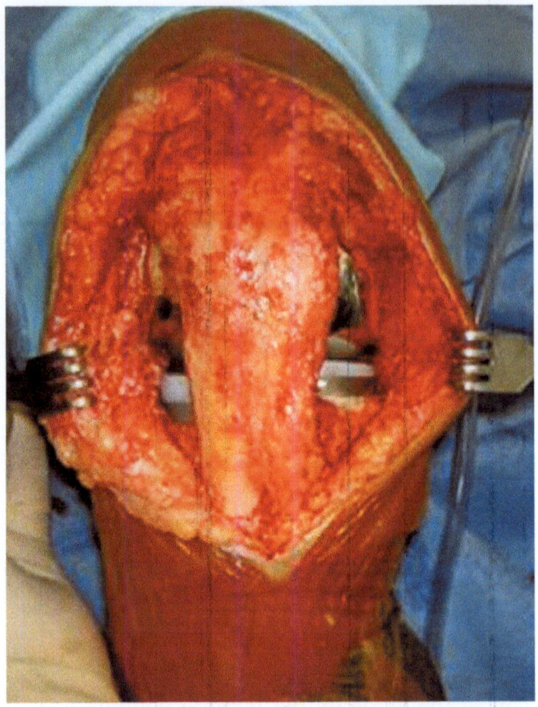

Fig. 12.5 Control of patellar tracking is also important

ylene insert is often thicker than for the medial side in case of femoral dysplasia even if the principle of under-correction of the deformity for all cases of lateral UKA remains the basis for successful long-term results (Fig. 12.4).

Patellar tracking should be checked before closing (Fig. 12.5) facilitated by the absence of patellar eversion during the procedure. The tourniquet is released before closure to allow adequate hemostasis. In our practice, one intra-articular drain is left in place for 36 h. Postoperative rehabilitation protocols include immediate weight-bearing protected by crutches during the first 2 or 3 weeks, according to patient tolerance and exercises focused on passive flexion immediately and then active recuperation of flexion and extension. All patients should receive routine prophylaxis with low-molecular-weight heparin preoperatively and postoperatively for 21 days.

12.4 Methods

During the study period from April 1972 to December 2000, of the 232 combined unicompartmental knee arthroplasties performed at our institution, 100 (43%) of them were combined medial and lateral UKAs. During the same study period, 4500 TKA and 870 isolated UKAs were performed at our institution.

We retrospectively reviewed all patients treated at our institution with a bicompartmental knee arthroplasty (100 knees) following a diagnosis of bicompartmental osteoarthritis of the knee. The 100 combined medial and lateral UKAs were performed in 84 patients by the two senior authors (JMA and JNA) between April 1972 and December 2000, using cemented prostheses. The inclusion criteria in this study were: a minimal clinical follow-up of 5 years and a complete follow-up with available X-rays. The exclusion criteria were a contemporary HTO, a contemporary or previous ACL reconstruction, or a revision arthroplasty. The etiologies of the osteoarthritis were primary osteoarthritis in 92 knees (92%) and post-traumatic osteoarthritis in eight (8%). The grade of arthritis involving the medial compartment according to the Ahlback classification [24] was grade 2 for three (3%) knees, grade 3 for 92 knees (92%), and grade 4 for five knees (5%). The grade of arthritis concerning the lateral compartment was: grade 2 for 30 (30%) knees, grade 3 for 65 knees (65%), and grade 4 for five knees (5%).

Among the 84 patients, 39 (48 knees) died before the final review (at a mean of 12 years postoperatively) but data were available from the last follow-up before their death (1 year before) and were used for the final analysis. Six patients were lost to follow-up. Thus, 94 knees in 78 patients were available for the final analysis. Approval of the institutional ethics committee was obtained.

All UKA components were cemented on the tibial and femoral sides. Between 1972 and 1989, Marmor-like (Zimmer, Warsaw, IN) or Alpina (Biomet, Bridgend, UK) implants were used in the UKA, whether of the medial or the lateral compartment. After 1989, Miller-Galante UKA (Zimmer, Warsaw, IN) prostheses were systematically implanted using modern dedicated instrumentation, including tibial and femoral cutting guides. The design characteristics and the surgical technique of this device were previously described [26, 27].

All patients were clinically evaluated preoperatively, at 3 months postoperatively, at yearly intervals postoperatively, and at the last follow-up by an independent observer using the Knee Society (KS) score and function score [14]. The arc of knee flexion was recorded preoperatively, during follow-up, and at the final evaluation. For patients operated on in the 1970s and 1980s, the KS score was calculated based on data collected on the standardized knee evaluation sheet used in the department [14]. Patient satisfaction regarding the procedure was assessed using the four-level scale (enthusiastic, satisfied, no change, not satisfied) previously used for evaluation of outcomes after UKA [15, 28-30]. Radiographic evaluation was performed by one independent observer (SP, Fellow in hip and knee reconstruction at the time of the evaluation) using long-leg radiographs and anteroposterior (AP), lateral, and skyline radiographs of the knee at last follow-up. Lower-limb alignment was assessed on long-leg radiographs performed using a standardized protocol in which the patient stood with the patella facing anteriorly. These images were used to preoperatively and postoperatively calculate the femoral angle (CH: condylar axis to hip center), the tibial angle (PA: plateau axis to ankle) and the articular deformation (CP: condylar axis and plateau axis) [30, 31]. The hip-knee-ankle angle was calculated as the sum of the three previously defined angles (HKA= CH+PA+CP), considering CP as positive in case of lateral convergence [30, 31]. Postoperative alignments of the femoral and tibial components as well as the postoperative alignment of the limb were assessed on long-leg radiographs according to the standardized protocol used preoperatively [30, 31]. The presence, extent, or progression of femoral, tibial, or patellar radiolucencies according to the KS roentgenographic score was evaluated on full tangential AP and lateral radiographs and on skyline radiographs [14]. Furthermore, progression of osteoarthritis was evaluated in the non-resurfaced compartment on AP radiographs and in the patellofemoral joint on skyline radiographs [7]. The Ahlback classification was used to evaluate osteoarthritis progression in the femoropatellar compartment [24].

Patient demographics were described using means and standard deviations or medians and ranges for continuous variables, and counts (percent) for categorical variables. Clinical improvement between the preoperative and postoperative evaluation as described by the mean KS knee and function score was analyzed using a t test for paired comparisons [32]. The radiographic outcomes were descriptively reported using means and standard deviations to describe preoperative and postoperative alignment. Finally, 17-year survival analysis was performed using the Kaplan-Meier technique (with 95% confidence intervals) for all patients, considering revision for any reason or radiographic loosening as the endpoint [33]. The data were analyzed using SPSS software (version 12; SPSS Inc., Chicago, IL). All calculations assumed two-tailed tests.

12.5 Results

The KS knee and function scores improved in both compartments ($p = 0.00034$ and $p = 0.00023$) between the preoperative and final evaluations (minimum follow-up of 5 years; mean, 11.7± 7

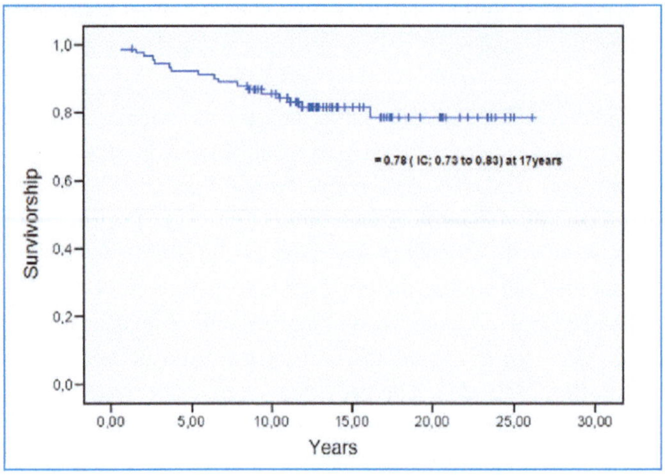

Fig. 12.6 The Kaplan-Meier survival curve, considering revision due to any cause as the endpoint, shows an expected survivorship of 0.78 (95% confidence interval 0.73–0.83) at 17 year

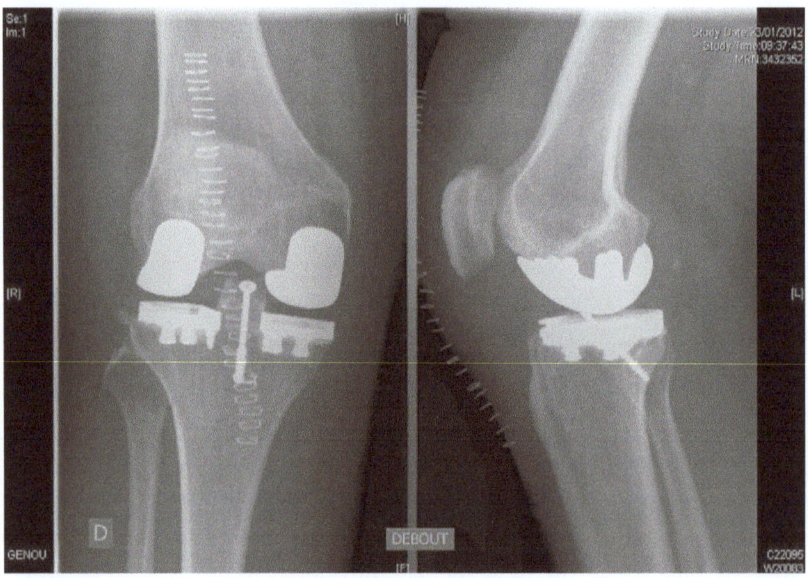

Fig. 12.7 Intraoperative avulsion of the tibial spine should be immediately treated. We recommend a composite fixation using a Fiber-Wire type suture anchored on a cancellous screw

years; range: 5–23 years) for the 94 knees available. Mean active knee flexion improved from 112° ± 5° (range: 100–45°) preoperatively to 136° ± 4° (range: 117–149°) at final follow-up. Among the bi-UKA patients at the time of the final follow-up, 31 (40%) were enthusiastic regarding the procedure, 40 were (51%) satisfied, and seven (9%) were not satisfied, but all of this last group required an early revision before 4 years for aseptic loosening.

The mean preoperative HKA angle was 176° (range: 170–180°) and 178°± 4° (range: 175–182°) after surgery. The mean AP axis of the tibial component was 89° ± 3° (range: 85–90°) on the medial side and 90° ± 2° (range: 88–93°) on the lateral side. The mean tibial slope was 3° ± 4° (range: 0–8°). The mean AP femoral axis was 92° ± 7° (range: 86–94°). Fourteen knees (15%) showed radiolucencies (< 1 mm) at the tibial bone–cement interface, but without any sign of progression after 5 years of follow-up. No femoral radiolucencies were observed. At final follow-up, 14 knees showed asymptomatic (without any change in the clinical score) osteoarthritis progression in the patellofemoral compartment. With revision for any reason as the endpoint, 17-year survivorship was 0.78 (95% confidence interval: 0.73–0.83) (Fig. 12.6). In four cases, avulsion of the anterior tibial spine was observed intraoperatively, requiring intraoperative fixation using synthesis by screw or/and non-absorbable suture. In these knees, there were no adverse effects on the final outcome (Fig. 12.7). No other intraoperative complication occurred. Twelve patients had postoperative deep venous thromboses and were treated with a therapeutic dose of low-molecular-weight heparin. For 17 knees, a revision was required at a mean of 6.5 years (range: 9 months to 12 years): 16 for aseptic loosening and one for a symptomatic progression of osteoarthritis in the patellofemoral compartment. Among the 16 cases of aseptic loosening, eight involved loosening of both the medial and lateral implants, five of the medial implant, and three of the lateral one. Ten knees were revised using a conventional postero-stabilized TKA with a tibial stem, and eight knees with a hinged prosthesis. One knee was revised for progression of osteoarthritis in the patellofemoral compartment at 10 years, by addition of a patellofemoral implant. In this patient, a good result was achieved at the final follow-up of 15 years.

12.6 Conclusions

Bicompartmental knee arthroplasty, as a bone- and ligament-sparing technique, provides good functional results and a high rate of satisfaction. In our series, excellent long-term clinical and radiological outcomes were achieved, with a survivorship similar to that of classic unicompartmental knee arthroplasty using the older generation of implants. Use of the newest implants and ancillaries may optimize long-term follow-up, even if the proper indications and an adequate surgical technique continue to be the main determinant of success. As the preservation of a functional ACL remains the key to success, particular care should be given to the tibial spines, which are at risk throughout the procedure.

References

1. Dennis MG, DiCesare PE (2003) Surgical management of the middle age arthritic knee. Bull Hosp Jt Dis 61:172-178
2. Flecher X, Parratte S, Aubaniac JM, Argenson JN (2006) A 12-28-year follow-up study of closing wedge high tibial osteotomy. Clin Orthop Relat Res 452:91-96
3. Hanssen AD, Stuart MJ, Scott RD, Scuderi GR (2001) Surgical options for the middle-aged patient with osteoarthritis of the knee joint. Instr Course Lect 50:499-511
4. Pagnano MW, Clarke HD, Jacofsky DJ, Amendola A, Repicci JA (2005) Surgical treatment of the middle-aged patient with arthritic knees. Instr Course Lect 54:251-259
5. Sohn DH, Toth AP (2008) Meniscus transplantation: current concepts. J Knee Surg 21:163-172
6. Stuart MJ, Lubowitz JH (2006) What, if any, are the indications for arthroscopic debridement of the osteoarthritic knee? Arthroscopy 22:238-239
7. Berger RA, Meneghini RM, Sheinkop MB, Della Valle CJ, Jacobs JJ, Rosenberg AG, Galante JO (2004) The progression of patellofemoralarthrosis after medial unicompartmental replacement: results at 11 to 15 years. Clin Orthop Relat Res 92-99
8. Fuchs S, Tibesku CO, Frisse D, Genkinger M, Laass H, Rosenbaum D (2005) Clinical and functional comparison of uni- and bicondylar sledge prostheses. Knee Surg Sports Traumatol Arthrosc 13:197-202
9. Confalonieri N, Manzotti A, Cerveri P, DeMomi E (2009) Bi-unicompartmental versus total knee arthroplasty: a matched paired study with early clinical results. Arch Orthop Trauma Surg 129:1157-63
10. Engh GA (2007) A bi-compartmental solution: what the Deuce? Orthopedics 30:770-771
11. Fuchs S, Tibesku CO, Genkinger M, Laass H, Rosenbaum D (2003) Proprioception with bicondylar sledge prostheses retaining cruciate ligaments. Clin Orthop Relat Res 148-154
12. Fuchs S, Tibesku CO, Genkinger M, Volmer M, Laass H, Rosenbaum D (2004) Clinical and functional comparison of bicondylar sledge prostheses retaining all ligaments and constrained total knee replacement. Clin Biomech (Bristol, Avon) 19:263-269
13. Insall J, Walker P (1976) Unicondylar knee replacement. Clin Orthop Relat Res 83-85
14. Insall JN, Dorr LD, Scott RD, Scott WN (1989) Rationale of the Knee Society clinical rating system. Clin Orthop Relat Res 13-14
15. Argenson JN, Chevrol-Benkeddache Y, Aubaniac JM (2002) Modern unicompartmental knee arthroplasty with cement: a three to ten-year follow-up study. J Bone Joint Surg Am 84:2235-2239
16. Argenson JN, Komistek RD, Aubaniac JM, Dennis DA, Northcut EJ, Anderson DT, Agostini S (2002) In vivo determination of knee kinematics for subjects implanted with a unicompartmentalarthroplasty. J Arthroplasty 17:1049-1054
17. Cloutier JM, Sabouret P, Deghrar A (1999) Total knee arthroplasty with retention of both cruciate ligaments. A nine to eleven-year follow-up study. J Bone Joint Surg Am 81:697-702
18. Goodfellow JW, O'connor J (1986) Clinical results of the Oxford Knee: surface arthroplasty of the tibi-

ofemoral joint with a meniscal bearing prosthesis. Clin Orthop Relat Res 21-42
19. Andriacchi TP, Galante JO, Fermier RW (1982) The influence of total knee-replacement design on walking and stair-climbing. J Bone Joint Surg Am 64:1328-1335
20. Komistek RD, Allain J, Anderson DT, Dennis DA, Goutallier D (2002) In vivo kinematics for subjects with and without an anterior cruciate ligament. Clin Orthop Relat Res 404:315-325
21. Rolston L, Bresch J, Engh G, Franz A, Kreuzer S, Nadaud M, Puri L, Wood D (2007) Bicompartmental knee arthroplasty: a bone-sparing, ligament-sparing, and minimally invasive alternative for active patients. Orthopedics 30:70-73
22. Stiehl JB, Komistek RD, Cloutier JM, Dennis DA (2000) The cruciate ligaments in total knee arthroplasty: a kinematic analysis of 2 total knee arthroplasties. J Arthroplasty 15:545-550
23. Banks SA, Fregly BJ, Boniforti F, Reinschmidt C, Romagnoli S (2005) Comparing in vivo kinematics of unicondylar and bi-unicondylar knee replacements. Knee Surg Sports Traumatol Arthrosc 13:551-556
24. Ahlback S (1968) Osteoarthrosis of the knee. A radiographic investigation. Acta Radiol Diagn 277:7-72
25. Gibson PH, Goodfellow JW (1986) Stress radiography in degenerative arthritis of the knee. J Bone Joint Surg Br 68:608-609
26. Argenson JN, Flecher X, Parratte S, Aubaniac JM (2005) Patellofemoralarthroplasty: an update. Clin Orthop Relat Res 440:50-53
27. Argenson JN, Guillaume JM, Aubaniac JM (1995) Is there a place for patellofemoralarthroplasty? Clin Orthop Relat Res 162-167
28. Argenson JN, Parratte S, Bertani A, Flecher X, Aubaniac JM (2008) Long-term results with a lateral unicondylar replacement. Clin Orthop Relat Res 466:2686-2693
29. Parratte S, Argenson JN, Dumas J, Aubaniac JM (2007) Unicompartmental knee arthroplasty for avascular osteonecrosis. Clin Orthop Relat Res 464:37-42
30. Cooke D, Scudamore A, Li J, Wyss U, Bryant T, Costigan P (1997) Axial lower-limb alignment: comparison of knee geometry in normal volunteers and osteoarthritis patients. Osteoarthritis Cartilage 5:39-47
31. Cooke TD, Scudamore RA, Bryant JT, Sorbie C, Siu D, Fisher B (1991) A quantitative approach to radiography of the lower limb.Principles and applications. J Bone Joint Surg Br 73:715-720
32. Petrie A(2006) Statistics in orthopaedic papers. J Bone Joint Surg Br 88:1121-1136
33. Kaplan E, Meier P (1958) Nonparametric observation from incomplete observations. J Am Stat Assoc 53:457-481

13 Arthrosurface Inlay Resurfacing: Indications, Surgical Technique, and Results

Anthony Miniaci

13.1 Introduction

Cartilage lesions in the knee are common [1] and can be highly symptomatic [2-4]. The biological treatment spectrum offers a wide range of cartilage procedures that address these lesions from different perspectives: Palliative interventions (debridement) aim at lesion stabilization and the removal of mechanical symptoms. Reparative (marrow stimulation techniques), restorative (chondral, osteochondral transplantation), and reconstructive (allograft, prosthetics) procedures target defect filling and surface reconstructions, while corrective procedures (osteotomy) take aim at the underlying disease process. All but palliative and prosthetic reconstructive measures require prolonged rehabilitation to ensure adequate biological response, remodeling, and healing.

In individuals of advanced age, with longer-standing symptoms and a surgical history, the transition from biological procedures to joint arthroplasty is not well established because prosthetic design concepts of conventional joint replacement do not fulfill the requirements of early intervention; rather, they provide a solution for delayed treatment. The fundamental goal is to maximize implant longevity. Very good long-term results have been published [5-8], yet conventional arthroplasty is not without controversy: onlay surface replacements introduce a non-native joint surface geometry, which has implications for pain relief, functional outcomes, and implant survivorship. High-demand patients, such as younger, more active populations as well as heavy and morbidly obese patients, have inferior clinical outcomes combined with higher revision rates [7-10]. While the delay strategy may work on an individual basis, today many patients are seeking solutions that allow them to return to work and active lifestyles.

First-intervention metallic prosthetics should follow the treatment concepts of biological procedures: a minimally invasive approach, joint preservation through maintenance of healthy soft tissues and bone stock, and biomechanical stability combined with a new contoured joint surface that counteracts lesion propagation.

Since 2003, a knee resurfacing platform (Arthrosurface, Franklin, MA) has been developed that is consistent with the paradigm of joint preservation. Moreover, it allows the surgeon to address joint arthrosis with a contoured metallic implant that is thin, sized to the lesion, and specific to the joint surface of the patient. The 66 different sizes and shapes (47 different metallic ones for the knee and a corresponding set of 19 polyethylene component choices) provide the first step in arthroplasty under the continuum of care for joint arthrosis and arthritis (Fig. 13.1). All metallic components are made of a CoCr alloy and have Ti coverage where they interface with bone (screw fixation, undersurface of the articular component); the polyethylene components are ultra-high-molecular-weight polyethylene (UHMWPE) and are cemented into the prepared implant bed.

A. Miniaci (✉)
Orthopedic Surgery
Cleveland Clinic Sports Health Center
Garfield Heights, OH, USA
E-mail: miniaca@ccf.org

N. Confalonieri, S. Romagnoli (eds.), *Small Implants in Knee Reconstruction*,
DOI 10.1007/978-88-470-2655-1_13, © Springer-Verlag Italia 2013

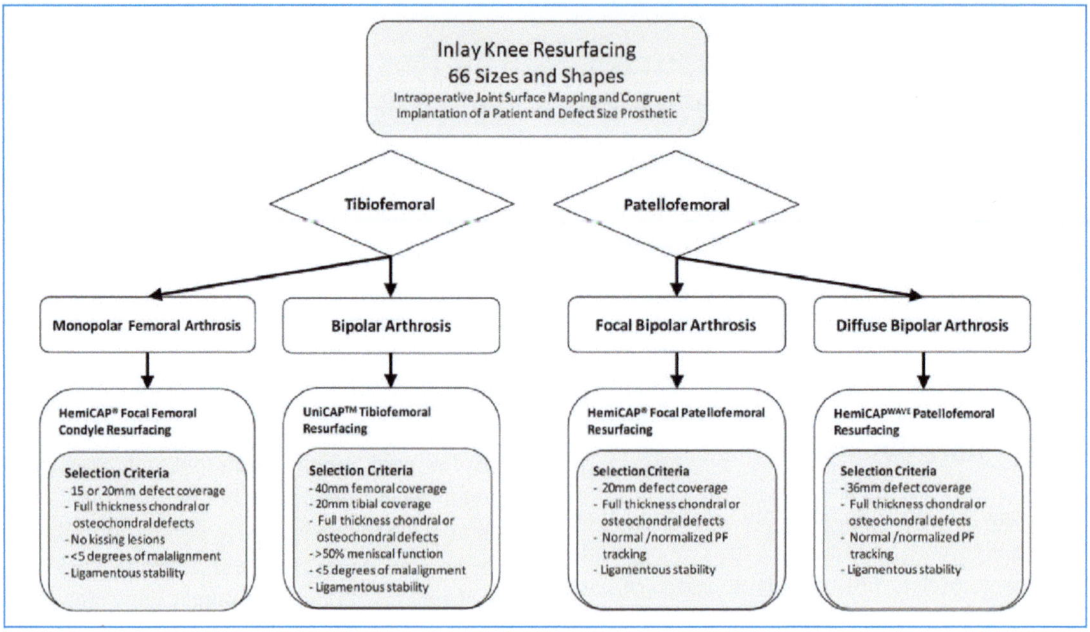

Fig. 13.1 Inlay knee resurfacing platform for tibiofemoral and patellofemoral mono- and bipolar arthrosis

Table 13.1 Technical pearls for inlay knee resurfacing

1.	Manage patient expectations and educate on early focal resurfacing vs. delayed total arthroplasty.
2.	Ensure adequate implant defect coverage.
3.	Recess implant components slightly below the articular surface (0.5–1.0 mm) to avoid damage to the opposing articular surfaces.
4.	Careful intraoperative mapping of the defect needs to be undertaken in order to match the prosthetic implant curvature to the native articular surface.
5.	Ensure uniform cement coverage surrounding components.
6.	Inlay components do not correct the mechanical tibiofemoral alignment.

Basic science [11-14] and clinical outcomes [15-18] complement each other and support this platform for the treatment of chondral and osteochondral defects. Inlay resurfacing is not a replacement of existing cartilage repair procedures; rather, it is an extension of reconstructive methods with the support of individual patient management. The key aspects that should be considered when performing inlay resurfacing are listed in Table 13.1.

13.2 Monopolar Focal Femoral Condyle Inlay Resurfacing

Focal femoral condyle prosthetic resurfacing continues localized management of full-thickness chondral and osteochondral lesions and expands the range of precursor biological treatment options. Successor procedures such as unicondylar knee replacement provide a sound clinical exit strategy when larger surface reconstruction is warranted.

This interim treatment solution for patients between 40 and 60 years of age provides a biomechanically stable, congruent defect-filling designed to protect the remaining normal cartilage. It consists of two components, an articular component and a fixation component (Fig. 13.2), joined by a morse taper interlock. The cobalt chrome 15- or 20-mm articular components are both available in a variety of incremental offset convexities corresponding to the surface curvature of the patient's condyle.

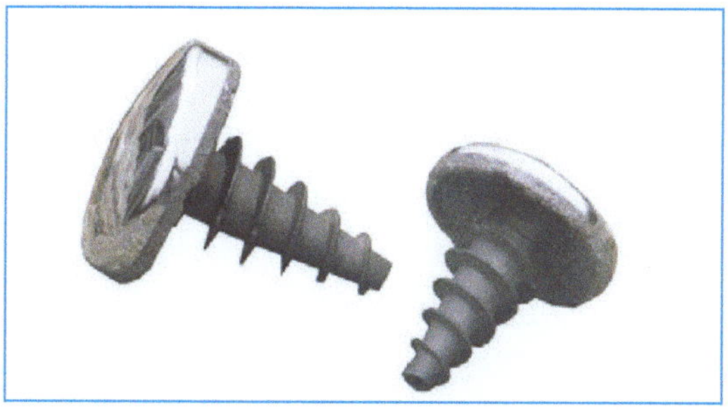

Fig. 13.2 Examples of HemiCAP focal inlay resurfacing prosthetics: high-pitched screw fixation component and modular, contoured articular component

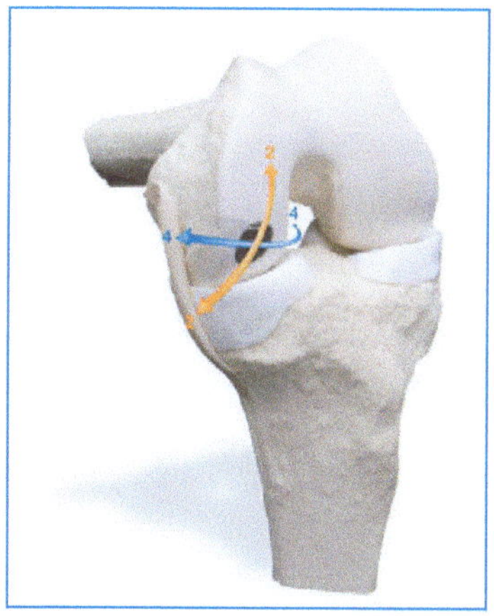

Fig. 13.3 Intraoperative 3-D surface mapping using the HemiCAP system

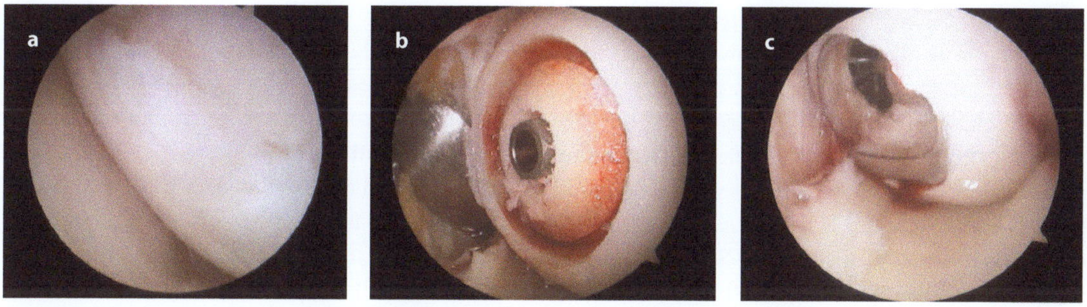

Fig. 13.4 Example of HemiCAP focal femoral condyle resurfacing after failed microfracture, medial femoral condyle. **a** Defect filling after prior microfracture, resulting in soft, fissured repair cartilage. **b** Implant bed with screw fixation in center. **c** HemiCAP focal resurfacing implant with slightly recessed implant margins

13.2.1 Surgical Technique

A small para-patellar incision is made over the defect through which the device is implanted on the medial or lateral femoral condyle. Using a drill guide and pin, the surgeon establishes a perpendicular working access to the joint surface and drives a cannulated step drill into the bone until the proximal shoulder of the drill is flush to the articulating surface. The fixation component is placed at the correct height under visual control and the patient-specific joint surface curvature is measured intraoperatively (Fig. 13.3). The implant socket is prepared using precision surface milling. A sizing trial allows for proper assessment of the cartilage–implant interface. The final articular component is aligned on the implant holder and inserted into the taper of the fixation component. Progressive tapping on the impactor engages the articular and fixation components. Final placement of the surface prosthetic is targeted slightly recessed (0.5–1.0 mm) to the surrounding articular cartilage to account for nearby cartilage thickness variations during weight-bearing, thereby avoiding any overloading or deleterious effects to the opposing side (Fig. 13.4).

13.2.2 Results

Kirker-Head et al. reported on the biocompatibility of this implant in the caprine model [11]. A continuous trabecular and subchondral bone interface was observed surrounding both the screw and the resurfacing unit. Cartilage flow from the adjacent native tissue covered the implant-cartilage interface. Several clinical studies of

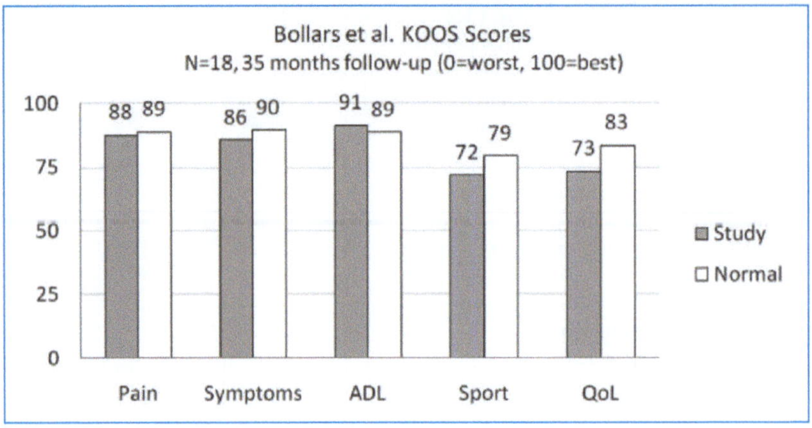

Fig. 13.5 35-month follow-up KOOS scores comparing focal femoral condyle resurfacing to normative, age-matched values (from [20])

the HemiCAP focal femoral condyle resurfacing prosthesis have been undertaken to date, showing encouraging results with a follow-up of up to 6 years.

Von Hasselbach and Witzel reported on 121 patients with a mean age 52.5 years in whom the HemiCAP resurfacing prosthesis was implanted, with a mean follow-up in this series of 14 months [19]. The follow-up Hospital for Special Surgery (HSS) score was high (95.3), with an increase of 12% from baseline. Second-look arthroscopies performed for non-device related indications showed no deleterious cartilage effects on opposing articular surfaces. Radiographs showed no peri-prosthetic radiolucency or implant subsidence.

Thirty-six patients in the prospective US phase II multicenter feasibility trial have completed their 2-year follow-up. Forty patients (26 males, 14 females), with an average age of 47 years, were treated with the device: 38 for isolated full-thickness defects of the medial femoral condyle and two for defects on the lateral side. Two patients were lost to follow-up, one died before the 2-year endpoint, and in one conversion to unicondylar knee replacement was necessary. The average preoperative WOMAC domains showed significant baseline pain (308) and functional deficiencies (999) that had improved remarkably by 3 months after the procedure (pain 68, function 246). The average results showed further improvement across all domains from 1 to 2 years postoperatively. The mean total WOMAC score was best at the 2-year follow-up time point and had improved from 1436 preoperatively to 341.

Bollars et al. studied 18 patients with an average age of 51 years in whom the study device was implanted and found excellent results at a follow-up of 35.3 months [16]. In these middle-aged patients, 83% had a normal or nearly normal IKDC score. Compared to normative age-matched scores, in the study patients there was a close match across all KOOS domains (Fig. 13.5).

Becher et al. studied 21 patients with a mean age of 54 years at the time of the initial focal resurfacing. The minimum follow-up was 5 years (range: 5–6 years) [15]. The authors demonstrated radiographic joint space preservation and statistically significant improvements across all KOOS score subdomains, Tegner score, and SF-36 score.

To date, examples from second-look arthroscopies have confirmed the preclinical results. The prosthetic appears to be well incorporated; the superficial cartilage layer from adjacent healthy margins covers the implant cartilage interface; and opposing tibial surfaces have not shown any apparent response to the contoured prosthetic.

13.3 Bipolar Tibiofemoral Inlay Resurfacing

Bipolar knee inlay resurfacing was introduced in 2008 to provide an option for patients with early tibiofemoral arthrosis (Fig. 13.6). It is minimally invasive, preserves the menisci and

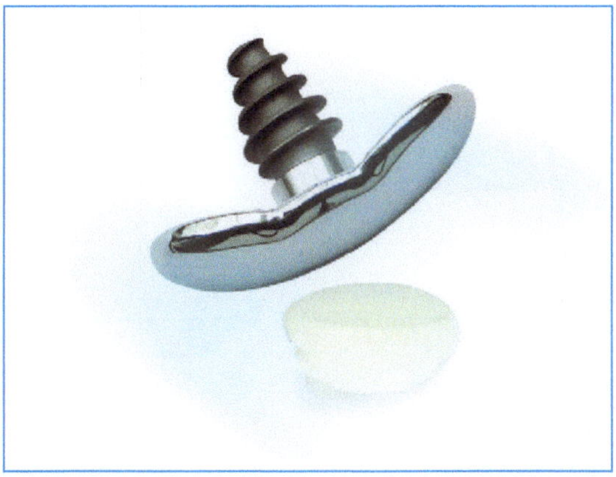

Fig. 13.6 The UniCAP meniscal-sparing unicondylar system

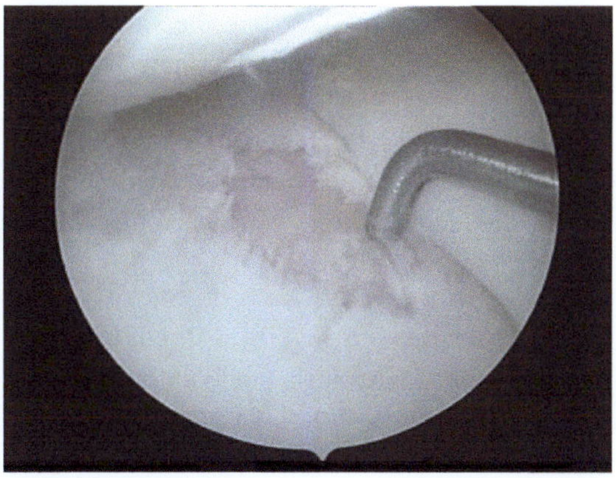

Fig. 13.7 Localized tibial defect

cruciate ligaments, and retains the bony architecture of the knee joint. Similar to the focal monopolar femoral condyle implants, the larger bipolar tibiofemoral implants come in a number of different surface convexities to allow for precise and contoured inlay resurfacing. Inherent to the technique, the tibiofemoral alignment cannot be changed with inlay implants. Therefore, the mechanical tibiofemoral axis has to be taken into consideration for indications and for surgical planning (Fig. 13.1).

13.3.1 Indications

The target population consists of middle-aged patients who have failed previous conservative treatment and/or surgical interventions and have re-developed significant pain, causing limitations in function and in the activities of daily living and requiring surgery for mono-compartmental arthrosis.

Preoperative clinical examination should show a stable knee with less than 5° of mechanical malalignment, range of motion with a deficit of less than 10° of flexion or 5° of extension, satisfactory meniscal function, and a normal to slightly overweight body mass index (BMI <30). If a patient considered for resurfacing has factors just outside these parameters, for example malalignment or ligamentous instability, these should be dealt with prior to or in conjunction with the UniCAP procedure. When more than one risk factor is present, consideration needs to be given to the compounding effect when determining patient indications and expectations.

Contraindications for the procedure include metabolic disorders affecting implant fixation, bony deformation, mechanical malalignment affecting the ipsilateral compartment, high BMI >30, and widespread degeneration that cannot be covered by the prosthesis. Patients need to be carefully selected, on an individual basis (Fig. 13.1), taking into account both their expectations and the demands of their activities.

13.3.2 Surgical Technique

The patient is positioned and prepared for standard knee arthroscopy allowing for deep knee flexion during femoral preparation. The anterolateral portal is established first, as it improves visualization of the medial compartment (Fig. 13.7). Once the proper indication is confirmed, a full-length anteromedial skin incision is placed vertically 1 cm medial to the patella tendon and extending proximally from the mid-pole of the patella down to 1 cm distal to the joint line. Capsular integrity is maintained by limiting the capsulotomy to the anteromedial portal for the arthroscopic tibial preparation. The full-length skin incision is made initially in order to aid in tissue dissection and avoid challenges associated with extravasation during arthroscopy. Extending the skin incision distally below the joint line facilitates exposure and avoids posterior pin deviation and skin interference during reaming of the posterior femoral implant bed. Once concomitant findings have been addressed, attention is directed towards the tibial defect.

13.3.2.1 Arthroscopic Tibial Resurfacing

Normal knee kinematics include a tibial rollback phenomenon during knee flexion whereby access to the tibial plateau can become challenging. Consequently, arthroscopically assisted tibial preparation greatly facilitates visualization and work flow.

With the knee in 20–30° of flexion and valgus stress, the tibial templates are trialed through the anteromedial incision until the underside curvature matches the plateau surface with full contact in all planes. An overly anterior or posterior placement of the tibial component should be avoided and a bony rim (≥ 5mm) maintained around the implant. This will protect tibial plateau stability and minimize the risk of reaming through the anterior cortex.

The tibial drill guide is attached and aligned front to back with the tibial plateau.

A small incision is made over the proximal anteromedial tibia, ensuring that the distal bullet is fully engaged into the cortical bone and that the tibial template is parallel to the tibial plateau. A drill pin is placed through the center of the tibial template, defining the axis of the tibial tunnel. Care must be taken to maintain the proper axis without excessive torque, to avoid pin deviation. The tibial pilot drill is advanced over the drill pin into the center of the tibial defect and then removed. The introducer, driver, and blade stop are assembled and advanced into the prepared tunnel until the tip of the introducer is flush with the tibial plateau. The introducer and driver are then removed, leaving the blade stop set at the appropriate depth for reaming the tibial implant. A blade drive shaft is moved through the tunnel and connected to the tibial cutting blade, which is introduced through the anteromedial portal.

A high speed drill is used with an initial counterclockwise rotation to ensure an even cutting engagement into the plateau. Preparation of the tibial implant bed through clockwise rotation is completed when the cutting blade reaches the proximal end of the blade stop. A congruent, slightly recessed fit of the tibial component is verified with the appropriate sizing trial while the tibial cutter remains in place. Proud margins are lowered by adjusting the blade stop clockwise with a wrench: a 90° turn lowers the blade stop and implant floor by 1 mm after re-reaming. Before the final tibial implant is placed, attention is directed to the preparation of the femoral component.

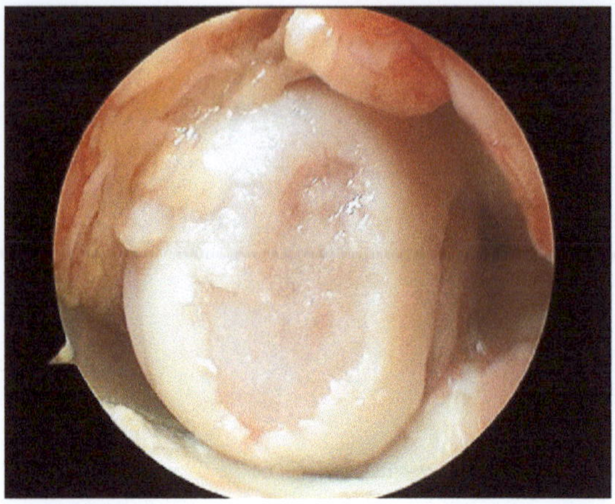

Fig. 13.8 Degenerative defect of the medial femoral condyle

13.3.2.2 Femoral Resurfacing

The femoral drill guide is placed over the defect (Fig. 13.8) with four points of contact to establish a perpendicular working axis to the joint surface. Adequate defect coverage is confirmed and a threaded pin is advanced into the bone. The femoral centering shaft is driven over the pin until the laser mark line is flush with the original articular surface. The 40-mm contact probe is placed over the femoral centering shaft to map the anterior-posterior (AP) curvature; medial-lateral (ML) mapping is repeated with the 20-mm contact probe. The average medial-lateral offset will determine the appropriate central femoral reamer, which is advanced over the centering shaft until it contacts the stop. All instruments are removed and the appropriate guide block is selected based on the average anterior-posterior offsets. The

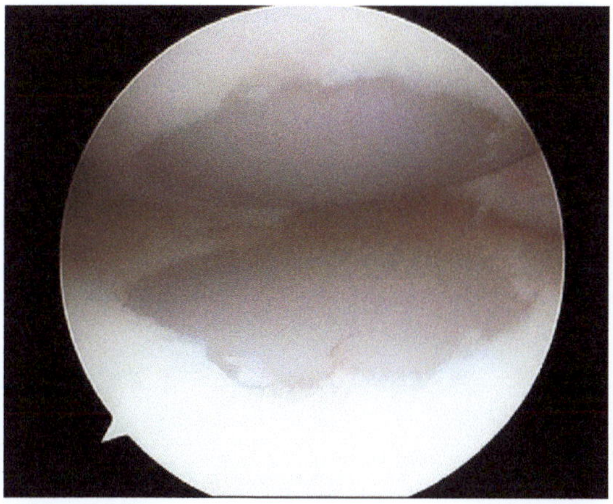

Fig. 13.9 Final tibiofemoral inlay resurfacing components

guide block is attached to the femoral drill guide and realigned on the distal femur under four points of contact to ensure accurate guide pin placement. Pin sleeves are inserted into the guide block. Both the anterior pin and subsequently the posterior short threaded pin are advanced into the bone to the level of the laser mark line. The guide block and pin sleeves are removed and proper pin alignment is confirmed. Analogous to the central reamer, the posterior implant bed is reamed based on the average medial-lateral offsets, followed by the anterior implant bed. Both reamers have a pin stop that is visible through the slotted window in the reamer shaft. Slightly recessed implant margins are confirmed with the corresponding femoral sizing trial. The femoral pilot drill is advanced through the sizing trial handle to the level of the laser mark line and left in place. The handle is removed and the femoral step drill is advanced over the femoral pilot drill down to the stop in the slotted window. The pilot hole is tapped and the fixation component is inserted into the sizing trial handle and advanced into the bone with the hex driver.

The final tibial implant is cemented first, before the final femoral component is implanted. The tibial component is inserted into the implant bed and both suture and suture retriever are passed through the tibial tunnel exiting on the distal drill hole. A slotted driver is used to adjust the final axial rotation of the tibial poly implant. A cement injector is advanced through the distal tibial tunnel. The tibial implant bed and tunnel are cemented under pressure, ensuring an even fixation and support column for the tibial component. A small amount of bone cement is applied to the underside of the femoral articular component and impacted engaging the morse taper between the components (Fig. 13.9).

13.3.3 Rehabilitation

Peri-operative narcotics and intra-articular local anesthetics can be used for immediate postoperative pain control [21, 22]. Cold compresses are helpful in reducing pain and swelling in the first 48 h following the procedure.

Weight-bearing as tolerated is encouraged for 2–6 weeks while slowly weaning off crutches. Range of motion exercises are started immediately, either through home exercise or formal physical therapy. A continuous passive motion machine several times a day for the first 2 weeks can also be used but is not required. Strengthening begins as soon as pain and swelling will allow. Patients should not return to sporting or other high-demand activities until a full range of motion is achieved, with no pain or swelling evident.

13.3.4 Results

Miniaci et al. presented the findings of their prospective series at the 2011 ISAKOS meeting [23]. Thirty-eight patients with a mean age of 48 years underwent surgery performed on an outpatient basis. The average follow-up was 19 months (range: 12–27 months). KOOS subcomponent scores showed statistically significant improvement on pain, symptoms, activities, and sports (Fig. 13.10). The average VAS pain score was reduced from 6.9 to 2.7 at the last follow-up. Postoperative range of motion returned to normal in 89% of the knees within the first 6 weeks postoperatively. No loosening or mechanical failure was observed during follow-up. Radiographically, there was no case of implant subsidence, prosthetic disengagement, or periprosthetic cyst formation.

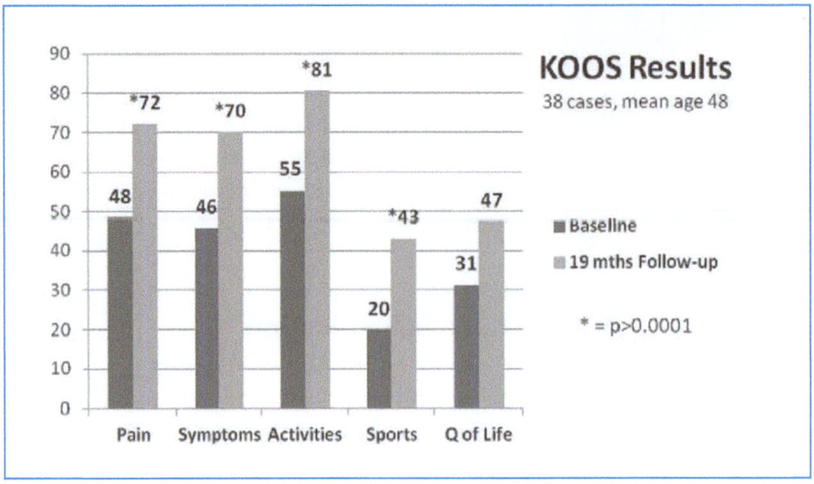

Fig. 13.10 Prospective KOOS component score improvement at 19 months follow-up after tibiofemoral UniCAP resurfacing

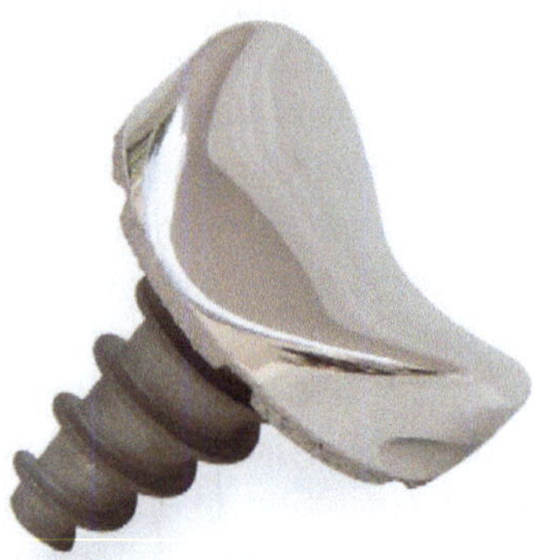

Fig. 13.11 Trochlear component of the focal HemiCAP patellofemoral resurfacing implant

13.4 Focal Bipolar Patellofemoral Inlay Resurfacing

The HemiCAP focal patellofemoral resurfacing prosthesis (Fig. 13.11) provides an extension of reconstructive procedures in patients with focal bipolar lesions in which patellofemoral arthroplasty would be too invasive.

Patellar and trochlear components are matched intraoperatively to the native geometry [14] and allow for congruent surface reconstruction in patients with focal traumatic or degenerative disease and failed prior biological procedures. A detailed description of the surgical technique was previously published [14,18]. The authors reported that the procedure allowed for restoration or maintenance of normal biomechanics while minimizing the amount of bony resection.

Patellofemoral (PF) kinematics were evaluated following inlay resurfacing of the trochlea on eight fresh-frozen cadaveric knee specimens using a real-time pressure sensor pad (Tekscan, Boston, MA) [17]. Each specimen was tested in three different conditions, intact, defect, and inlay resurfacing, which were assessed for PF contact area, peak contact pressure, and peak force. In the defect state, peak contact force increased from 13 to 18 N and peak contact pressure from 23 to 31 kg/cm^2. Edge loading and peak contact forces were highest in the periphery of the lesion. Following resurfacing, peak contact force and pressure were restored to 88% and 90% compared to the intact state while contact area was restored to 85% of normal. Results from this investigation support the importance of a congruent defect-filling in the patellofemoral joint. The authors concluded that, despite the inherent challenges, limited trochlear resurfacing achieved anatomic re-approximation of the PF surface and knee contact pressures. Clinical studies are ongoing, evaluating 2- to 5-year results.

13.5 HemiCAP^{Wave} Resurfacing Arthroplasty

Due to the complex surface morphology of the PF joint and the high transarticular pressures,

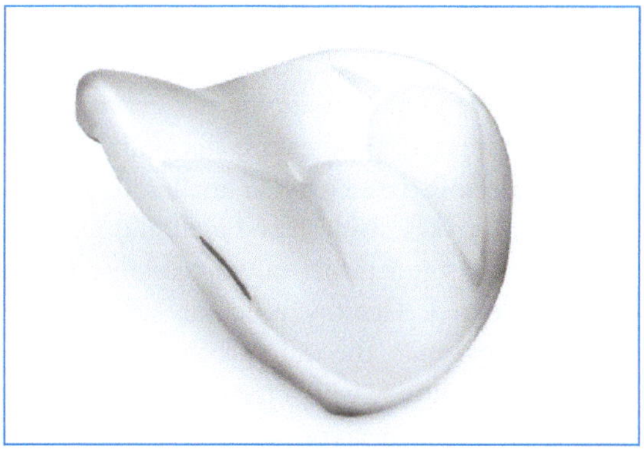

Fig. 13.12 HemiCAP^{Wave} trochlear component

biological treatment options have not achieved consistent results. Onlay versus inlay PF arthroplasty continues to be a source of controversy, despite the advantages of native joint surface geometry with inlays. In order to achieve successful outcomes with any type of PF arthroplasty, the underlying pathology has to be carefully assessed and should be taken into account in the treatment plan. The goal remains to avoid overstuffing the PF joint and to re-establish normal PF tracking in a smooth and congruent central compartment.

The HemiCAP^{Wave} resurfacing provides a thin, anatomical implant with a lateral flange and no overstuffing, due to congruent inlay implantation with curvatures measured specifically for each patient (Fig. 13.12). Despite its relatively recent introduction, the technique has gained rapid acceptance among knee surgeons treating patients with PF disease. Ongoing studies continue to evaluate the clinical benefits and the durability of the procedure.

13.5.1 Surgical Technique

13.5.1.1 Trochlear Resurfacing

With the knee in extension, the offset drill guide is used to establish a perpendicular working axis to the central trochlear surface. A guide pin is advanced into the bone to accommodate the contact probe for surface mapping and measurement of superior/inferior and medial/lateral offsets. The latter determines the corresponding central reamer, which is advanced until the outer edge mark

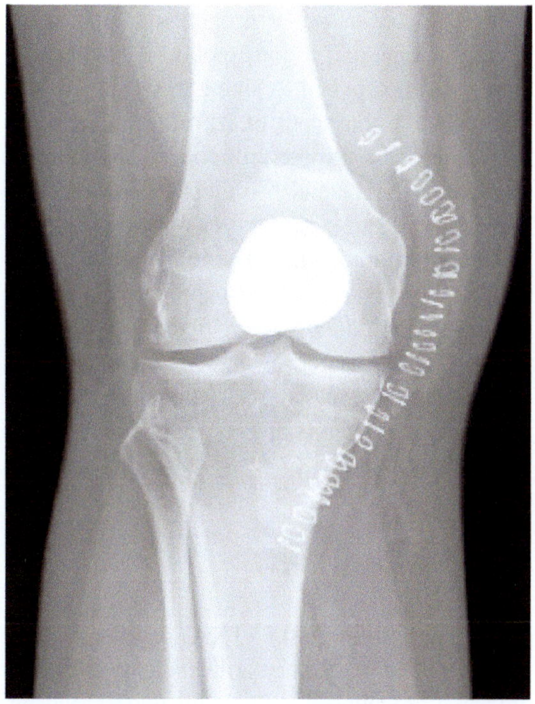

Fig. 13.13 Postoperative AP radiograph following HemiCAP^{Wave} resurfacing

is flush with the medial and lateral facets. The results of superior/inferior mapping determine the appropriate guide block, which is secured in the trochlear groove. A set of guide block reamers prepares the implant bed. The fit of the congruent inlay to the surrounding articular surface is confirmed with a sizing trial. A step drill prepares the pilot hole for the insertion of the tapered screw fixation. The femoral resurfacing component is aligned on the implant holder and inserted into the prepared socket. The fixation and articular components are connected with the aid of the impactor, and the prosthetic is firmly seated in the trochlea (Fig. 13.13).

13.5.1.2 Patellar Resurfacing

An alignment guide provides target placement for the patellar component while the surgeon monitors the range of motion. The drill guide is placed over the marked location on the patella and a guide pin is inserted to establish a normal working axis. A cannulated drill is advanced over the guide pin to form a pilot hole into which the patellar centering shaft is placed with a power drill. The contact probe provides patellar offset measurements and a corresponding reamer prepares the implant bed. A sizing trial is again used to confirm a congruent fit with the implant cartilage interface. Proper component alignment is marked at the 12 and 6 o'clock positions. Two different contour configurations can be trialed to ensure optimal tracking. The inlay patellar component benefits from cement application onto the implant rather than cement placement into the socket. This ensures even cement distribution surrounding the patellar component. The final patellar component is aligned and cemented into the implant bed.

13.6 Discussion

Total knee arthroplasty (TKA) is an excellent choice in end-stage knee arthritis. However, less invasive procedures are gaining widespread acceptance, as evidenced by the rapid increase over the past decade in the number of unicompartmental knee arthroplasties (UKAs) performed each year. Riddle et al. [24] reported an average increase in UKAs of 32.5% from 1998 to 2005, while TKAs had increased by only 9.4%. Yet, UKAs only account for 8% of all knee arthroplasty procedures. The use of UKAs in the younger population is a matter of debate as the revision rate is reportedly twice as high as in TKAs [4, 25, 26]. In a study by Furnes et al. [25], the proportion of patients ≤ 60 years of age receiving a UKA was 29%; the 7-year implant survival rate was 75.7% compared to 86% for patients between the ages of 61 and 69 and 91.3% for those > 70 years of age. While a good option for older (>65 years), less active patients, those under 65 and those with an active lifestyle would benefit from a less invasive procedure that would retain UKA or TKA as a primary exit strategy.

The availability of custom-fitting implants specific to the defect size and contoured to fit the native surface geometry of the patient has opened new treatment strategies, thus avoiding an interruption or delay during the transition from biologic to metallic joint resurfacing. Inlay resurfacing has several biomechanical and clinical advantages: Important structures for normal knee kinematics, such as menisci, cruciate ligaments, and the native joint contour, are preserved. Transarticular pressure profiles are normalized, thus keeping the soft-tissue tension unaltered [12-14]. As a result, overstuffing is avoided and pain relief as well as functional outcomes are accordingly improved. Healthy articular surfaces are preserved and share the weight-bearing load with the implant contour, which has positive implications for implant survivorship. The cartilage loss in limited arthrosis is addressed with a new, contoured prosthetic surface that is secured within the implant bone bed and anchored with a high-pitched screw fixation, in turn reducing the risk of lesion propagation through the offloading effect at the defect perimeter.

This concept has been validated in several basic science studies. Kirker-Head et al. [11] assessed the functional and biological responses of focal femoral condyle resurfacing. One year after implantation, the histological data confirmed the biocompatibility of the device and its incorporation into the femoral condyle. Becher et al. evaluated transarticular tibiofemoral pressure profiles in a variety of settings and reported the biomechanical safety of the device [12, 13]. Provencher et al. studied PF kinematics after limited trochlear resurfacing and concluded that the prosthesis provides a unique and favorable alternative to earlier implant designs by re-establishing anatomic PF surface and knee contact pressures [14].

13.7 Conclusions

The introduction of small knee implants over the past decade has stimulated the discussion on the continuum of care for knee arthrosis and arthritis. Established biological procedures for focal cartilage repair have been expanded through new reconstructive procedures utilizing patient-specific prosthetic inlays that simultaneously address the pathology and preserve healthy tissues. These treatment strategies follow surgeon-driven joint preservation goals that are consistent with localized repair in early-intervention cartilage repair. The 2- to 5-year clinical results support

HemiCAP resurfacing as a viable treatment option, although larger patient series with long-term follow-up are needed to establish the full spectrum of clinical performance criteria and related outcomes.

References

1. Curl WW, Krome J, Gordon SE, Rushing J, Smith BP, Poehling G (1997) Cartilage Injuries: A Review of 31,516 Knee Arthroscopies. Arthroscopy 13:456-60
2. Wluka A, E, Ding, Jones G, Cicuttini FM (2005) The clinical correlates of articular cartilage defects in symptomatic knee osteoarthritis: a prospective study. Rheumatol 44:1311-1316
3. Davis-Tuck ML, Wluka AE, Wang Y et al (2008) The natural history of cartilage defects in people with knee osteoarthritis. Osteoarthritis Cartilage 16:337-342
4. Heir S, Nerhus TK, Røtterud JH, Løken S, Ekeland A, Engebretsen L, Arøen, A (2010) Focal Cartilage Defects in the Knee Impair Quality of Life as Much as Severe Osteoarthritis A Comparison of Knee Injury and Osteoarthritis Outcome Score in 4 Patient Categories Scheduled for Knee Surgery. Am J Sports Med 38(2):**231-237**
5. Lastad Lygre SH, Espehaug B, Havelin LI, Furnes O, Vollset SE (2010) Pain and function in patients after primary unicompartmental and total knee arthroplasty. J Bone Joint Surg 92A(18):2890-2897
6. Loughead JM, Malhan K, Mitchell SY, Pinder IM, McCaskie AW, Deehan DJ, Lingard EA (2008) Outcome following knee arthroplasty beyond 15 years. Knee 15(2):85-90
7. Rand JA, Trousdale RT, Ilstrup DM, Harmsen WS (2003) Factors Affecting the Durability of Primary Total Knee Prostheses. J Bone Joint Surg 85A: 259-265
8. Rand JA, Ilstrup DM (1991) Survivorship analysis of total knee arthroplasty. Cumulative rates of survival of 9200 total knee arthroplasties. J Bone Joint Surg 73A:397-409
9. Amin AK, Clayton R, Patton JT, Gaston M, Cook RE, Brenkel IJ (2012) Total knee replacement in morbildly obese patients: results of a prospective, mathed study. J Bone Joint Surg 94-B:Supp 6 in press
10. Julin J, Jämsen E, Puolakka T, Konttinen YT, Moilanen T (2010)Younger age increases the risk of early prosthesis failure following primary total knee replacement for osteoarthritis; a follow-up study of 32,019 total knee replacements in the Finnish Arthroplasty Register. Acta Orthopaed 81 (4):413-419
11. Kirker-Head CA, Van Sickle DC, Ek SW, McCool JC (2006) Safety of, and biological and functional response to, a novel metallic implant for the management of focal full- thickness cartilage defects: Preliminary assessment in an animal model out to 1 year. J Orthop Res 24(5):1095-1108
12. Becher C, Huber R, Thermann H, Paessler HH, Skrbensky G (2008) Effects of a contoured articular prosthetic device on tibiofemoral peak contact pressure: a biomechanical study. Knee Surg Sports Traumatol Arthrosc 16(1):56-63
13. Becher C, Huber R, Thermann H, Ezechieli L, Ostermeier S, Wellmann M, von Skrbensky (2011) Effects of a surface matching articular resurfacing device on tibiofemoral contact pressure: results from continuous dynamic flexion-extension cycles. Arch Orthop Trauma Surg 131:413-419
14. Provencher M, Ghodadra N, Verma N, Cole BJ, Zaire S, Shewman E, Bach B (2009) Patellofemoral Kinematics After Limited Resurfacing of the Trochlea. J Knee Surg 22:310-316
15. Becher C, Kalbe C, Thermann H, Paessler HH, Laprell H, Kaiser T, Fechner A, Bartsch S, Windhagen H, Ostermeier S (2011) Minimum 5 – year results of focal articular prosthetic resurfacing for the treatment of full-thickness articular cartilage defects in the knee. Arch Orthop Trauma Surg 131:1135-1143
16. Bollars P, Bosquet M, Vandekerckhove B, Hardeman F, Bellemans J (2012) Prosthetic inlay resurfacing for the treatment of focal, full thickness cartilage defects of the femoral condyle: a bridge between biologics and conventional arthroplasty. Knee Surg Sports Traumatol Arthros 20(9):1753-9
17. Davidson PA, Rivenburgh D (2008) Focal anatomic patellofemoral inlay resurfacing: theoretic basis, surgical technique, and case reports. Orthop Clin North Am 39(3):337-46
18. Cannon A, Stolley M, Wolf B, Amendola A (2008) Patellofemoral resurfacing arthroplasty: Literature review and description of a novel technique. Iowa Orthop J 28:42-8
19. von Hasselbach C, Witzel U (2007) Biomechanics and clinical results of focal HemiCAP® resurfacing in the femoral condyle. Poster Presentation. German Congress for Orthopaedics and Traumatology, Berlin
20. Paradowski et al (2006) Knee complaints vary with age and gender in the adult population: population-based reference based data for the knee injury and osteoarthritis outcome score (KOOS). BMC Musculoskelet Disord 7:38–45
21. Weiss JM, Noble PC, Conditt MA, Kohl HW, Roberts S, Cook KF, Gordon MJ, Mathis KB (2002) What Functional Activities Are Important to Patients With Knee Replacements? Clin Ortho Rel Res 404:172-188
22. Chirwa SS et al (1989) Intra-articular bupivacaine (Marcaine) after arthroscopic meniscectomy: a randomized double blind controlled study. Arthroscopy 5:33-35
23. Miniaci A, Arneja S, Jones M (2011) Clinical results of a novel knee resurfacing arthroplasty for focal osteoarthritis of the knee. ISAKOS
24. Riddle DL, Jiranek WA, McGlynn FJ (2008) Yearly incidence of Unicompartmental Knee Arthoplasty in the United States. J Arthroplasty 23(3):408-412

25. Furnes O, Espehaug B, Lie SA, Vollset SE, Engesaeter LB, Havelin LI (2007) Failure mechanisms after unicompartmental and tricompartmental primary knee replacement with cement. J Bone Joint Surg Am 89:519-25
26. Koskinen E, Eskelinen A, Paavolainen P, Pulkkinen P, Remes V (2008) Comparison of survival and cost-effectiveness between unicondylar arthroplasty and total knee arthroplasty in patients with primary osteoarthritis: a follow-up study of 50,493 knee replacements from the Finnish Arthroplasty Register. Acta Orthop 79:499-507

14 Isolated Patellofemoral Replacement

John Newman

14.1 Introduction

Isolated symptomatic patellofemoral arthritis (PFOA), which was considered rare in the past, has been reported in 8% of women and 2% of men over the age of 55 [1]. In addition, radiological changes in the absence of severe symptoms are even more frequent, despite the fact that many physicians do not take skyline radiographs. [2]. However the number of cases in which isolated patellofemoral replacement (PFR) is indicated remains small, probably about 1% of the cases that come to any form of knee replacement, despite the fact that anterior knee pain is the most common condition seen in a general knee clinic. This condition, which is usually benign and self limiting, should be managed primarily with physiotherapy, although some surgeons suggest that subtle instability can be corrected. However, the condition is definitely not an indication for PFR, which should almost always be reserved for patients with radiological evidence of arthritic change.

14.1.1 Diagnosis of PFOA

There is an amazing variation in the magnitude of the symptoms caused by established PFOA. Just as severe patellofemoral pain can be experienced by youngsters who seem to have pristine joints, many patients with gross radiological changes may suffer little in the way of pain though many have catching, even if pain is not a symptom. More commonly, patients present with anterior knee pain that tends to be aggravated by activity; particularly when it involves weight-bearing on a flexed knee. Stair climbing is usually painful and generally associated with grinding; kneeling and squatting are often impossible. Frequently the complaint is of locking or giving way and night pain is more common than in pure tibiofemoral arthritis. Often, however, it is in the relatively early stages of PFOA that patients experience the most pain, which may be intense and cause disability even if radiologically the disease is not particularly severe.

The diagnosis can usually be made on clinical grounds, with marked quadriceps wasting and other signs of retropatellar disease supporting the clinical history. Most patients will have retropatellar tenderness or pain on patellar compression either actively or passively. In addition, attempts to squat will usually cause pain and a full squat will be impossible to achieve. Radiological confirmation is usually easy as the disease can frequently be seen on the lateral X-ray, but this is not invariably the case; skyline views at around 30° give a better assessment [3]. In addition, it is sometimes useful to take skyline views in various degrees of flexion because the pathology may be much more obvious in one position than another (Fig. 14.1).

Infrequently, patients will have a convincing history and appropriate physical signs but still the pathology is difficult to demonstrate. In such cas-

J. Newman (✉)
Litfield House Medical Centre
Bristol, UK
E-mail: newmancorner@doctors.org.uk

N. Confalonieri, S. Romagnoli (eds.), *Small Implants in Knee Reconstruction*,
DOI 10.1007/978-88-470-2655-1_14, © Springer-Verlag Italia 2013

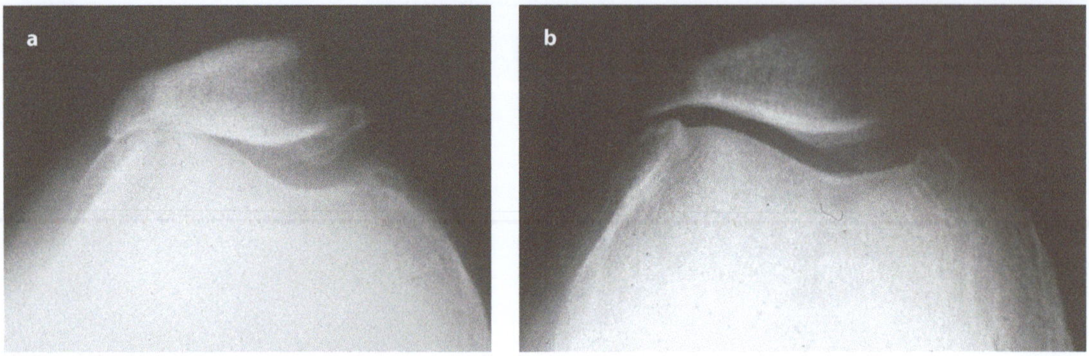

Fig. 14.1 **a, b** Skyline X-rays taken in different degrees of flexion, demonstrating the more obvious pathology in one knee than in the other

es, when confirmation is needed prior to surgery, magnetic resonance imaging can be useful, or the cartilage loss can be confirmed by preoperative arthroscopy [4]. Furthermore, severely dysplastic trochleas may create technical problems; in such cases 3D imaging of the trochlea might be helpful [5].

14.1.2 Alternative Treatments of PFOA

Non-operative treatment in the form of quadriceps-strengthening exercises can help since patients frequently have gross weakness and wasting. However, it is often impossible to build up wasted quadriceps musculature since attempting to do so aggravates the pain and prevents maximal effort.

As the disease usually affects the lateral facet of the patellofemoral joint, medialising the patella by taping or bracing can help, although this is usually not a satisfactory long-term solution. Articular steroid injections can alleviate exacerbations but do little for the long-term; likewise, hyaluronic acid injections seem only to have a short-lived benefit [6].

Multiple non-arthroplasty surgical treatments have been tried for PFOA . These include arthroscopic debridement, re-alignment procedures with or without anteriorisation, cartilage repair procedures, lateral facetectomy and patellectomy. A fairly recent review found these procedures to be largely unsatisfactory [7]. All have their advocates but there are few long-term reports or control studies, which makes evaluation difficult. However, it has been known for many years that patellectomy for isolated PFOA is unsatisfactory [8] and that extensor mechanism re-alignment for instability can result in arthritic changes [9]. Thus, as yet no conservative surgical treatment has proved universally satisfactory. It is against this background that the indications for isolated patellofemoral replacement must be viewed.

14.1.3 Indications for PFR

Precise indications are hard to define since PFOA presents in a variety of ways and patients with different stages of the disease will seek medical attention. In general, patients will have significant anterior knee pain that interferes with important activities, although many cope by avoiding aggravating activities and using a banister when on stairs. This, however, may not be acceptable to younger patients. All should have undergone a course of non-operative treatment, but it will frequently have failed. Whether conservative surgical treatments should be tried first in well-defined PFOA is a matter of opinion. In general, good quality results are less often achieved than with isolated PFR and patients often have a longer period of rehabilitation. Fortunately, such procedures, other than patellectomy, which should be avoided, do not compromise a subsequent arthroplasty option.

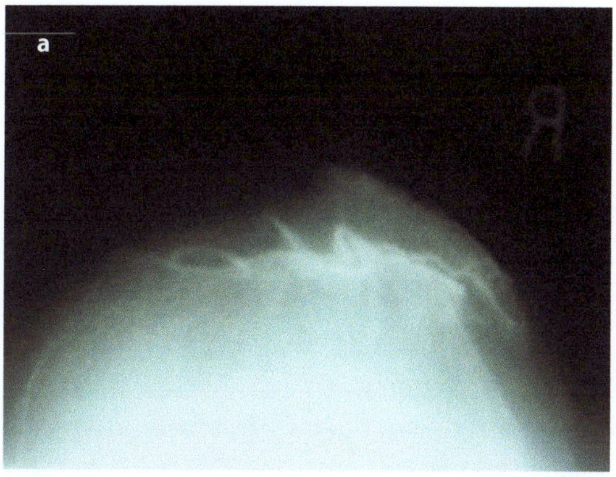

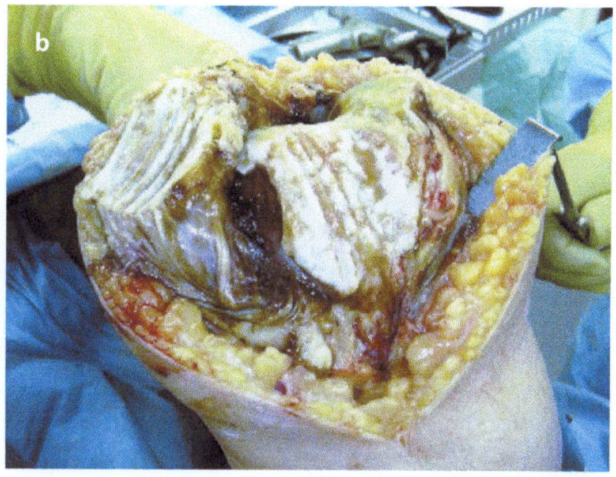

Fig. 14.2 a, b Skyline X-ray and operative picture of an elderly woman with gross ridging of the patellofemoral joint. The tibiofemoral joint was well preserved

There are thus several groups of patients with indications for isolated PFR but in all cases there should be a complete loss of articular cartilage on one, or preferably, both sides of the patellofemoral joint.

1. Severe PFOA in the elderly with excellent preservation of the tibiofemoral joint. If the patellofemoral disease is symmetrical this may be the first part of tricompartmental arthritis, such that accurate assessment of the tibiofemoral joint is essential if arthritic changes are not to develop at this site within a few years. Sometimes extremely severe disease can develop in the patellofemoral joint without tibiofemoral involvement (Fig. 14.2).
2. Lateral facet PFOA in the middle aged; probably the most common indication.
3. PFOA with associated extensor mechanism instability. These are usually cases of trochlear dysplasia in which the extensor mechanism tracks abnormally and wears out the lateral trochlear articular cartilage although no true dislocation has occurred.
4. PFOA with a chronically dislocated extensor mechanism, whether or not a patellectomy has been performed [10, 11] (Fig. 14.3).
5. Continuing pain after failed conservative surgery. In most series some 30% of patients have undergone previous surgery, usually involving an attempt to realign the extensor mechanism.

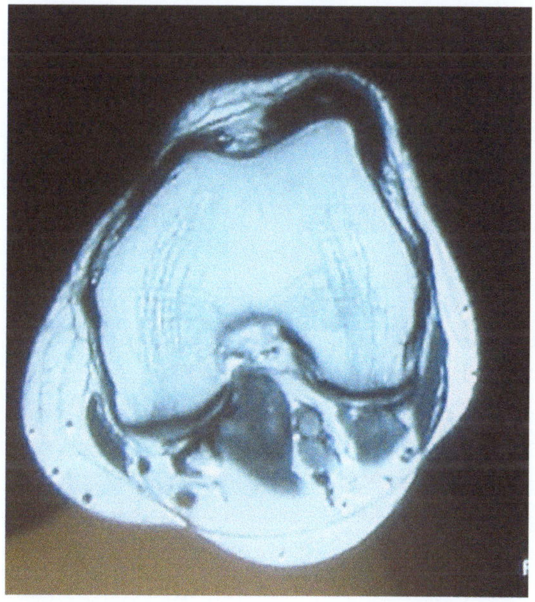

Fig. 14.3 Magnetic resonance imaging shows persistent subluxation of the patellar tendon following patellectomy. The tendon snapped painfully across the lateral femoral condyle with flexion and extension of the knee. The insertion of a trochlear component provided a groove and solved the problem

Indications 2–5 probably all have trochlear dysplasia as the underlying basis for the development of the arthritic change. Despite being well-described by the Lyon group [12], this condition was poorly recognised in the UK and USA until fairly recently. In Bristol, where the knee

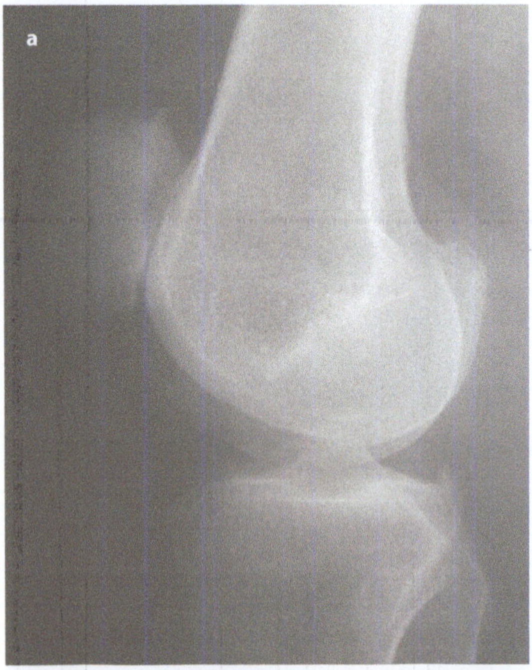
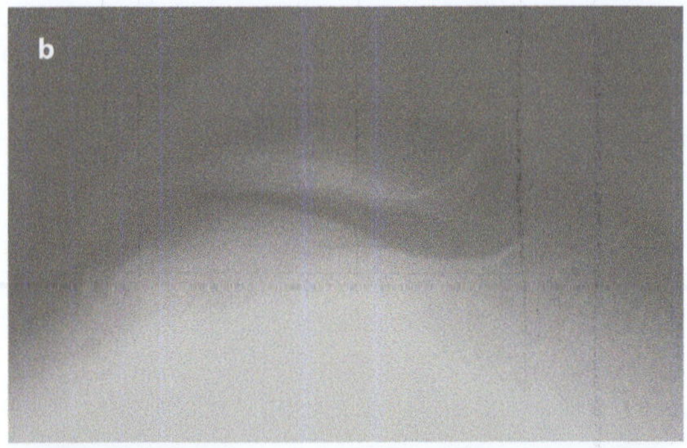
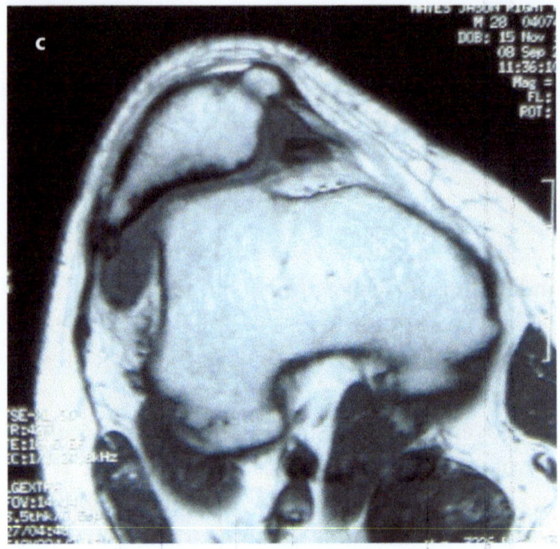
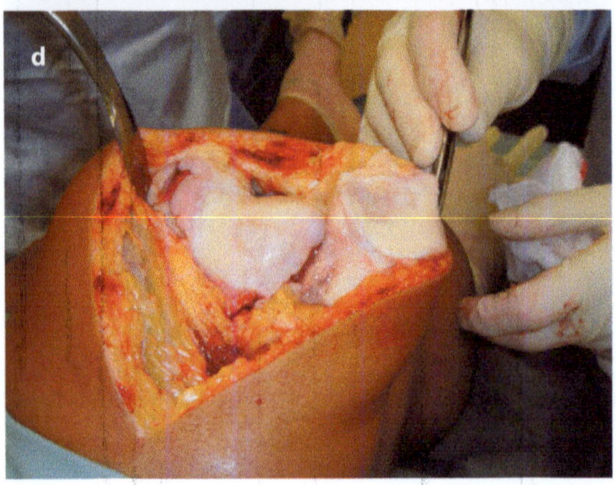

Fig. 14.4 **a, b** Lateral and skyline X-rays from a 29-year-old man with a severe patellofemoral disability who had undergone three previous realignment procedures. Mild subluxation persists but the severity of the lateral compartment cartilage damage is unclear. **c** Magnetic resonance imaging confirmed the subluxation and suggested both dysplasia and cartilage wear. **d** Intraoperatively, gross cartilage loss and wearing extending around onto the lateral aspect of the lateral femoral condyle were seen. Note also the mild trochlear bump and dysplasia. Note also that a lateral approach has been used to aid correction of the maltracking. Despite his extremely young age, he did well with a patellofemoral replacement

database now contains pathological data on over 700 knees that have undergone isolated PFR, the most frequently recorded pathological diagnosis is lateral facet osteoarthritis. This probably follows some instability or mal-tracking usually associated with a degree of dysplasia. However, up until the last few years trochlear dysplasia frequently went unnoticed, with the result that the diagnosis was not recorded [13]. In contrast, previous dislocation was recognised, because for many years it was known to be associated with PFOA, whether or not it had been treated by a realignment procedure [9]. However in recent years it has become apparent that trochlear dysplasia is a common precursor in patients requiring PFR. In fact, it is now regarded as the prime cause of PFOA, with the articular cartilage becoming worn due to the variable instability of the extensor mechanism associated with the dysplasia [14] (Fig. 14.4). It is also probable that this condition accounts for the not insignificant number of patients who have adolescent anterior knee pain and eventually go on to develop PFOA [15].

6. PFOA following fracture. Although patellar fracture is an important cause of isolated PFOA the number of cases seen is small considering the frequency with which patellar fractures occur. The Bristol Knee Database showed that in only 17 of the over 600 cases of PFR had there been a prior patellar fracture, so that clearly symptomatic arthritis rarely developed. This is probably because in young people the patellar is covered with a layer of articular cartilage that is thicker than in any other joint, which may help to avoid the rapid development of arthritic changes.
7. Persistent pain after patellectomy; this is not infrequent and is perhaps to be expected since removal of the patella addresses only one side of the joint and the extensor mechanism continues to rub against the often rough, arthritic trochlear surface.
8. Persistent anterior knee pain associated with posterior cruciate ligament deficiency that results in increased pressure on the patella. If possible, the posterior sag should be corrected but until recently surgery for posterior cruciate ligament deficiency was not universally successful, in which case persistent anterior knee pain can then be helped by PFR.
9. In association with a unicompartmental knee replacement in bicompartmental arthritis. There is an increasing trend towards preservation of the cruciate ligaments in order to improve knee function. Since the lateral compartment is seldom involved early in the arthritic process, merely replacing the medial and patellofemoral compartments either with two separate implants or a combined implant (Deuce) has some logic. The former has been done for many years in mainland Europe, often with satisfying results [16], while the latter procedure is gaining credence but long-term results are awaited.

Finally, it must again be stressed that isolated PFR is definitely not indicated for crippling anterior knee pain in young adults who have normal-looking articular cartilage. Moreover, no deformity can be corrected; the procedure should therefore be confined to patients who have normal limb alignment and no significant fixed flexion deformity.

14.2 Operative Technique

14.2.1 Incision

While the PFR can be performed through any standard knee replacement incision, the majority of surgeons utilise the medial parapatellar approach, as it is the one with which they are typically most familiar with. Mid or subvastus approaches can also be used if preferred. The incision should be based slightly proximal to that used for total knee replacement (TKR) and care must be taken to avoid damaging the meniscus or tibiofemoral articular cartilage. Although helpful, the patella does not need to be everted and a minimally invasive approach can be used; however, this is not recommended unless the surgeon is familiar with the technique of both minimally invasive incisions and PFR. The entire joint should be inspected. If necessary, the approach can easily be extended to allow a TKR in case unexpected damage to the tibio femoral joint is found.

A lateral incision should also be considered since most patients present with lateral patellofemoral disease that is often associated with extensor mechanism subluxation. This approach gives slightly less satisfactory access but in such circumstances seems sensible as the capsular incision performs the lateral release and can be left open if necessary. In addition, the need for a medial incision is avoided thus preserving quadriceps function. The skin incision can also be placed more laterally, thereby preserving normal sensation over the front of the knee. This is appreciated by patients when they must kneel, although following PFR few patients kneel with ease [17].

The disadvantages of a lateral incision are that most surgeons are less familiar with it; the approach is less satisfactory should a TKR be required; there is an increased risk of bleeding from the lateral genicular vessels; and a less well-defined capsular layer makes closure, when required, more difficult. For these reasons cross-marking of the capsule is recommended to aid alignment during closure. Furthermore, despite the relatively rare need for transfusion following PFR [18], it is probably wise to release the tourniquet before closure and to use a drain, depending on one's normal practice. In spite of these disadvantages, the use of a lateral incision can make dealing with a badly subluxed or dislocated extensor mechanism very much easier.

14.2.2 Implantation

The precise technique of implantation will vary with the implant being used but accurate alignment of the trochlear component must be achieved, paying particular attention to rotation. This is probably best assessed by using the long axis of the tibia as in TKR [19], although navigation or robotic systems may eventually prove beneficial [20]. It is important to preserve as much femoral bone as possible and to bear in mind that the lateral ridge may be relatively deficient, a factor that must be considered when setting the component rotation. There are as yet no reports of leaving the patella un-resurfaced, so this should not be done. The thickness of the patella should always be measured since a misshapen and extremely thin patella is frequently encountered. While it is desirable to leave 14 mm of bone this is not always possible. Care must be taken to avoid an asymmetric cut. Not infrequently, the button will need to be supported on a peripheral rim thus leaving a central defect that can be filled with bone graft or cement. In this way virtually all patellae can be resurfaced. The use of a patella augmentation button would be an option in an excessively thin patella. In patients who have undergone a previous patellectomy it is unnecessary to attempt reconstruction.

The ideal shape of the patellar button has yet to be determined. Most systems use an onlay button but inlay may prove to be at least as satisfactory although many arthritic patellae are extremely sclerotic such that achieving optimal seating may be difficult.

The vital part of the operation is ensuring that correct tracking occurs. A lateral release will be required in many more cases than in TKR. During exposure of the patella for resurfacing it is probably sensible to do a routine peripatellar release but more may be required. Two tests are useful to check that no lateral tracking persists. Firstly, the patella should track normally during flexion and extension of the knee (the rule of no thumb). Secondly, it should be possible to hold the patella in the middle of the trochlear groove, having turned it up through 90° (the flip test). If these criteria are not met, further releases are required laterally; this may only mean releasing the tight lateral band, which can often be palpated, but a full release of the capsule and synovium may be required.

If problems persist, it may be possible to overcome them by advancing the vastus medialis oblique during closure; this can be predicted either by hanging a forceps on the medial edge of the patellar retinaculum or by inserting two or three temporary sutures before again testing the tracking. It is rare for malalignment to persist after these methods have been used. Should this happen, then medialisation of the tibial tubercle will be needed but before doing so the rotation of the trochlear component should be checked very carefully to ensure that it is in a few degrees of external rotation. By whatever means, the necessary perfect tracking must be achieved or the patient will suffer catching and lateral pain. This is so important that the operation can indeed be considered as a soft-tissue procedure in which an implant happens to be inserted.

14.3 Postoperative Care and Rehabilitation

This follows the same lines as in a TKR, i.e. with antibiotic and thrombo-embolic prophylaxis. The physiotherapist should mobilise the patient in the usual way but the process may be slower than anticipated, with the patient often needing several days to regain quadriceps control and satisfactory knee flexion. If there has been extensive medial reefing or advancement of the vastus medialis oblique, it is probably wise to aim to regain flexion more slowly than usual. Continuous passive motion is not used routinely but can be helpful if slow progress with flexion is being made.

14.4 Complications

These are the same as with any form of knee replacement but two potential early problems should additionally be mentioned.

Firstly, the high incidence of lateral release means that there is more likely to be bleeding. For this reason, following lateral release the tourniquet should be deflated before closure and drains should be used; nonetheless, the knee will appear swollen laterally because of the lack of a capsular closure. This will subside with time but can cause initial anxiety.

Secondly, there may be problems with patellar tracking. This means that either the problem was not addressed adequately at the time of surgery or the medial repair has given way. In either case the problem must be corrected, giving due consideration to the state of the soft tissues as recurrent surgery in the region of the patellar tendon can lead to devascularisation and rupture!

The specific late complication that might occur is lateral catching or pain. This again may be due to inadequate realignment of the extensor mechanism or, more likely, to incorrect placement of the trochlear component. Errors of flexion or extension can easily be seen on the lateral X-ray but rotational errors are harder to define and are more frequent. If this problem is encountered, the patient should have a computed tomography scan to check component rotation (Fig. 14.5), which can sometimes be corrected with benefit [21].

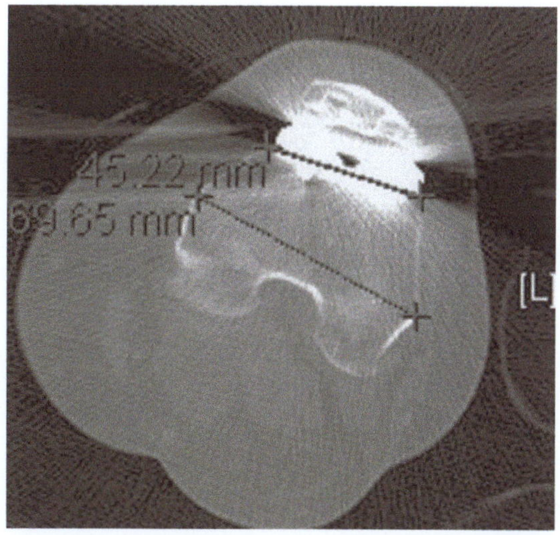

Fig. 14.5 A computed tomography scan from a patient who had persistent lateral pain. The trochlear component is internally rotated; this could not be detected radiologically

14.5 Results

14.5.1 Survivorship

The results of PFR are difficult to report in any meaningful way since different series have treated different groups of patients and the implants have undoubtedly evolved massively from the patellar cap, first introduced by McKeever [22], with substantial improvements made over the years. In addition, it is frequently impossible to be confident of the survivorship from the figures quoted in the literature. However, a number of series have been reported [23-28], generally with acceptable results in the short- to medium-term although none were particularly outstanding. Nonetheless, survivorship figures are sufficiently good to warrant continued interest in the procedure. They do not necessarily imply that the remaining cases were a clinical success. Conversely, it must of course be appreciated that some compartmental replacements are easily revised, often without any clear indication, and doing so does not guarantee improvement. Since revision is an easy procedure and is at times undertaken without any clear indication, the survivorship figures for any compartmental replacement will always compare badly to those of a TKR, which is much harder to revise [29]. It should also be noted that in most cases the revision was not for failure of the prosthesis itself as in general authors report a very low rate of loosening or other prosthetic problems. Instead, progression of arthritis and recurrent or persistent subluxation are the most frequent causes of failure. These problems can be at least in part resolved by better patient selection and improved surgical technique, accompanied by prosthetic design modifications.

14.5.2 The Richards Prosthesis

Three articles [30-32] have reported longer term results with the Richards prosthesis and demonstrated that most patients had continuing good function after a decade. However, in all of them the complication rate was relatively high and a considerable number of surgical procedures were required following the PFR, including patellectomy, extensor mechanism re-alignment, lateral release for lateral pain, and prosthetic revision, usually to a TKR. Most commonly, this was because of arthritis progression in the tibiofemoral joint, especially the medial compartment. Polyethylene wear and trochlear loosening were not major problems despite the deep groove in the trochlear component, which has the aim of constraining the V-shaped polyethylene patellar button. Similar problems were reported after 7 years with the Lubinus prosthesis, which is also sculpted into the trochlea [33]. It therefore seems that despite the many good short-term results, survivorship at around 15 years was only in the region of 75%, which does not match that seen following modern TKR. However, it was felt by some authors to be an appropriate procedure for those patients who were significantly disabled by isolated PFOA and yet were too young for TKR, and as a less destructive option for the older patient [34].

14.5.3 The Avon Prosthesis

More recently, the Bristol Knee Group reported a 96% 5-year survivorship of the first 100 Avon (Fig. 14.6) PFRs done, with excellent pain relief [35]; this is a marked improvement compared to their performance with the older Lubinus implant [33]. Over 400 procedures have now been done; inevitably some problems have been noted as re-

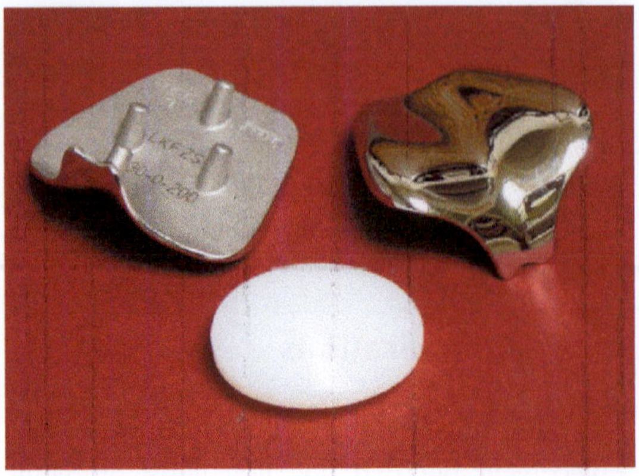

Fig. 14.6 The broad Avon prosthesis resects a minimal amount of anterior bone but a somewhat variable amount from the notch. This symmetrical prosthesis has a shallow trochlear groove

flected in the 8% revision rate over a 10-year period. All of these were straightforward revisions to a standard TKR [21]. The major cause of failure was arthritis progression in the tibiofemoral joint. While this can occur in either the medial or lateral compartment [36], it was uncommon in the younger group, in whom the primary diagnosis was trochlear dysplasia, a fact that had previously been noted [37]. This implant has now been in widespread use for well over 10 years and other centres are reporting results comparable to those from Bristol [38, 39]. Thus, it may well be that the procedure has come of age, although perfection has definitely not been achieved.

14.5.4 Other Prostheses

More recently, a variety of other prostheses, e.g. Leicester, FPV, Hermes, Performance, LCS, and Journey (Fig. 14.7), have come on the market and they aim to address some of the persisting problems. Most of these newer implants are sided rather than symmetrical, which seems logical. The Journey and Hermes prostheses maintain the broad trochlea. The former has a slightly deeper S shaped trochlear groove, which in theory should help address maltracking problems. As yet, few results are available for these implants although disappointing results with a high revision rate were recently reported for the LCS [40].

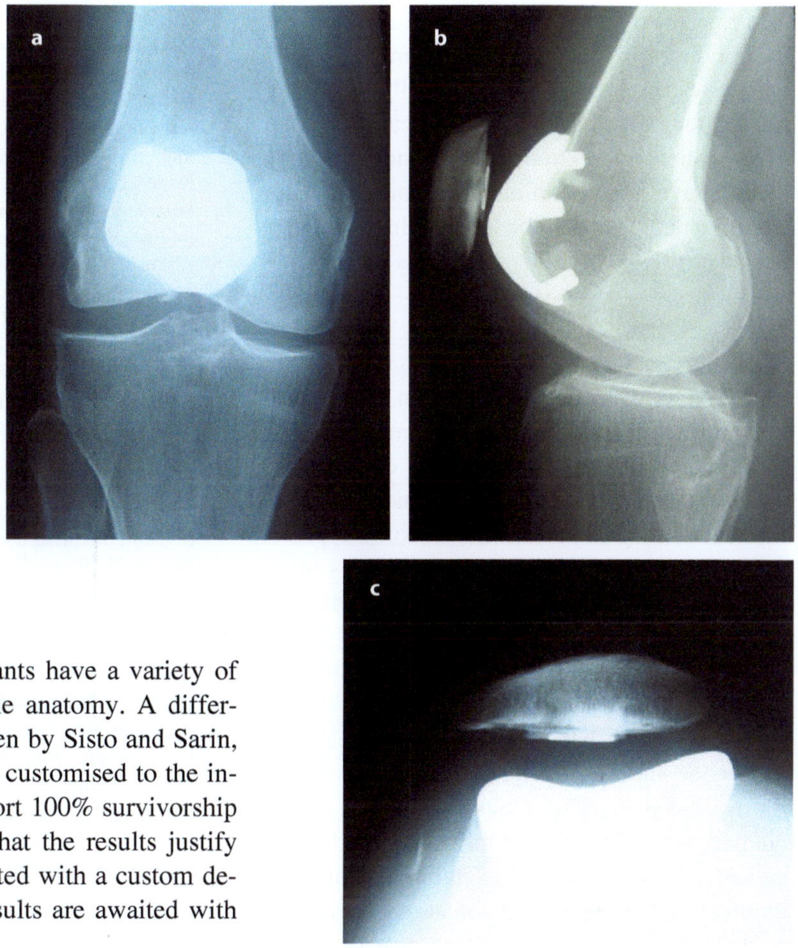

Fig. 14.7 X-rays showing a satisfactorily placed Journey prosthesis. This implant has a broad asymmetric trochlea, which requires a minimal flat resection of the anterior femur. The relatively deep S-shaped groove aids patellar capture and is made of Oxinium, to reduce wear in younger patients. **a** Note the well-preserved tibiofemoral joint on the anteroposterior view. **b** The lateral view shows correct flexion and extension alignment. **c** The skyline view shows good tracking of the patella although there is a mildly asymmetric cut, which can be difficult to avoid with some worn thin patellae

All of the above implants have a variety of sizes to cope with variable anatomy. A different approach has been taken by Sisto and Sarin, who have used an implant customised to the individual patient. They report 100% survivorship at 6 years and conclude that the results justify the additional cost associated with a custom device [41]. Longer term results are awaited with interest.

14.6 Patellofemoral or Total Knee Replacement for Isolated PFOA

During the evolution of TKR many surgeons were reluctant to use the procedure for the treatment of isolated PFOA and instead relied on non-implant solutions. In addition, some were of the opinion that TKR for isolated PFOA was not satisfactory, especially with respect to rehabilitation [42], while others noted that obtaining extensor mechanism balancing could be technically demanding [43]. However as TKR became a more standard procedure, surgeons who were unhappy with the outcome of isolated PFR used a TKR in such circumstances. Mont et al. concluded that doing so was a viable treatment option in patients the over the age of 55 [44]. A dichotomy of opinion has therefore evolved, with some surgeons choosing to use a familiar TKR and others a less invasive PFR. Thus, the authors of one report decided that isolated PFR yields comparable results to those of TKR and may be a less invasive option [45], whilst a meta-analysis of 28 observational studies concluded that although the PFR group had a higher overall complication rate this was largely implant-related [46]. Fortunately, it seems to be agreed that should an isolated PFR require revision this is a straightforward procedure and the outcome is not compromised by the prior arthroplasty [21, 47].

My personal view is that either procedure may well prove satisfactory in relatively elderly patients although it is absolutely essential that the surgeon is confident that there is no involvement of the tibiofemoral joint, since arthritis progression remains the major cause of failure. The real indication for isolated PFR is in younger patients who have crippling symptoms, usually secondary to a degree of instability and trochlear dysplasia. These patients do extremely well and since they tend to have pristine tibiofemoral joints the successful outcome should be long lasting.

14.7 Conclusions

For many years patellofemoral pain proved difficult to alleviate although it is now recognised as a common problem that frequently does not respond well to conservative management, whether medical or surgical. It has also become appreciated that a variable degree of dysplasia is often causative and can lead to severe symptoms due to the presence of eburnated bone in the lateral compartment of the patellofemoral joint, often at an early age.

Isolated PFR has been used as a treatment for a wide variety of patellofemoral pathologies for over 50 years. The results have been variable but better understanding of the disease and better patient selection have led to improvement. Furthermore, major design modifications have been made in the last decade such that, provided strict selection criteria are applied, excellent results can now be expected, at least in the mid-term. The procedure is here to stay but in small numbers. Further developments in prosthetic design and instrumentation will no doubt occur and should result in further improvements in outcome.

References

1. McAlindon TE, Snow S, Cooper C, Dieppe PA (1992) Radiographic patterns of osteoarthritis of the knee joint in the community. Ann Rheum Dis 51:844-849
2. Davies AP, Vince AS, Shepstone L, Donell ST, Glasgow MM (2002) The radiologic prevalence of patellofemoral osteoarthritis. Clin Orthop 402:206-212
3. IwanoT, Kurasawa H, Tokuyama H, Hoshikawa Y (1990) Radiographic and clinical findings of patellofemoral arthrosis. Clin Orthop 252:190-197
4. Gao X, Xu ZJ, He RX, Yan SG, Wu LD (2010) A preliminary report of patellofemoral arthroplasty in isolated patellofemoral arthritis. Chin Med (Eng) 123:3020-3
5. Biedert R, Sigg A, Gal I, Gerber H (2011) 3D representation of the surface topography of normal and dysplasic trochlea using MRI The Knee 18:340-346
6. Clark S, Lock V, Duddy J, Sharif M, Newman JH, Kirwan JR (2005) Intra-articular hylan in the management of patellofemoral osteoarthritis of the knee. The Knee 12:57-62
7. Donell and Glasgow MMS (2007) Isolated patellofemoral osteoarthritis. The Knee 14:169-176
8. Ackroyd CE, Polyzoides AJ (1970) Patellectomy for osteoarthritis. J Bone Joint Surg 60-B:353-357
9. Crosby BE, Insall JH (1976) Recurrent dislocation of the patella:Relation of treatment to osteoarthritis. J Bone Joint Surg 58-A:9-13
10. Ackroyd CE, Smith EJ and Newman JH (2004) Trochlear resurfacing for extensor mechanism instability following patellectomy. The Knee 11:109-111
11. Hau RCY and Newman JH (2008) Knee replacement for osteoarthritis secondary to chronic patella dislocation and trochlear dysplasia. The Knee 15:447-450
12. Dejour H, Walch G, Neyret PH, Adeleine P (1990) Dysplasia of the femoral trochlea. Rev. Chir. Orthop 76.45-54
13. Hendrix M and Newman JH (2006) Trochlear dysplasia-an under recognised cause of patello femoral arthritis. J Bone Joint Surg 88B:251
14. Newman JH (2007) Patellofemoral arthritis and its management with isolated patellofemoral replacement. Orthopedics 30:58-61
15. Utting MR, Davies G, Newman JH (2005) Is anterior knee pain a predisposing factor to patellofemoral osteoarthritis? The Knee 12:362-365
16. Heyse TJ, Khefacha A, Cartier P (2010) UKA in combination with PFR at average 12 year follow-up. Arch Orthop Trauma Surg 110:1227-1230
17. Hassaballa MA, Porteous AJ, Newman JH, Rogers CA (2003) Can knees kneel. Kneeling ability after total, unicompartmental and patellofemoral knee arthroplasty. The Knee 10:155-160
18. Henderson MS, Newman JH and Hand GCR (1999) Blood loss following knee replacement surgery use it don't lose it. The Knee 6:125 -129
19. Shakespeare D, Dikko B (2005) A simple precise technique for making the anterior cut in patellofemoral resurfacing. The Knee 12:454-455
20. Cossey AJ and Spriggins AJ (2006) Computer-assisted patellofemoral arthroplasty a method for optimising rotation. J Arthroplasty 2006 21 420-427
21. Mulford JS, Eldridge JD, Porteous AJ, Ackroyd CE and Newman JH (2009) Revision of isolated patellofemoral arthroplasty to total knee replacement. Current Orthop Prac 20:437- 441
22. McKeever DC (1955) Patellar prosthesis. J Bone Joint Surg 37:1074-1084
23 Arcerio RA, Toomey HE (1988) Patellofemoral arthroplasty: A 3 to 9 year follow-up study. Clin Orthop 236:60-71
24. Blazina ME, Fox JM, Pizzo D, BroukhimB, Ivey FM (1979) Patellofemoral replacement. Clin Orthop 144:98-102

25. Argenson J-N A, Guillaume J-M, Aubaniac J-M (1995) Is there a place for patellofemoral arthroplasty? Clin Orthop Relat Res 321:162-167
26. Cartier P, Sanouiller JL, Grelsamer R (1990) Patellofemoral arthroplasty. J Arthroplasty 5:49-55
27. Lubinus HH (1979) Patella glide total replacement. Orthopaedics 2:119-127
28. Aglietti P, Insall JN, Walker PS, Trent P (1975) A new patella prosthesis design and application. Clin Orthop. 1975 107 175-187
29. Goodfellow JW, O'Connor JJ, Murray DW (2010) A critique of revision rate as an outcome measure. J Bone Joint Surg 92B:1628-1631
30. de Winter WE, Feith R, Van Loon CJ (2001) The Richards type II patellofemoral arthroplasty: 26 cases followed for 1-20 years. Acta Orthop Scand 72:487-490
31. Kooijman HJ, Driessen AP, Van Horn JR (2003) Long-term results of patellofemoral arthroplasty. A report of 56 arthroplasties with 17 years follow-up. J Bone Joint Surg 85-B:836-840
32. Cartier P, Sanouiller JL, Khefacha A (2005) Long-term results with the first patellofemoral replacement. Clin Orthop Relat Res 436:47-54
33. Tauro B, Ackroyd CE, Newman JH, Shah NA (2001) The Lubinus patellofemoral arthroplasty-a five to ten year prospective study. J Bone Joint Surg 83-B:696-701
34. Merchant AC (2004) Early results with a total patellofemoral joint replacement arthroplasty prosthesis. J Arthroplasty 19:829-836
35. Ackroyd CE, Newman JH, Evans R, Eldridge JD, Joslin CC (2007) The Avon patellofemoral arthroplasty: five year survivorship and functional results. J Bone Joint Surg 89-B:310-315
36. Nicol SG, Loveridge JM, Weale AE, Ackroyd CE, Newman JH (2006) Arthritis progression after patellofemoral joint replacement. The Knee 13:290-295
37. De Cloedt P, Lagaye J, Lokietek W (1999) Femoropatella prosthesis. Acta Orthop Belg 65:170-175
38. Starks I, RobertsS, White SH (2009) The Avon patellofemoral joint replacement. J Bone Joint Surg 91B:1579-1582
39. Sarda PK, Shetty A, Maheswaran SS (2011) Medium term results of Avon patellofemoral joint replacement. Indian J Orthop 45:439-444
40. Charalambous CP, Abiddin Z, Mills SP, Rogers S, Sutton P Parkinson R (2011) The low contact stress patellofemoral replacement. J.Bone Joint Surg 93B:484-489
41. Sisto DJ, Sarin VK (2006) Custom patellofemoral arthroplasty of the knee. J Bone Joint Surg 88A:1475-1480
42. Kolettis GT, Stern SH (1992) Patella resurfacing for patellofemoral arthritis. Orthop Clin N. America 23:665-673
43. Parvizi J, Stuart MJ, Pagnano, Hanssen AD (2001) Total Knee Arthroplasty in patients with isolated patellofemoral arthritis. Clin Orthop 392:147-152
44. Mont MA, Haas S, Mullick T, Hungerford DS (2002) Total knee replacement for patellofemoral arthritis. J. Bone Joint Surg 84A:1977-1981
45. Dahm DL. Al-Rayashi W, Dajani K, Shah JP, Levy BA, Stuart MJ (2010) Patellofemoral arthroplasty versus total knee arthroplasty in patients with isolated patellofemoral osteoarthritis. Am. J Orthop 39:487-491
46. Dy CJ, Franco N, Ma Y, Mazumdar M, McArthy MM, Gonzalez DVA (2011) Complications after patellofemoral versus total knee replacement in the treatment of isolated patellofemoral arthritis. A meta-analysis. Knee Surg Sports Trauma Arthrosc [E-pub ahead of print]
47. Lonner JH. Jasko JG, Booth RE (2006) Revision of a failed patellofemoral arthroplasty to a total knee replacement. J.Bone Joint Surg 88A:2337-2342

Partial Knee Arthroplasty

15

Lindsay Rolston

15.1 Introduction

Total knee arthroplasty (TKA) continues to be a safe and effective surgical procedure for arthritis of the knee and is in fact the current gold standard for treatment [1, 2]. However, based on this author's experience of performing TKA for over 15 years, several observations are apparent. First, not all TKA patients are satisfied with their postoperative function. The work of Noble et al. [3] suggests that upwards of 50% of TKA patients describe some form of functional deficit, particularly during side-to-side movement. Such outcomes highlight the necessity of the anterior-cruciate ligament (ACL) and its important role in functional satisfaction subsequent to TKA. The second observation is that the ACL and the posterior-cruciate ligament (PCL) are often times healthy and undamaged at the time of the surgery. It is unsettling to realize that contemporary surgical techniques required the undue resection of these structures. The final observation is the previously documented combination of wear of the medial and patellofemoral joint (PFJ) compartments, coupled with a non-symptomatic lateral compartment [4]. Resection of the entire articular surface is a further example of the unnecessary sacrifice of healthy tissue.

The idea of partial knee arthroplasty, with retention of the lateral compartment and the cruciate ligaments, is not new. Unicompartmental knee arthroplasty (UKA) and patellofemoral arthroplasty have both been performed for nearly 30 years [5, 6]. Replacing the medial compartment alone during UKA while ignoring arthritic changes at the PFJ has been recognized as a satisfactory surgical option [7]. However, there is significant evidence that osteoarthritis may progress postoperatively and thereby compromise the clinical outcome [8, 9]. One potential solution is the addition of a patellofemoral arthroplasty to an existing UKA implant. However, combining these two implants can be technically challenging, as three discontinuous zones are introduced between the articular cartilage and the implant [10]. In addition to technical considerations, the cost of the procedure must also be considered. The use of two procedures instead of one to address bicompartmental knee disease unnecessarily increases surgical costs. This modular unlinked arthroplasty is not a new concept. Parratte et al. [11] looked at 77 knees in which 27 failures had occurred at a mean of 8 years. Twenty of the revisions were associated with cementless trochlear failure. While there are more recent studies with unlinked arthroplasty, the follow-up in most is < 2 years and the sample sizes include fewer than 30 patients [12-14].

Eight years ago, a monolithic implant (Journey Deuce bi-compartmental knee system, Smith and Nephew, Memphis, Tennessee, USA) was designed to simultaneously replace the medial and PFJ compartments of the knee (Fig. 15.1). This device conserves both the ACL and the PCL, in addition to sparing the non-symptomatic lateral compartment. The metal-backed medial

L. Rolston (✉)
Henry County Center for Orthopedic Surgery
& Sports Medicine
New Castle, IN, USA
E-mail: lrolston@hcmhcares.org

N. Confalonieri, S. Romagnoli (eds.), *Small Implants in Knee Reconstruction*,
DOI 10.1007/978-88-470-2655-1_15,

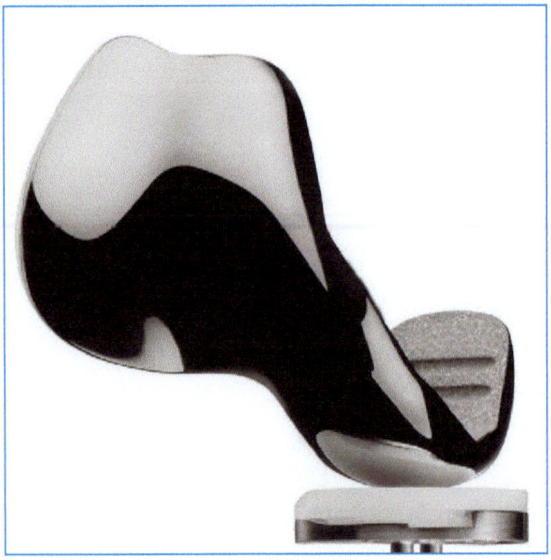

Fig. 15.1 Journey Deuce bi-compartmental knee system (Smith and Nephew, Memphis, Tennessee, USA)

tibial base plate is unicompartmental. Initial expectations include a smaller incision, potentially shorter recovery times postoperatively, less pain, reduced blood loss, and improved stability and function.

15.2 Approach

The development of less invasive arthroplasty techniques has been of interest for many years, despite concerns of reduced surgical visualization [15]. Based on the relative ease of implant insertion and the acceptable clinical outcomes, it is the author's opinion that minimally invasive procedures are preferred. With the Deuce knee, there is no need to visualize the lateral compartment, other than momentarily to assess its integrity. In addition, the surgical technique allows for a relatively small incision and ease of insertion.

Standard medial-parapatellar arthrotomy has been used for 80% of our patients. Typically, this only involves a 1-inch split into the quadriceps. In 20% of patients, the author has used a midvastus approach without difficulty. This approach is typically reserved for patients who have not undergone surgery previously, are less muscular, and are more flexible. When the exposure associated with a TKA is compared with that of the Deuce knee, the potential benefits of the latter are less dependent on incision length. Rather, the conservation of healthy tissue appears to be the most important advantage. Specifically, exposure of the lateral compartment and the lateral geniculate artery, which increase pain and reduce postoperative function if not coagulated, respectively, is avoided. Approximately 50% less bone is excised with the Deuce knee than in a traditional TKA. Moreover, forward subluxation of the tibia is also avoided, by placing a retractor in the lateral gutter or everting the patella. The resulting reduction in blood loss and tissue tension may further improve postoperative surgical outcome. Nonetheless, surgeons are encouraged to create whatever exposure is necessary to perform the procedure without added difficulty, as incision length and violation of the quadriceps are not of primary concern in terms of recovery. Furthermore, a liberal incision length may reduce the risk of mal-alignment, skin slough, and retained cement [16, 17]. A comparison of standard TKA exposure with that of the Deuce knee is provided in Fig. 15.2.

15.3 Technique

The technique for Deuce implantation begins with tibial preparation, which is similar to that of UKA. The Deuce tibial cutting block utilizes one pin to fixate the cutting block to the tibia, and a second pin for fixation extending under the lateral tibial condyle. The initial pin is placed as a negative stop for the vertical and horizontal resections. This prevents stress risers under the tibial spine or in a vertical direction, which in turn helps to prevent fracture (Fig. 15.3). The two pins in these locations not only fixate the block but also avoid the need for the placement of pins in the subchondral bone, which could result in subchondral collapse of the tibial base plate and subsequent failure of the procedure. A conservative tibial cut of 2–4 mm is made. In most instances, a resection of 2 mm off the lowest point of the tibial articular surface is ideal. If a neutrally aligned knee shows wear of the medial

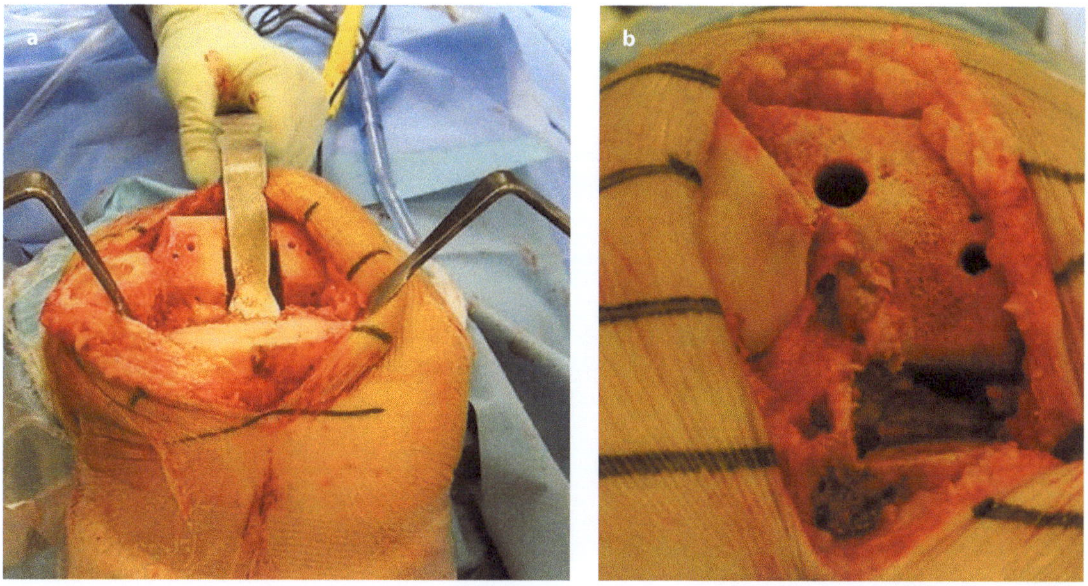

Fig. 15.2 Comparison of TKA (**a**) and Deuce knee (**b**) exposures

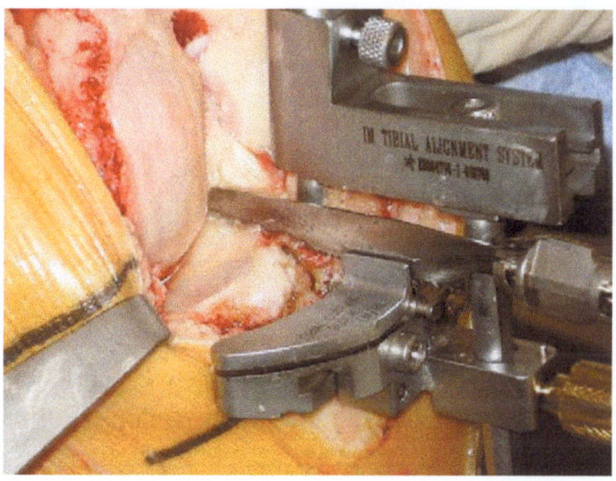

Fig. 15.3 Deuce tibial cutting block

and PFJ compartments, a 4-mm cut on the tibia is utilized to prevent over-correction and overloading of the lateral compartment. A conservative tibial cut is recommended as it allows for neutral varus/valgus placement, with a slope of 2–4°. Bicompartmental knee arthroscopy (BKA) with the Deuce knee has been shown to support the restoration of knee alignment [18].

As with UKA, it is important to place the tibial base on the cortical rim without overhang and to position the component as far laterally as possible without violating the ACL attachment on the tibia. This allows the maximal load to be distributed across the tibia. Spacer blocks are used to determine proper knee flexion and extension. Bone cuts similar to those in TKA are made in order to correct an extensive varus deformity. In contrast to UKA, balancing the knee in extension can be performed independent of flexion, supporting extensive deformity correction (Fig. 15.4) [18, 19].

Mating the transition zone between the trochlear and lateral femoral condyle is the largest initial technical concern. With revised instrumentation, this can be done reproducibly (Fig. 15.5). After the cuts have been made, trial implants are used just as in TKA (Fig. 15.6). The patellar component and its preparation are the same as that utilized for TKA. A lateral retinacular peel and partial lateral facetectomy balance the PFJ articulation. It is even more critical with BKA to properly balance the PFJ articulation, in order to prevent contact of the lateral facet of the patella with the native lateral femoral condyle at the transition zone. The technical considerations relevant to TKA regarding balancing the PFJ need to be highlighted with BKA. In addition to balancing the soft-tissue restraints of the lateral retinaculum, shifting the monolithic implant laterally as far as possible without overhang is essential for

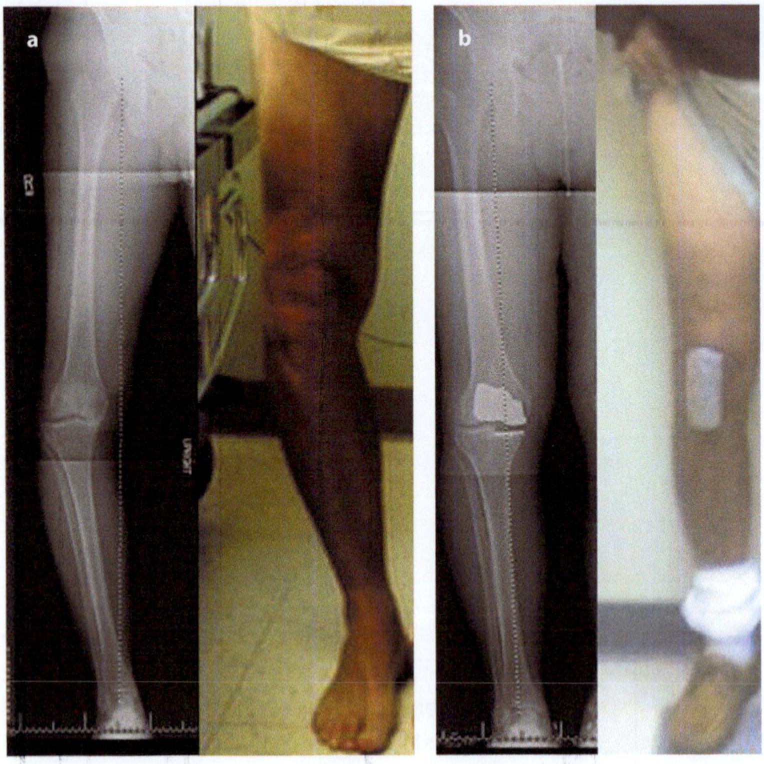

Fig. 15.4 Restoration of knee alignment before and after implantation of the Deuce knee: preoperative (**a**) and postoperative (**b**)

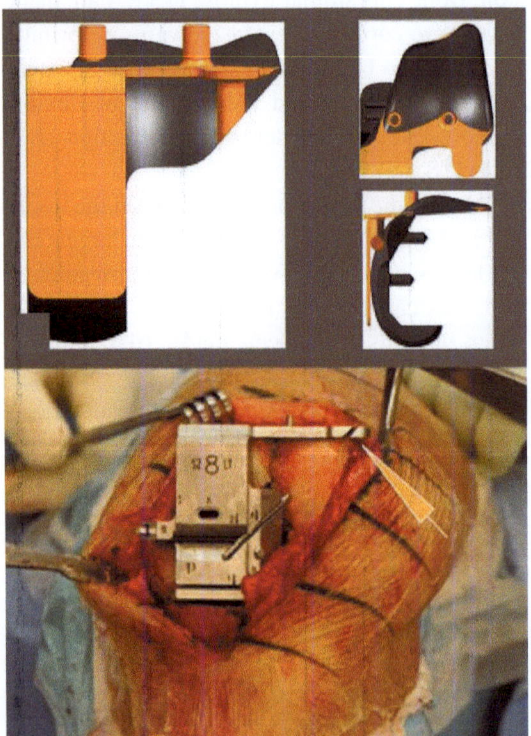

Fig. 15.5 Deuce sizing templates and new 4-1 cutting blocks

proper tracking of the patella within the trochlear groove. The trochlear groove is the same as the Genesis II total knee system (Smith and Nephew), an implant with a proven track record for PFJ function and excellent clinical outcomes [20, 21]. Both onlay and inset patellar components have been used with good results, although this author's preference is to use a 9.0-mm thickness three-peg onlay patella. While at our center there is a small subset of implants with the patella non-resurfaced that have reached the 5-year mark, currently we routinely resurface the patella since by definition, the PFJ is arthritic.

Rotation of the femoral component is also an important aspect of PFJ mechanics. Maintaining proper rotation or adding a degree or two of external rotation enables the optimization of PFJ function. Since the femoral component is monolithic, the consequence of implant rotation needs to be considered, as it relates to medial vs. PFJ compartment balancing. This increased external rotation can potentially place the tibiofemoral contact area more medially, whereas internal rotation of the implant can adversely affect PFJ

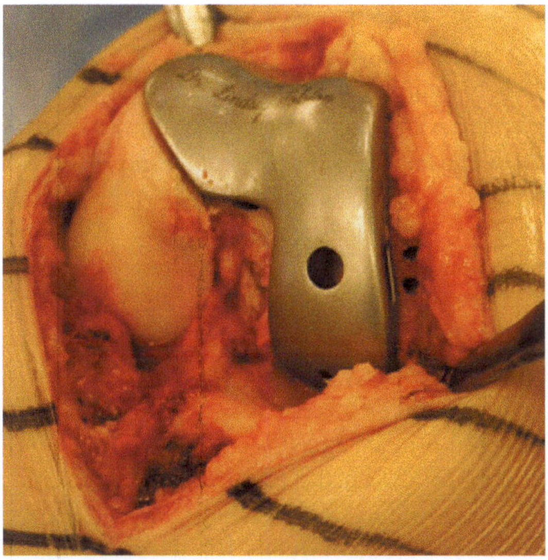

Fig. 15.6 Deuce knee trial implants in situ

mechanics. The rotation of the femoral implant is determined by the anterior posterior line of the trochlear groove and by the medial epicondylar axis. Since identifying the epicondylar axis remains difficult, the AP line is the mainstay for determining femoral implant rotation.

15.4 Special Considerations, Indications, and Patient Selection

First and foremost, a symptomatic lateral compartment is a contraindication to Deuce implantation. The patient's history and physical examination results are critical in identifying the origin of lateral knee pain. Pain at the lateral facet of the patella is often related to PFJ arthritis and can be successfully treated. However, true lateral joint line pain will not be addressed by this procedure, regardless of how pristine the lateral compartment may look radiographically. These patients may benefit from preoperative magnetic resonance imaging and/or arthroscopy to address lateral compartment pathology. An intact ACL is preferred. However, the author has a series of patients without an ACL in whom successful outcomes have been obtained. ACL deficiency is observed in 6.38% of patients. If patients present with symptomatic instability, it is preferable to either perform ACL reconstruction at the time of surgery or to convert to TKA. For patients who are ACL-deficient but have lower activity levels and are asymptomatic, proceeding with a BKA will not affect clinical outcome. Finally, as in UKA or patellofemoral arthroplasty, inflammatory arthritis is an additional contraindication.

In difficult cases in which flexion contracture is > 10°, conversion to TKA may be necessary. Flexion contracture can be improved with release of the hamstring tendons medially, the capsular tissue posteriorly, and the excision of posterior osteophytes in the medial aspect of the knee. Adequate bone quality is preferred. There are minimal limits on the extent of varus deformity that can be corrected, in contrast to UKA. Since actual bone cuts are made and the knee can be balanced in flexion independent of extension, a medial release up to 20° of varus is possible while achieving good stability and functional outcome, postoperatively.

One frequent question revolves around patient selection. Who is the ideal candidate? Is it the young active patient who can appreciate the stability of the knee gained by retaining the cruciate ligaments in addition to the reduced bone resection? Alternatively, is it the elderly patient fearful of the pain and rehabilitation following TKA? After performing 1,000 of these procedures, it is the opinion of the author that age and activity level are not critical in determining candidacy. Each of these patient groups can benefit equally from BKA with the Deuce knee.

Appropriate preoperative physical examination is critical. The location of the pain is the most important factor. As patients typically refer to a lateral aspect of the knee, it is essential to pinpoint whether this is the lateral facet of the patella, or whether this is true lateral joint-line tenderness. Patients with the former are still candidates for Deuce, as the PFJ is resurfaced. In those with the latter, the pain will not be addressed if the lateral compartment is not resurfaced. Lack of radiographic evidence of lateral osteoarthritis will not help determine candidacy if any lateral pain exists. In such cases, it is appropriate to consider magnetic resonance imaging or arthroscopy prior to determining the implant choice. ACL integrity, flexion contracture, patellar tracking, and lateral compartment narrowing must also be considered during the physical examination.

Clearly, a lateral notch osteophyte on the lateral condyle can and should be excised in each and every case. The necessary excision of this kissing-type lesion is not a contraindication to Deuce implantation. Full-thickness lesions of the weight-bearing rail of the lateral femoral condyle should not be accepted. In this case, conversion to TKA is recommended regardless of the symptomatology of the lateral joint.

Additional special considerations include the neutrally aligned knee with medial compartment arthrosis and an open lateral compartment. Most medial compartment arthritic knees result in varus deformity. Occasionally, based on the anatomy of the femur and tibia, X-ray may reveal medial and PFJ arthritis with a non-symptomatic lateral compartment. In such cases, it is critical to resect more bone on the distal femur or tibial to avoid over-correction. Patella baja may result from high tibial valgus osteotomy. In this instance the patella is brought into contact with the native cartilage in the transition zone, which is not optimal. Moreover, the closing wedge high tibial osteotomy results in a neutrally aligned medial compartment that is at risk for over-correction. In both cases, conversion to TKA is necessary. It is this author's recommendation to avoid bicompartmental replacement in those patients with patella baja.

15.5 Post-surgical Follow-Up

As previously noted, one of the potential benefits of Deuce implantation is better recovery. By conserving healthy tissue and minimizing joint trauma during surgery, postoperative function may be improved. Early evidence supports this hypothesis. In a gait study of eight BKA patients and ten controls, BKA knees were found to support normal frontal plane mechanics and extensor moments about the knee during walking [22]. At 1.2 years following surgery, Deuce patients had largely returned to normal function.

Regarding clinical outcomes, this author collected postoperative data during a single surgeon survey of 166 Deuce and 46 TKA procedures (Legion, Smith and Nephew). Age and BMI were controlled between groups. The length of hospital stay was 2.5 days for Deuce vs. 3.5 days for TKA. The average tourniquet time was 7 min shorter for Deuce than for TKA. Only 4.6% of patients with Deuce but 29% of those with TKA required a blood transfusion. At a minimum 24 months follow-up, there was a 1.3% revision rate. The average total Knee Society Score (KSS) for the Deuce group currently has exceeded that of the TKA group at every interval through 2 years, surpassing a score of 90 by 6 months (Fig. 15.7). Moreover, at every interval Deuce patients have had a range of motion greater than that of the standard TKA group (Fig. 15.8). Complications have included the following: 3 manipulations, 3 cases of infection (1 acute, 2 chronic), 1 loose all-polyethylene tibial component, 1 partial lateral meniscectomy, 1 medial tibial plateau fracture, 1 loose patella, 2 liner locking mechanism failures, and 3 tibial base plate fractures. The risk of fracture was attributed to the base plate design, which has since been revised by the manufacturer. To date, over 5,000 Deuce knees, including 1000 by this author, have been implanted over the course of 7 years. While the early postoperative clinical outcomes have been acceptable, in order to verify the long-term safety and efficacy of the Deuce knee additional studies are necessary.

In addition to clinical outcomes, the author assessed early functional performance in a survey that included the number of days the patient utilized any assistive devices, time to return to driving, discontinuation of all pain medicine, length of hospital stay, length of incision, average tourniquet time, and the need for a blood transfusion. In the author's experience, compared to TKA patients Deuce patients discontinued their use of assistive devices 10 days earlier, were able to return to driving 10 days earlier, and discontinued their pain medicine 7 days earlier.

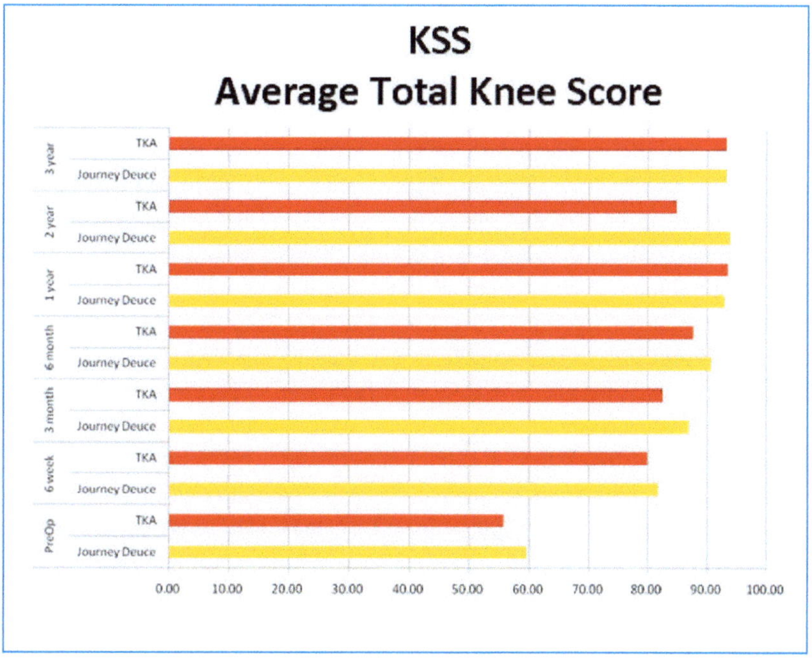

Fig. 15.7 Knee Society Score (KSS) results of a postoperative surgeon survey

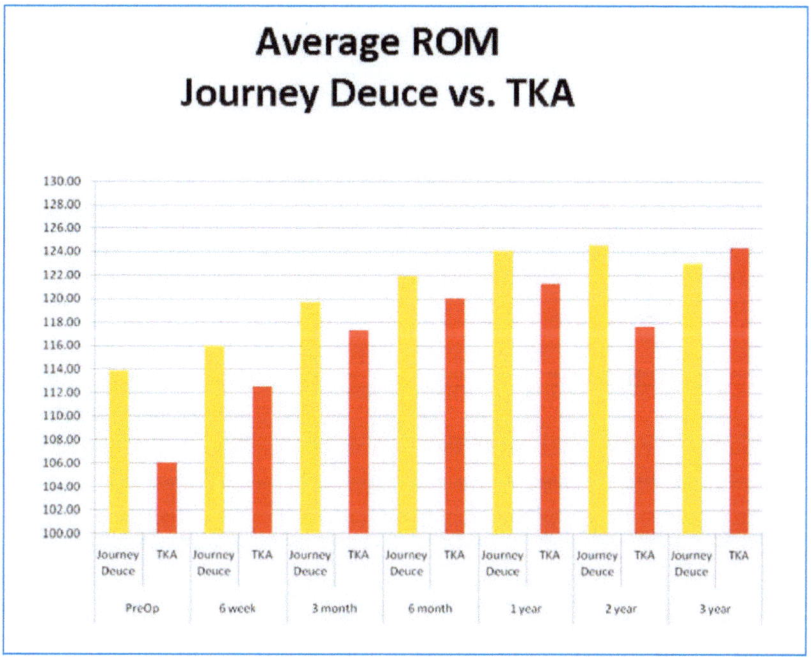

Fig. 15.8 Range of motion (ROM): results of a postoperative surgeon survey

15.6 Tips and Pearls

Optimal results with any type of partial knee arthroplasty procedure are dependent upon a multitude of factors. After performing 1,000 Deuce procedures, in this author's experience there have been no femoral failures. This largely parallels the TKA literature. In UKA or BKA, the tibial side of the arthroplasty seems to be the weak link. The first recommendation is to minimize the depth of the tibial resection. The reasons for this include the fact that the subchondral bone plate is a more rigid structure on which to apply a base plate. The proximal tibia below 4 mm becomes softer and thus less able to resist the forces on the medial aspect. In addition, a partial knee arthroplasty is often performed in younger patients, who may be at risk for future revision arthroplasty, in which the preservation of tibial bone is critical to the success of the procedure.

The importance of balancing the knee is essential in reducing excessive stress on the medial tibial base plate. Therefore, correction of a large varus deformity is recommended, in contrast to the common instruction in UKA, in which the release and correction of this deformity is avoided. However, in the author's experience during BKA, it is also important not to over-correct the deformity and place the weight-bearing line onto the lateral joint.

Recovery following partial knee arthroplasty is multifactorial. Appropriate pain management is critical. In our center, a pain cocktail has been most useful. Femoral and/or sciatic nerve blocks are a recommended method of pain management. However, blocks can compromise weight-bearing in the affected limb for 1–2 days, potentially increasing the risk of a fall during ambulation. Often times these patients are discharged during this same period, such that a femoral and/or sciatic nerve block may inhibit proper therapy and recovery.

15.7 Conclusions

The author's experience with the Deuce knee suggests that this device can be effectively utilized patients with symptomatic medial and PFJ compartments who are candidates for BKA. While TKA is an effective treatment for bicompartmental disease, recent evidence supports improved functional outcomes following BKA with Deuce [22]. This appears to be due primarily to ACL preservation and reduced bone resection, tissue distress, and blood loss during implantation. Moreover, a survey of 1,000 Deuce patients supports the stability of the Deuce knee at a minimum follow-up of 2-years. The same survey found that aseptic loosening of the femoral component does not seem to occur nor has there been a failure of the femoral component, either in the author's series or in other published series. Furthermore, blood loss appears to be less in BKA than in TKA, while the complication of postoperative dislocation is largely eliminated. The finding of an early return of movement following BKA is consistent in our series and in other published series [23].

Progression of lateral osteoarthritis is unlikely as long as the initial postoperative alignment is neutral or slightly varus. BKA is a viable procedure for a significant number of osteoarthritis patients [8, 9]. Although additional studies are necessary to address mid- to long-term outcomes, the current procedure will likely have a place in the orthopedics reconstructive market for years to come. Recommendations for the future of this device may include a porous tibial base design with improved durability. The cemented UKA tibia is currently an unsolved matter in orthopedics. Specifically, Palumbo et al. [24] reported 61% radiolucency of the tibial tray and 14% aseptic loosening of the tibial requiring revision at 2 years. Other authors have also described an increased tibial lucency rate with unicompartmental devices [25, 26].

The transition zone in BKA, either linked or unlinked, remains technically demanding. Therefore, custom cutting blocks and an increased number of femoral sizes may help improve patellar tracking and reduced anterior knee pain. Tria et al. [27] reported a 25% incidence of anterior knee pain following Deuce BKA. It must be noted that the authors used first-generation instrumentation on all of their patients, which did not allow for a reproducible symmetric and flush transition zone between the lateral flange of the femoral component and the native cartilage laterally. This would clearly have been the cause of pain at the patellofemoral articulation. New sizing templates and 4-1 cutting blocks now allow for a reproducible transition zone and seem to have dramatically reduced the incidence of anterior knee pain, with improved overall results. However, these blocks became available in a limited fashion in the USA in 2008 but have never been available elsewhere. Furthermore, increasing the number of sizes undoubtedly maximizes coverage of the native trochlea and reduces technical errors related to rotation and sizing of the femoral component.

Much has been learned regarding the capabilities and liabilities of a monolithic BKA design over the last 9 years. Clearly, medial and patellofemoral joint osteoarthritis is common and comprises the typical pattern of osteoarthritis encountered by joint surgeons [4]. The importance of a less invasive approach and the integrity of the cruciate ligaments are paramount. The first generation experience provides the knowledge needed to pursue improvements in implant design and in the associated surgical techniques, with the aims of tissue conservation and the maintenance of native knee biomechanics.

References

1. Hart JA (2004) Joint replacement surgery. Med J Aust 180(5 Suppl):S27-30
2. Kurtz S, Mowat F, Ong K, Chan N, Lau E, Halpern M (2005)Prevalence of primary and revision total hip and knee arthroplasty in the United States from 1990 through 2002. J Bone Joint Surg Am 87(7):1487-1497
3. Noble PC, Conditt MA, Cook KF, Mathis KB (2006) The John Insall Award: Patient expectations affect satisfaction with total knee arthroplasty. Clin Orthop Relat Res 452:35-43
4. Ledingham J, Regan M, Jones A, Doherty M (1993) Radiographic patterns and associations of osteoarthritis of the knee in patients referred to hospital. Ann Rheum Dis 52(7):520-526
5. Borus T, Thornhill T (2008) Unicompartmental knee arthroplasty. J Am Acad Orthop Surg 16(1):9-18
6. Leadbetter WB, Ragland PS, Mont MA (2005) The appropriate use of patellofemoral arthroplasty: an analysis of reported indications, contraindications, and failures. Clin Orthop Relat Res (436):91-99
7. Kendrick BJ, Rout R, Bottomley NJ et al (2010) The implications of damage to the lateral femoral condyle on medial unicompartmental knee replacement. J Bone Joint Surg Br 92(3):374-379
8. Berger RA, Meneghini RM, Sheinkop MB et al (2004) The progression of patellofemoral arthrosis after medial unicompartmental replacement: results at 11 to 15 years. Clin Orthop Relat Res (428):92-99
9. Hernigou P, Deschamps G (2002) Patellar impingement following unicompartmental arthroplasty. J Bone Joint Surg Am 84-A(7):1132-1137
10. Lonner JH (2009) Modular bicompartmental knee arthroplasty with robotic arm assistance. Am J Orthop (Belle Mead NJ). Feb 38(2 Suppl):28-31
11. Parratte S, Pauly V, Aubaniac JM, Argenson JN (2010) Survival of bicompartmental knee arthroplasty at 5 to 23 years. Clin Orthop Relat Res 468(1):64-72
12. Argenson JN, Parratte S, Bertani A et al (2009) The new arthritic patient and arthroplasty treatment options. J Bone Joint Surg Am 91 Suppl 5:43-48
13. Heyse TJ, Khefacha A, Cartier P (2010) UKA in combination with PFR at average 12-year follow-up. Arch Orthop Trauma Surg 130(10):1227-1230
14. Lonner JH, John TK, Conditt MA (2010) Modular Bicompartmental Arthroplasty. Presented at The Knee Society Closed Meeting, Rochester, MN
15. Khanna A, Gougoulias N, Longo UG, Maffulli N (2009) Minimally invasive total knee arthroplasty: a systematic review. Orthop Clin North Am 40(4):479-489
16. Berend KR, Lombardi AV, Jr (2005) Avoiding the potential pitfalls of minimally invasive total knee surgery. Orthopedics 28(11):1326-1330
17. Dalury DF, Dennis DA (2005) Mini-incision total knee arthroplasty can increase risk of component malalignment. Clin Orthop Relat Res 440:77-81
18. Rolston L, Siewert K (2009) Assessment of knee alignment after bicompartmental knee arthroplasty. J Arthroplasty 24(7):1111-1114
19. Emerson RH, Jr., Higgins LL (2008) Unicompartmental knee arthroplasty with the oxford prosthesis in patients with medial compartment arthritis. J Bone Joint Surg Am 90(1):118-122
20. Bourne RB, Laskin RS, Guerin JS (2007) Ten-year results of the first 100 Genesis II total knee replacement procedures. Orthopedics 30(8 Suppl):83-85
21. Crockarell JR Jr, Hicks JM, Schroeder RJ, Guyton JL, Harkess JW, Lavelle DG (2010) Total knee arthroplasty with asymmetric femoral condyles and tibial tray. J Arthroplasty 25(1):108-113
22. Wang H, Dugan E, Frame J, Rolston L (2009) Gait analysis after bi-compartmental knee replacement. Clin Biomech (Bristol, Avon) 24(9):751-754
23. Morrison TA, Nyce JD, Macaulay WB, Geller JA (2011) Early adverse results with bicompartmental knee arthroplasty: a prospective cohort comparison to total knee arthroplasty. J Arthroplasty 26(6 Suppl):35-39
24. Palumbo BT, Henderson ER, Edwards PK, Burris RB, Gutierrez S, Raterman SJ (2011) Initial experience of the Journey-Deuce bicompartmental knee prosthesis: a review of 36 cases. J Arthroplasty 26(6 Suppl):40-45
25. Tibrewal SB, Grant KA, Goodfellow JW (1984) The radiolucent line beneath the tibial components of the Oxford meniscal knee. J Bone Joint Surg Br 66(4):523-528
26. Gulati A, Chau R, Pandit HG et al (2009) The incidence of physiological radiolucency following Oxford unicompartmental knee replacement and its relationship to outcome. J Bone Joint Surg Br 91(7):896-902
27. Tria AJ Jr (2010) Bicompartmental arthroplasty of the knee. Instr Course Lect 59:61-73

Revision of UKR

16

Sergio Romagnoli, Francesco Verde,
and Sara Zacchetti

16.1 Introduction

In the last 10 years, the use of unicompartmental knee replacement (UKR) instead of total knee replacement (TKR) has increased, especially in young patients. This surgical technique can be used if ligament stability is maintained and the femoropatellar joint and medial or lateral femorotibial compartment are intact. UKR is less invasive than total replacement in terms of tissue sparing and it permits a more physiologic articular restoration. As good results in terms of survival rate continue to be reported in the literature, the number of unicompartmental implants has increased but so has the revisions rate [1, 2].

From 2001 to 2010, at the Istituto Ortopedico Galeazzi, we performed 189 unicompartmental revisions. These have been classified according to the type of the failed implant, the cause of failure, and the type of implant used for the revision.

16.2 Causes of Failure

Five main causes of failure can be recognized:

1. Incorrect indications: R.A. (Rheumatoid Arthritis)-chondrocalcinosis, contralateral compartment degeneration, lateral meniscus degeneration, symptomatic degeneration of the patellofemoral joint, cruciate ligament deficiency, and collateral ligament instability.
2. Incorrect surgical technique: mechanical axis over-correction, incorrect tibial resection (frontal plane or slope), incorrect prosthesis dimensions or alignment (and thus wrong position during extension or flexion), incorrect fixation (cement or cementless), and ligament instability.
3. Polyethylene-metal wear.
4. Capsuloligamentous instability.
5. Infections.

16.3 Revision Classifications

Revisions can be early or late, depending on the time between the first implant and the revision. An early revision is one that takes place less than two years after the first implant while late revisions are those carried out thereafter (Fig. 16.1).

The need for an early revision can arise from:

- Aseptic loosening: This is the main cause of revision and usually involves the tibial component. It is caused by the incorrect position or cementation mistakes.
- Opposite compartment degeneration: This reflects over-correction of the mechanical axis.
- Incorrect component positioning. Both the tibial and the femoral compartments can be involved. Errors in tibial positioning include: oblique varus, which causes tibial loosening and secondary polyethylene (PE) wear; oblique valgus and subsidence; varization; and secondary PE wear. Among the errors in femoral positioning are: incorrect anteropos-

S. Romagnoli (✉)
Galeazzi Orthopedic Institute
Milan, Italy
E-mail: sergio.romagnoli@libero.it

N. Confalonieri, S. Romagnoli (eds.), *Small Implants in Knee Reconstruction*,
DOI 10.1007/978-88-470-2655-1_16, © Springer-Verlag Italia 2013

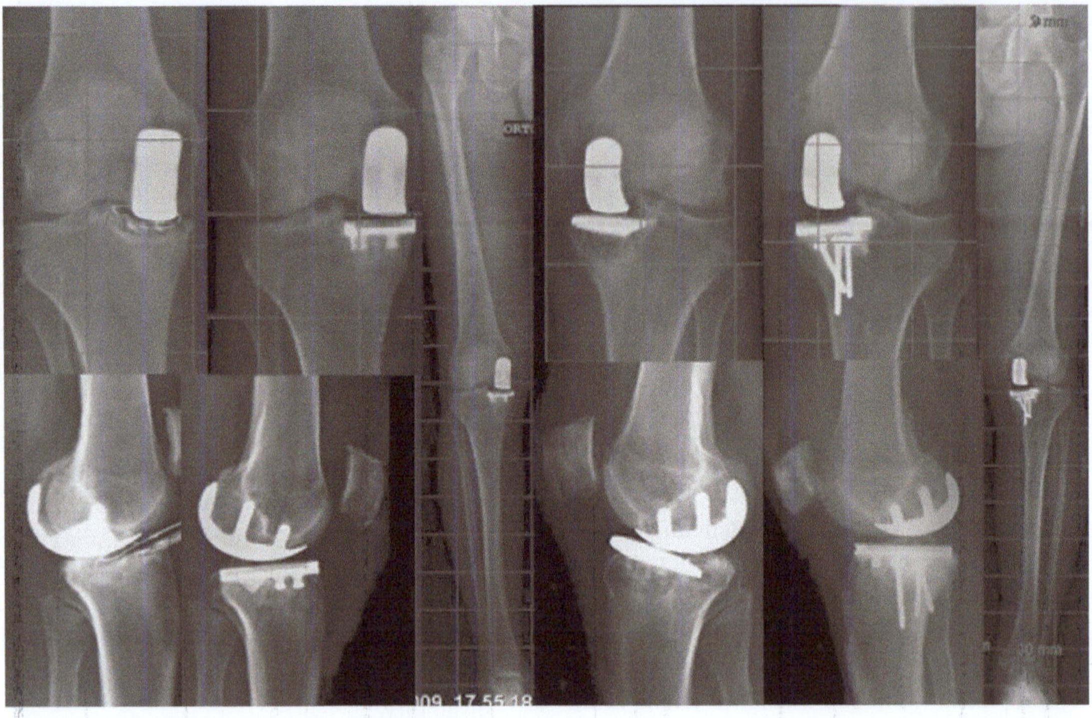

Fig. 16.1 *On the left*: an early revision at 1.6 years due to tibial loosening; *on the right*: a late revision at 10.2 years due to tibial subsidence and osteolysis

terior position and sizing (and thus incorrect contact in extension between the femour over the prosthetic component and tibial plateau, pain and lack of extension), and peripheral in flexion (causing tibial loosening and PE wear).

- Infections: Even if statistically relevant, they are not as frequent and complicated as septic total implants.
- Pain.

The causes of late revision are:

- Aseptic loosening.
- Opposite compartment degeneration (Fig. 16.2).
- P.F. (patellofemoral) degeneration (rare complication): This is due to an incorrect indication for UKR; it frequently develops in obese women, with secondary evolution of arthritis. The severe FR pathology is a contraindication for an isolated unicompartmental implant if malalignment and overpressure are present or if chondropathy (III–IV°) is determined intraoperatively.
- Capsuloligamentous instability: This often develops after loosening and/or PE wear or after incorrect component positioning. Incorrect femoral positioning is generally a late cause of failure.
- Polyethylene wear: either linear or volumetric, depending, respectively, on whether a fixed or mobile platform insert is used.
- Component fracture: Either component can be involved; fracture is often associated with PE wear.
- Pain.

UKR revisions can also be classified with respect to the prosthesis used during surgery. In general, revision involves replacement with another UKR, or a TKR. However, the final decision depends on the cause of the failure, the bone defect, ligament stability, the contralateral compartment and patellofemoral integrity, PE-metal debris migration, and the patient's age.

Generally, we prefer another UKR implant in revisions due to incorrect positioning or prosthetic loosening, if the patient's is < 65 years

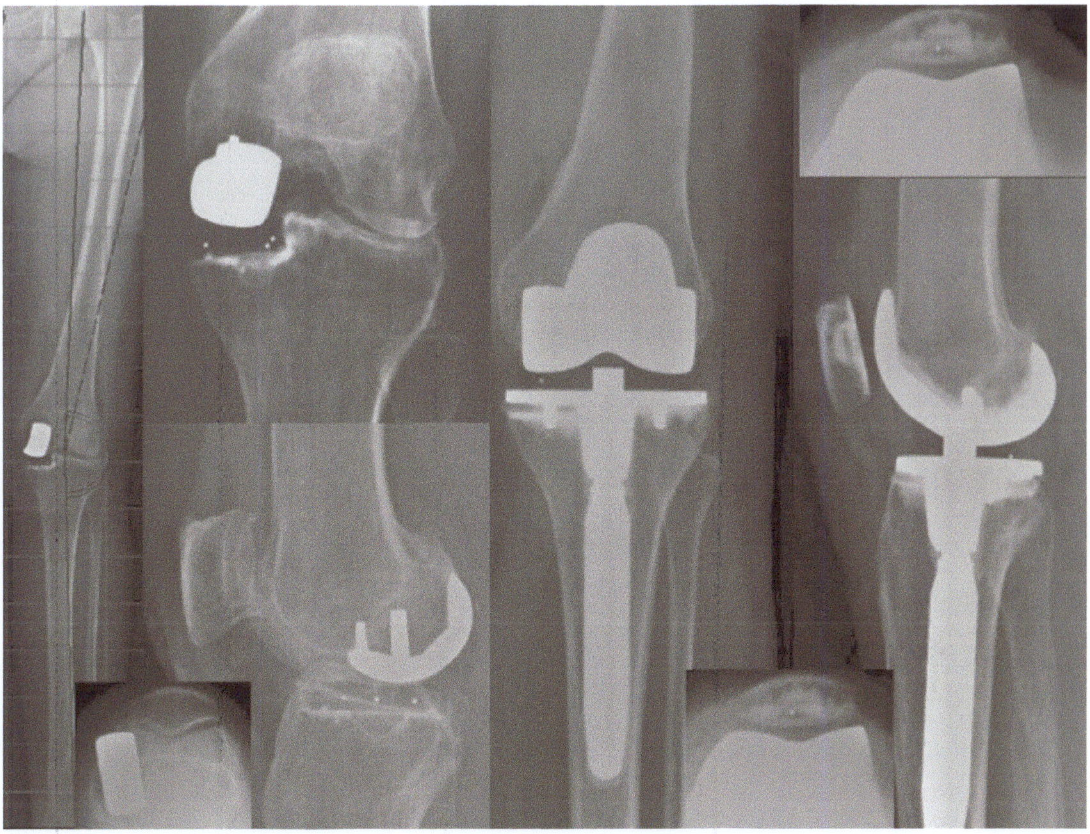

Fig. 16.2 UKR-TKA revision at 3.7 years due to lateral compartment degeneration

of age, has a minimal tibial bone defect, undamaged contralateral compartment, cruciate ligaments and patellofemoral joint, and is asymptomatic and without PE-metal-cement debris migration.

A TKR is advisable if the indication was incorrect or an infection occurred, the patient is > 65 years of age, has a severe tibial bone defect, evident contralateral compartment degeneration, a deficiency of the cruciates or collateral ligaments, PE-metal debris migration, or symptomatic patellofemoral degeneration (Fig. 16.3).

In case of septic loosening we prefer a two-stage revision technique.

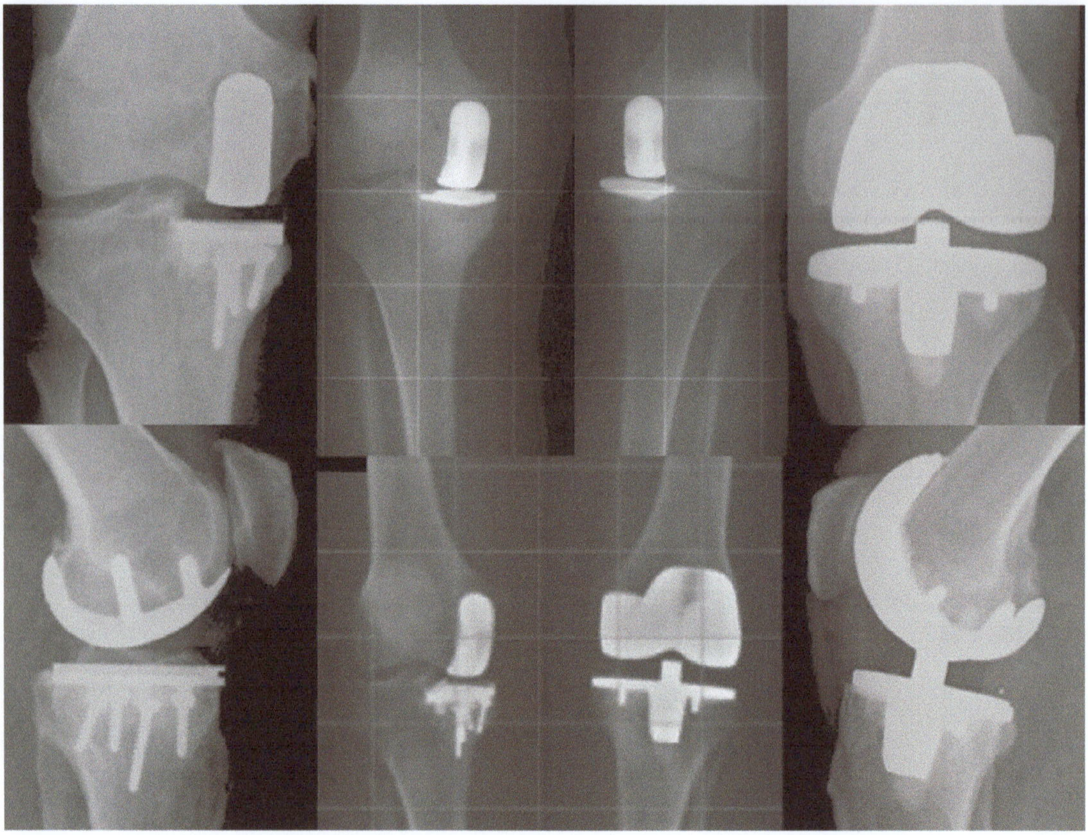

Fig. 16.3 Bilateral UKR revision after 18 years due to tibial loosening consequent to a fall from a tree: revision with another UKR in the right knee and a TKA in the left knee

16.4 Patients and Methods

From February 2001 to December 2010, at the Istituto Ortopedico Galeazzi, 189 unicompartmental revisions in 182 patients (7 were bilateral nonsimultaneous implants) were performed. Eleven of these patients (12 knees) later died for unrelated reasons. The initial sample comprised 137 women and 45 men with an average age at surgery of 68 years (range: 39–88 years). The mean weight was 76 kg (range: 46–115 kg) and the mean height was 172.7 cm (range: 158–176 cm).

All patients were contacted by phone. Twenty-four were unable to attend a physical examination and thus were telephone-interviewed and their X-rays were analyzed. The remaining 108 patients (3 bilateral cases) underwent clinical and X-ray examination (Fig. 16.4).

Clinical examination included skin incision, soft-tissue condition, range of movement (ROM), ligamentous stability, extensor mechanism integrity, and neurovascular structures.

The radiographic analysis examined the mechanical axis, component position in the frontal and sagittal planes (slope), signs of component loosening, such as radiolucencies, bone stock defect, and joint line level.

16.5 Surgical Technique

The main considerations associated with revision are preoperative planning, the previous incision, removal of the prosthetic components, correction of the bone defect, fixation of the new components, and obtaining joint stability and the joint line level [3].

If possible, the skin incision should be made at the previous scar and possibly enlarged lon-

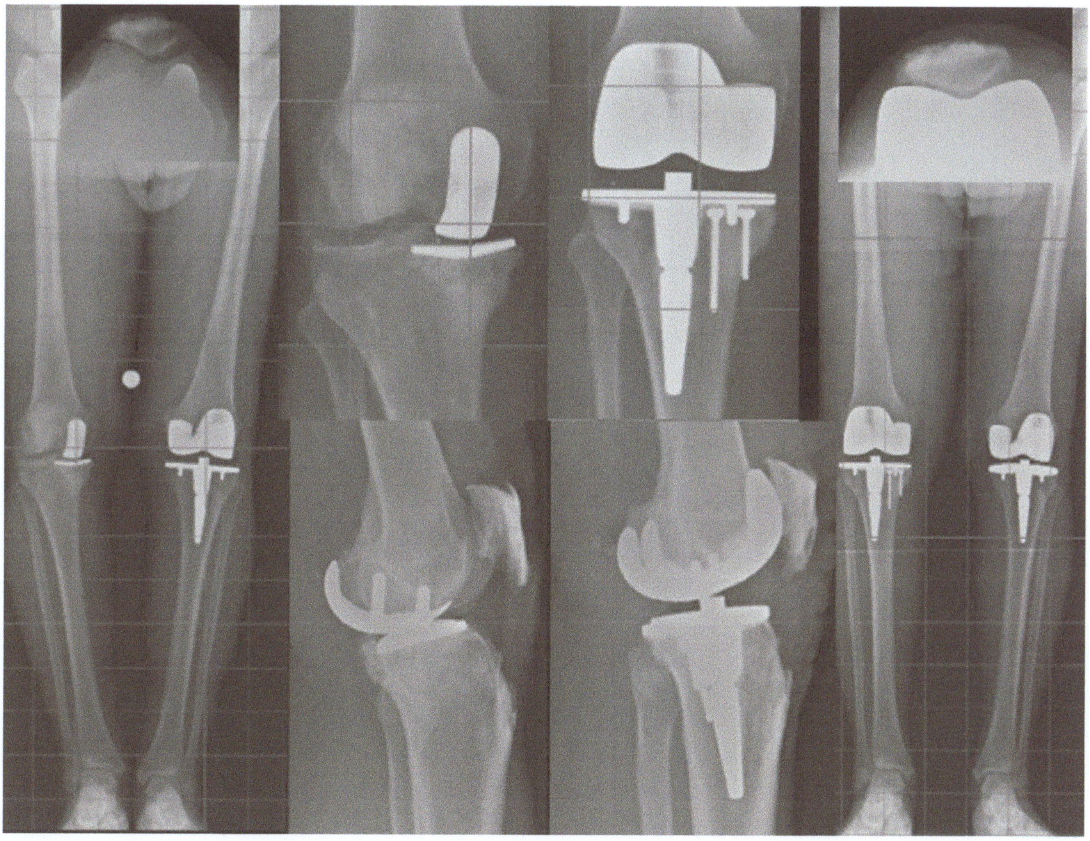

Fig. 16.4 UKR revision (broken tibial component) with a TKA stem and screws to repair a tibial defect

gitudinally. Less skin invasiveness will reduce both bleeding and the amount of damage to the quadriceps muscle, thus improving the functional recovery.

The new prosthesis is chosen based on the dimension of the bone defect, capsuloligamentous stability, and contralateral and patellofemoral compartment integrity. The migration of PE and metal debris must also be taken into account.

When another UKR is indicated, there is the option to replace all of the components or, as is more frequently the case, if the femoral component is stable, only the tibial component will be substituted. In the presence of a limited bone defect, the tibial cut must correct the previous component position, i.e., frontal obliquity and slope, and reproduce the correct joint line. These aims are achieved by using a tibial component with thicker modular PE inserts, but preferably not more than 12 mm. If the defect requires a component thickness > 12 mm, this is a contraindication to another UKR. Alternatively, the bone defect can be treated with screws and cement to avoid exchange of the bearing or, albeit less often, with bone graft. It is mandatory that the defect engage only the cancellous bone. Not more than 20% of the peripheral cortex can be deficient. In all cases, an anatomical component that achieves complete cortical coverage is needed.

In some cases the problem is incorrect positioning and sizing of the femoral component; failure in such cases is due to the conflict between the tibial component and the femoral cartilage. In the case of a mobile-bearing prosthesis, complete revision with TKA is advisable, whereas with a fixed-bearing implant we prefer a femoral component with the availability of two series in relation to the distal thickness. Thicker components are needed for revisions involving a femoral bone defect.

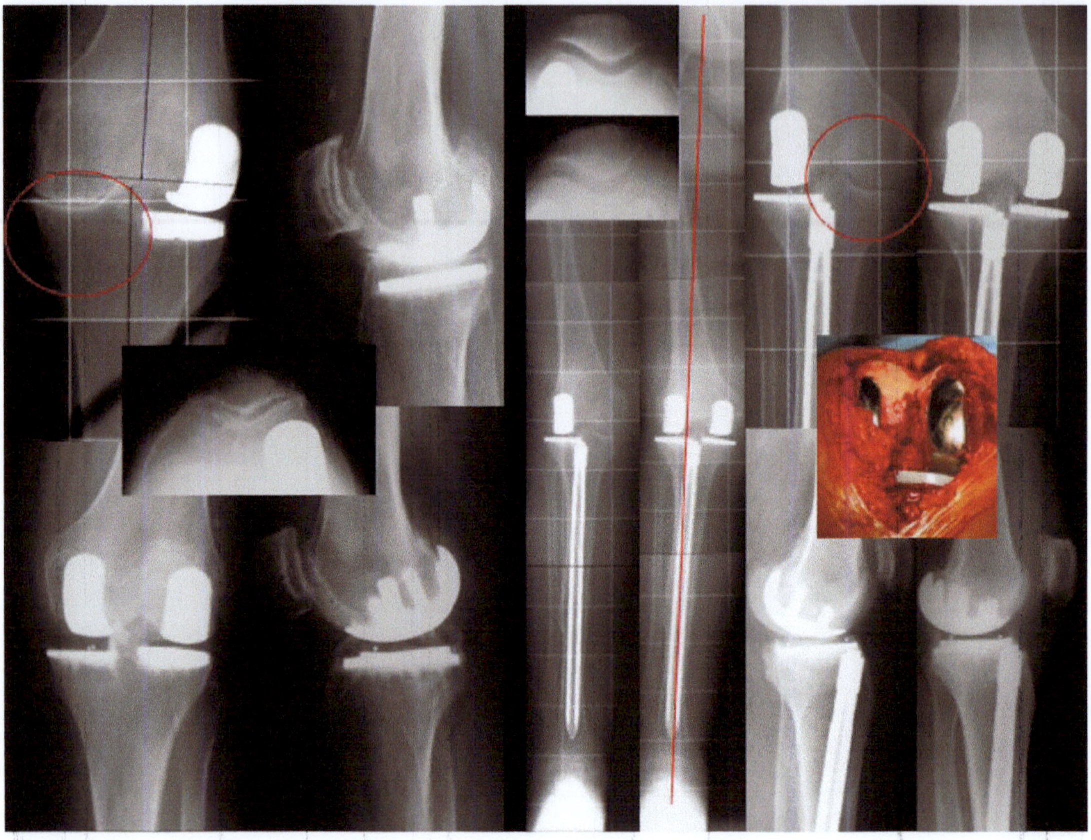

Fig. 16.5 *On the left*: revision after 16 years with another UKR in the medial compartment. *On the right*: in 1995, a lateral UKR implant and in 2003 treatment of a tibial fracture with a nail were followed in 2005 by a revision with another UKR in the medial compartment

Another possibility is a revision consisting of another UKR in the opposite degenerated compartment. This is possible only if the components of the previous prosthesis are stable, the patellofemoral compartment and cruciate ligaments are undamaged and asymptomatic, and PE wear is minimal. If the other degenerated compartment is the patellofemoral one and the patient is undergoing a revision due to chronic anterior knee pain, then a patellofemoral component can be implanted as well. In these cases, the result is a bi-compartmental implant (Fig. 16.5) [4].

If the bone defect is limited and the choice is a TKA, a standard cut can be made at the level of the wear and a primary implant performed.

Component fixation may be standard (cement or cementless), depending on the bone stock and bone quality. In case of a bone defect > 12 mm, we prefer to use a stem (cement or cementless) often joined to a wedge. Another option is to correct the bone defect using bone grafts, or screws and/or cement. The aim is to achieve the correct height and obliquity of the joint line.

In women, even if the defect is < 12 mm we prefer to use a stem in case of low-quality bone, with the exception of patients < 55 years (Fig. 16.6).

In case of a severe bone defect and capsuloligamentous instability, a constrained prosthesis is necessary.

In revisions due to sepsis, we prefer a two-stage procedure, as in these patients it is associated with a low rate of re-infection and fewer complication than TKA.

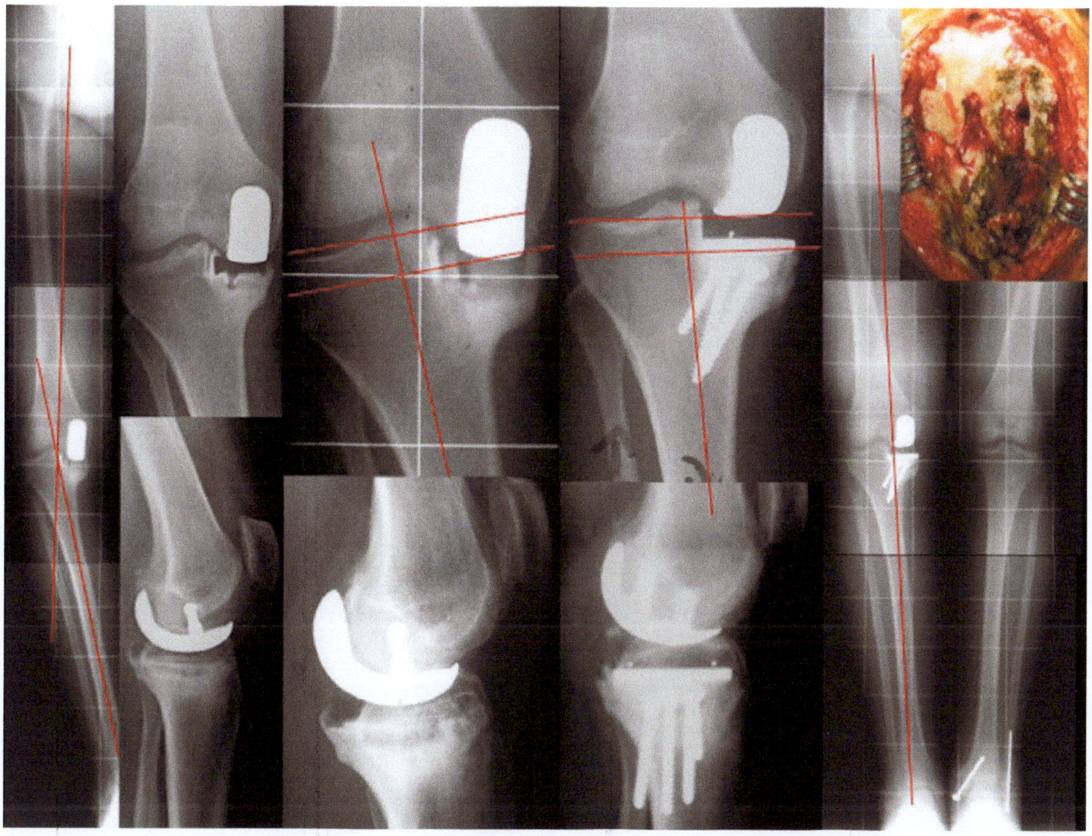

Fig. 16.6 Revision at 7 years with another UKR, using cement and screws, in a 53-year-old man

16.6 Results

The average follow-up of the 189 knees was 6.8 years. In 123 (65.1%), the revision consisted of a TKA and in the remaining 66 (6%) with another UKR.

In the UNI-TKA group, in 106 (86.2%) we used standard implants, with a tibial stem in 60 of these cases. In the other 17 (13.8%) cases a semi-constrained prosthesis was used (Fig. 16.7).

In 11 knees a two-step revision due to septic loosening was necessary.

Among the 66 (34.9%) knees in which the revision consisted of UKR, in 19 (28.8%) cases only the tibial component was replaced, in six (9.1%) cases only the femoral component, and in one (1.5%) case only the patellar component. In 37 (56.1%) knees, a complete UKR substitution was necessary. Of the three other knees, one (1.5%) was revised with a patellofemoral prosthesis due to joint degeneration and in the other two (3%) another UKR was performed but in the opposite compartment, resulting in a bi-compartmental implant.

In the 123 cases of TKA revision there were 13 (10.5%) failures: nine (7.3%) aseptic and four (3.2%) septic; the latter included one knee in which a previous revision was performed due to septic loosening. In the aseptic knees, the average age of the prosthesis at failure was 3.7 years (Fig. 16.8). All of the patients in this group were female (100%): five (55.6%) younger and four (44.4%) older than 65 years.

In 66 revisions with UKR, there were four aseptic failures (6%), with failure occurring after an average of 5.5 years. Three of the failures occurred in men (75%). Three of the patients were under the age of 65 years (75%) (Fig. 16.9). There were no septic failures.

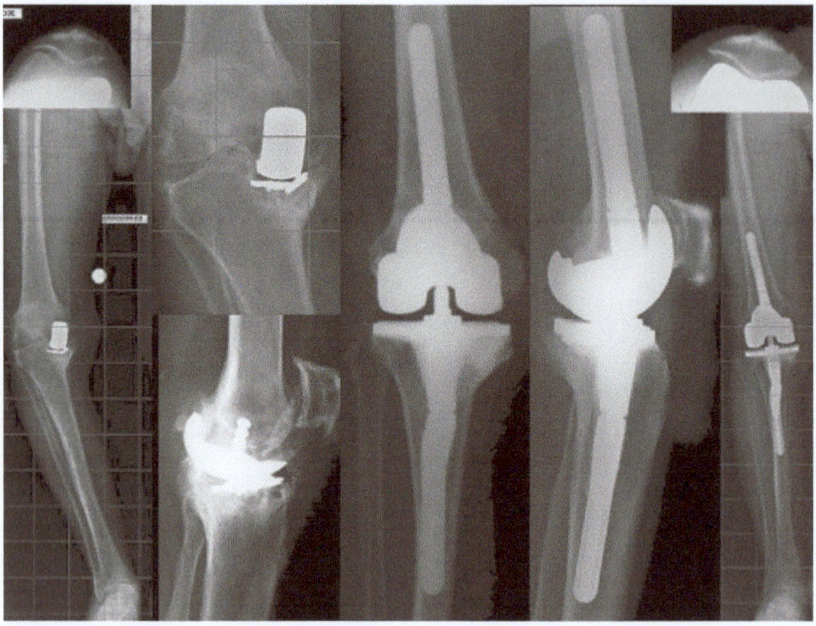

Fig. 16.7 Revision after 22 years with a semi-constrained prosthesis due to severe bone defect

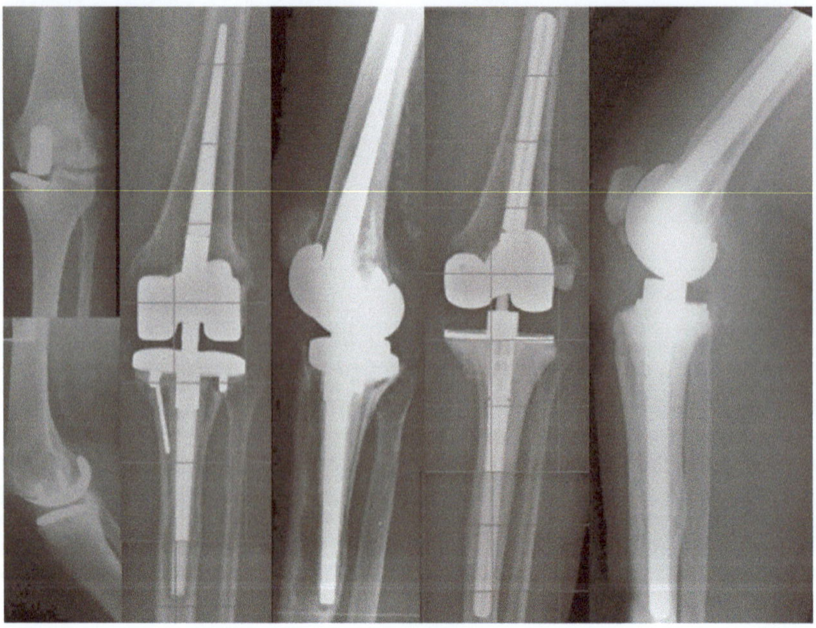

Fig. 16.8 TKA revision of a UKR due to failure at 2.4 years

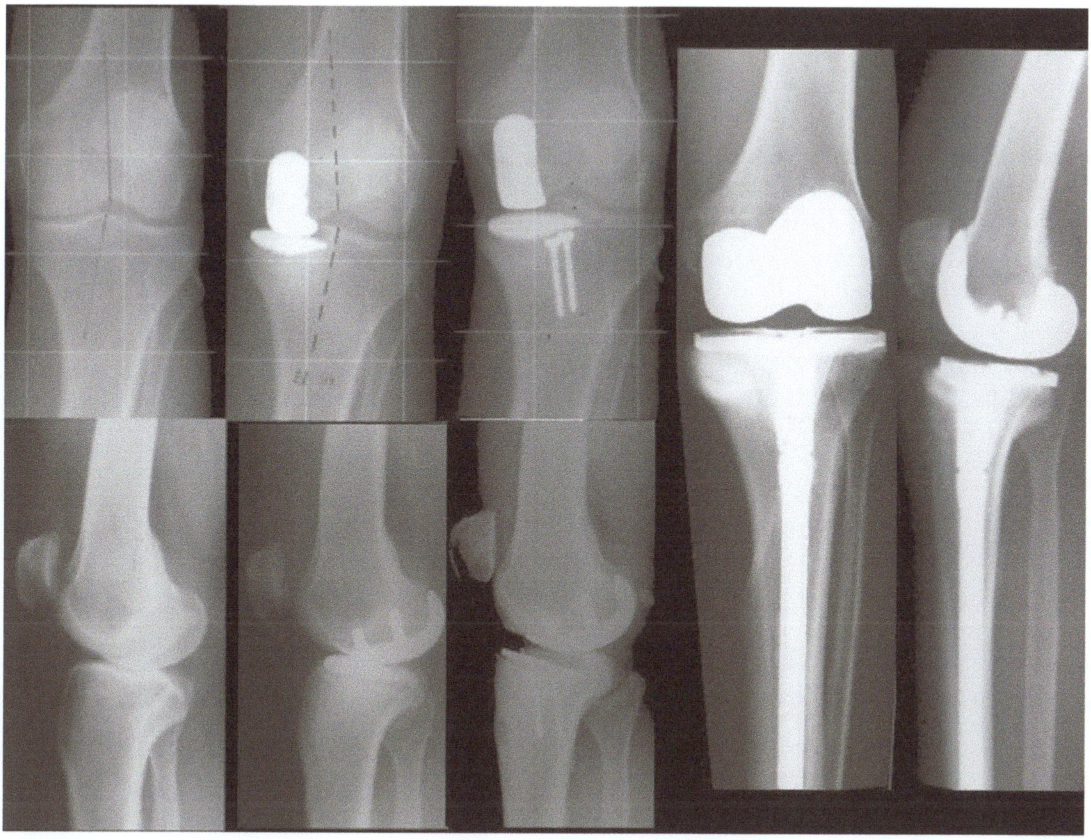

Fig. 16.9 TKA stemmed in second Uni revision due to recurrent tibial loosening

16.7 Conclusions

In our experience, the results of a revision procedure primarily depend on the correct indications. In many cases, partial or complete unicompartmental substitution is a relatively simple procedure. When all the conditions are respected, a UKR implant in the opposite compartment or the implant of a patellofemoral prosthesis results in a successful bi-compartmental prosthesis. The advantages of this strategy are based on the mini-invasiveness of the procedure and consequently on the rapid functional recovery.

When a TKA is indicated. the results will depend on the characteristics of the patient, the quality of the bone and the nature of the bone defect. In most cases, the bone defect is manageable with a graft, wedges, screws, and/or cement. In these cases the use of a stem is mandatory and perhaps also a semi-constrained prosthesis.

In our series, there was a clear difference between the two groups regarding gender and age. In fact, all of the patients in the UKR-TKA group were women compared to only 25% in the UKR-UKR group. In addition, 44% of the patients in the UKR-TKA were > 65 years of age compared to 25% in the UKR-UKR group. The large percentage of men under the age of 65 in the UKR-UKR group likely accounts for the high physical functional impact, as determined in other studies as well [5-7]. Aseptic failures were only slightly higher in the UKR-TKA than in the group UKR-UKR group (7.3% vs. 6%, respectively).

However, TKA and UNI revisions did not significantly differ with respect to the survival rate, with rather little advantage conferred by the latter approach. Nonetheless, the average survival rate of the failed implants was higher in UKR-UKR revisions than in UKR-TKA revisions (5.5 years vs. 3.7 years). Also none of the 66 UKR revisions had septic complications, which did occur in four of 123 of the TKA revisions.

Among the 112 TKA revisions in which aseptic failure occurred, three (2.7%) involved septic loosening while among the 11 cases of TKA revision that resulted in septic failure there was one (9.1%) recurrence. These findings can be explained by a simple surgical rule: for the same appropriate indication and surgical technique, there is less risk of complications in less invasive surgeries.

References

1. Romagnoli S, Verde F, Eberle RW (2006) 10 year minimum follow-up of medial unicompartmental knee arthroplasty with the allegretto prosthesis. J Bone Joint Surg Br 88-B(Supp I) 100
2. Romagnoli S, Verde F, Eberle RW (2008) 10-year follow-up of lateral unicompartmental knee arthroplasty with the Allegretto. Poster presentation (P205), AAOS, San Francisco
3. Romagnoli S, Bibbiani E, Castelnuovo N, Cusmà G, Verde F (2008) The problem of UKR revisions. J Bone Joint Surg Br 90-B (Supp. I) 182
4. Romagnoli S, Bibbiani E, Castelnuovo N, d'Amario F (2009) Bi-unicompartmental knee prostheses. In: Scuderi GR, Tria AJ (eds) Minimally invasive surgery in orthopaedics. Springer New York, pp- 327-340
5. Pearse AJ, Hooper GJ, Rothwell A, Frampton C (2010) Survival and functional outcome after revision of a unicompartmental to a total knee replacement: the New Zealand National Joint Registry. J Bone Joint Surg Br. 92(4):508-12
6. Goodfellow JW, O'Connor JJ, Murray DW (2010) A critique of revision rate as an outcome measure: re-interpretation of knee joint registry data. J Bone Joint Surg Br. 92(12):1628-31
7. Johnson S, Jones P, Newman JH (2007) The survivorship and results of total knee replacements converted from unicompartmental knee replacements. Knee 14(2):154-7

Index

N. Confalonieri, S. Romagnoli (eds.), *Small Implants in Knee Reconstruction*,
DOI 10.1007/978-88-470-2655-1, © Springer-Verlag Italia 2013

V

W

MIX
Papier aus verantwortungsvollen Quellen
Paper from responsible sources
FSC® C105338

If you have any concerns about our products,
you can contact us on
ProductSafety@springernature.com

In case Publisher is established outside the EU,
the EU authorized representative is:
Springer Nature Customer Service Center GmbH
Europaplatz 3, 69115 Heidelberg, Germany

Printed by Libri Plureos GmbH
in Hamburg, Germany